Cultures of Neurasthenia

I0036554

THE WELLCOME SERIES IN THE HISTORY OF MEDICINE

The Wellcome Series in the History of Medicine
series editors are
V. Nutton, M. Neve and R. Cooter.
Please send all queries regarding the series to
Michael Laycock,
The Wellcome Trust Centre for the History of
Medicine at UCL,
210 Euston Road, London NW1 2BE, UK.

Cultures of Neurasthenia
From Beard to the First World War

Edited by
Marijke Gijswijt-Hofstra and Roy Porter

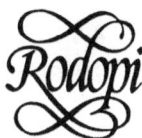

Rodopi

Amsterdam - New York, NY 2001

Transferred to digital printing 2014

Cover image: www.dreamstime.com

The paper on which this book is printed meets the
requirements of "ISO 9706:1994, Information and
documentation - Paper for documents - Requirements for
permanence".

ISBN: 978-90-420-0921-9
E-Book ISBN: 978-94-012-1114-7
© Editions Rodopi B.V., Amsterdam – New York, NY 2001

Contents

Notes on Contributors

Nelleke Bakker is a historian who teaches history of education at the University of Groningen, The Netherlands. Her Ph.D. on the history of child-rearing literature in the Netherlands (1845-1925) was published in 1995. She has contributed to several volumes and journals, *Paedagogica Historica, History of Education Quarterly* and the *Journal of Social History* among them.

Christopher E. Forth teaches European intellectual and cultural history at the Australian National University. He is the author of *Zarathustra in Paris: The Nietzsche Vogue in France, 1891-1918*, and is currently preparing a book-length study of the crisis of French manhood and co-editing a volume entitled *Body Parts: Critical Explorations in Corporeality.*

Marijke Gijswijt-Hofstra is Professor of Social and Cultural History at the University of Amsterdam. She has published on the granting of asylum in the Dutch Republic, deviance and tolerance (16th-20th centuries), witchcraft and cultures of misfortune (16th-20th centuries), the reception of homoeopathy in the Netherlands (19th-20th centuries), and on women and alternative health care in the Netherlands (20th century). She has recently edited in English, with Hilary Marland and Hans de Waardt, *Illness and Healing Alternatives in Western Europe* (London: Routledge, 1997), and, with Roy Porter, *Cultures of Psychiatry and Mental Health Care in Postwar Britain and the Netherlands* (Amsterdam: Rodopi, 1998). She is currently working on the history of psychiatry and mental health care in the Netherlands in the twentieth century.

Doris Kaufmann has been Professor of Modern History in the Department of History at the University of Bremen since 2000. Previously at the Max Planck Institute for the History of Science in

i

Berlin; 1998-2000 research director of the project of the Max Planck Society "History of the Kaiser Wilhelm Society during the National Socialist period, 1933-45". Member of the School of Social Science at the Institute for Advanced Study in Princeton in 1992-93. She is author of *Katholisches Milieu in Münster, 1928-33* (1984); *Frauen zwischen Aufbruch und Reaktion. Protestantische Frauenbewegung in der ersten Hälfte des 20. Jahrhunderts* (1988); *Aufklärung, bürgerliche Selbsterfahrung und die "Erfindung" der Psychiatrie in Deutschland, 1770-1850* (1995); (editor) *Geschichte der Kaiser-Wilhelm-Gesellschaft im Nationalsozialismus. Bestandsaufnahme und Perspektiven der Forschung* (2000).

Tom Lutz is the author of *American Nervousness, 1903: An Anecdotal History* (Cornell 1991) and *Crying: The Natural and Cultural History of Tears* (Norton 1999; Norton UK 2000, Europa 2000, Ambos/Anthos 2001). He is at work on a history of anti-work-ethic subcultures in America and an ethnography of the Los Angeles blues scene.

Hilary Marland is Senior Lecturer at the Department of History and Director of the Centre for the History of Medicine at the University of Warwick, England. She is former editor of *Social History of Medicine*, and has published on midwifery, infant and maternal welfare, nineteenth-century medical practice and alternative healing. She is currently writing a monograph with the working title *Dangerous Motherhood: Insanity of Childbirth in the Nineteenth Century*.

Michael Neve is Senior Lecturer at the Wellcome Trust Centre for the History of Medicine at University College London. He teaches and publishes on the history of psychiatry and on European writings on degeneration from around 1860 to the 1920s. Among his publications is *1900: A fin-de-siècle reader*, co-edited with Mike Jay (Penguin, 1999).

Roy Porter is Professor of the Social History of Medicine at the Wellcome Trust Centre for the History of Medicine at University College London. Recent books include *Doctor of Society: Thomas Beddoes and the Sick Trade in Late Enlightenment England* (London: Routledge, 1991); *London: A Social History* (Hamish Hamilton, 1994); '*The Greatest Benefit to Mankind': A Medical History of Humanity* (London: HarperCollins, 1997); and *Enlightenment:*

Britain and the Creation of the Modern World (Harmondsworth: Allen Lane, 2000) and *Bodies Politic: Disease, Death and the Doctors in Britain: 1650-1914* (London: Reaktion Books, 2001). He is co-author of *The History of Bethlam* (London: Routledge, 1997) and of *Gout: The Patrician Malady* (New Haven and London: Yale University Press, 1998)

Joachim Radkau is Professor of Modern History at the University of Bielefeld. His research is moving within a triangle of history of technology, environment and medicine, based upon the conviction that these three sub-disciplines of history can give mutual inspirations. His main book publications: *Aufstieg und Krise der deutschen Atomwirtschaft* (1983); *Holz - Ein Naturstoff in der Technikgeschichte* (1987, together with Ingrid Schäfer); *Technik in Deutschland - Vom 18. Jahrhundert bis in die Gegenwart* (1989); *Das Zeitalter der Nervosität - Deutschland zwischen Bismarck und Hitler* (1998); *Natur und Macht - Eine Weltgeschichte der Umwelt* (2000).

Volker Roelcke is Professor in the History of Medicine and Science at the Medizinische Universitäet Lûebeck. His main research interests are in the history of psychiatry in Germany from the late 18th to the 20th century, the history of ,diseases of civilization', and the history of medical anthropology. His publications include *Krankheit und Kulturkritik. Psychiatrische Gesellschaftsdiagnosen im bürgerlichen Zeitalter, 1790-1914* (1999). He is currently working on a project about Anglo-American-German relations in psychiatry, 1871-1945.

Heinz-Peter Schmiedebach is Professor of Medical History and head of the Institute for Medical History of the University of Greifswald. His main research interests are in the history of psychiatry, the development of public health in rural regions, the history of deontology, and the history of medical theories and clinical disciplines in the nineteenth and twentieth centuries in Germany. His publications include *Psychiatrie und Psychologie im Widerstreit* and *Medizin und Krieg* (together with Johanna Bleker). He is currently working on a project about the social integration of mentally ill patients (1900-1995).

Chandak Sengoopta is Wellcome Research Lecturer in the History of Medicine at the University of Manchester. His research interests lie in the history of the life and behavioral sciences in modern Europe. His monograph, *Otto Weininger: Sex, Science, and Self in*

Imperial Vienna was published in 2000 by the University of Chicago Press. He is currently working on the history of sex-gland research in early-twentieth-century Central Europe and Britain.

Sonu Shamdasani is a Research Associate at the Wellcome Trust Centre for the History of Medicine at UCL. He is the author of *Cult Fictions: C.G. Jung and the Founding of Analytical Pscyhology* (Routledge, 1998) and has edited a number of volumes.

Jessica Slijkhuis studied Arts and Culture at the University of Maastricht. She is currently working on her PhD thesis on *'Dutch psychiatry in the fin-de-siècle'* in the Department of History, Maastricht. She is interested in nineteenth and twentieth century history of Western civilisation and science in general and the history of psychology and psychiatry, crime, illness and deviance in specific.

Mathew Thomson is a Lecturer in the Department of History at the University of Warwick in England. His previous publications include *The Problem of Mental Deficiency: Eugenics, Democracy and Social Policy in Britain, 1870-1959* (Oxford: Oxford University Press, 1998). He is currently working on a social and cultural history of the category of the psychological in twentieth-century Britain.

Joost Vijselaar (historian) worked extensively on the history of psychiatry in the Netherlands and on the reception of Mesmerism. His thesis, *De magnetische geest. Het dierlijk magnetisme 1770-1830* ('The magnetic spirit. Animal magnetism 1770-1830') (Nijmegen: SUN, 2001). In recent years he wrote in co-operation with others a number of books on the history of psychiatric hospitals, the famous asylum Meerenberg amongst them. Apart from being a senior researcher at the Trimbos-institute (the National Institute for Mental Health) in Utrecht, he is currently working as a postdoctoral fellow at the University of Amsterdam on a study of the psychiatric patient in the Dutch psychiatric hospital in the twentieth century.

Introduction:
Cultures of Neurasthenia from Beard to the First World War

Marijke Gijswijt-Hofstra

Although the New York neurologist and electrotherapist George Miller Beard may not have coined the term,[1] contemporaries certainly called him the father of neurasthenia. From 1869 until 1883, the year that Beard died, he 'promoted' neurasthenia through his publications, the two most influential being *A Practical Treatise on Nervous Exhaustion (Neurasthenia): Its Symptoms, Nature, Sequences, Treatment* of 1880, appearing already the year after in German, and *American Nervousness: Its Causes and Consequences* of 1881. Beard interpreted neurasthenia, which literally means nerve weakness, as a disorder of modernity, caused by the fast pace of urban life. What is more, he presented it as a truly American disease, the inevitable, yet quite acceptable by-product of American civilisation. While this American stamp may have somewhat tempered the British interest in neurasthenia,[2] it by no means formed an obstacle to neurasthenia's reception and appropriation in Germany from the early-1880s onwards. The Dutch - relying on Beard in German – were to follow more slowly and hesitantly. In France it was thanks to Jean-Martin Charcot and his students that the issue of neurasthenia got disseminated from the late 1880s onwards.[3] A French translation of Beard's *Practical Treatise* belatedly appeared in 1895.

Neurasthenia's heyday in America and Europe continued into the first decade of the twentieth century. The First World War marked the more or less final retreat of neurasthenia. That is to say, the diagnosis of neurasthenia gradually became outdated, not that the types of condition which had been associated with the term no longer occurred. Indeed, conditions similar to the ones that used to be called 'neurasthenia', were, towards the end of the twentieth century, provided with a different label: chronic fatigue syndrome.[4] Moreover, as Tom Lutz indicates in this volume, the diagnosis of neurasthenia still enjoys a great deal of popularity in countries like

1

Japan and China, after having been introduced there in, respectively, the 1900s and the 1920s.

Beard and his followers applied the label of neurasthenia to a whole range of physical and mental symptoms, varying from, amongst others, anxiety, despair, phobias and insomnia to inattention, extreme fatigue, palpitations, migraine, indigestion, and impotence. Neurasthenic symptoms were thought to be caused by a lack of nerve force, which in its turn was supposed to stem from excess demands on the brain, the digestive organs and the reproductive system, while these excess demands were attributed to the fast pace of modern life. Moreover, in the European context heredity and degeneration figured more or less prominently as explanatory concepts. The therapeutic repertoire was likewise varied. Beard himself showed a preference for treatment with electricity. Quite famous was the rest cure of the American physician Silas Weir Mitchell, consisting of seclusion, bed-rest, electrical treatment, a nutritious diet, and massage. It was successfully adopted across the Atlantic, for instance by the London obstetrician William Smout Playfair and the Amsterdam physician B.H. Stephan. Other types of cures consisted of visits to spas, seaside resorts, or the mountains, and various forms of psycho-therapy possibly in combination with a stay in a sanatorium or (mental) hospital.

The history of neurasthenia makes a fascinating topic, not in the least because of its protean character, its floating diversity in the course of time, in different regions and in different groups. Its many-sided history encompasses sufferers or patients, the medical and psychiatric professions, pedagogues and other professional advisers, and novelists, to mention but the most important groups involved. Except for being appropriated in many different ways, neurasthenia's 'popularity' as a diagnosis varied significantly, as did the popularity of the available therapies. These differences in popularity not only manifested themselves through the years and between regions or even countries, but also along lines of class, gender, age, and religion. Moreover, the extent to which neurasthenia was regarded as a serious problem of modern civilization may well reflect the particular, more or less pessimistic, nature of the *fin de siècle* in different societies.

This being said, there is every reason to speak of cultures of neurasthenia in the plural, each with their own, more or less specific histories, each being embedded in broader cultural histories, and each involved with the crossing of boundaries: national, regional, socio-cultural, as well as conceptual and therapeutical. A full reconstruction and interpretation of these histories requires a comparative approach. Yet, the historiography of neurasthenia has so far tended to have a national focus. America, Britain, and Germany have received the most attention.[5] Only George F. Drinka has offered a cross-national perspective, covering both America and Europe in his *The Birth of Neurosis* of 1984.[6] However, his account of neurasthenia's vicissitudes, though useful, is brief and practically limited to medical ideas and practice. In the wake of Roy Porter's plea for doing medical history from below,[7] some attention has been paid to the perspective of patients who were diagnosed or even diagnosed themselves as neurasthenic, notably by Tom Lutz and Joachim Radkau.[8] Still, it hardly needs saying that the uncovering of the patient's view requires an ongoing effort.

Centred around late nineteenth and early-twentieth-century cultures of neurasthenia, a workshop titled 'Neurasthenia and Society' was held in June 2000 in Amsterdam. The event was co-organised by the Dutch Huizinga Institute for Cultural History, The Wellcome Trust Centre for the History of Medicine at UCL, the Department of History of the University of Warwick, and the Institute for the History of Medicine of the Robert Bosch Foundation (Stuttgart). Although it was the workshop's central aim to analyse and compare cultures of neurasthenia in Britain, Germany and the Netherlands, attention was also paid to developments in America and France, and to nervous disorders in Britain before the coming of neurasthenia. The articles contained in this volume are based on the pre-circulated papers presented at the workshop, mediated by the contributions of the invited commentators and participants.[9] What hereafter follows is an account of the questions and themes that were addressed, an introduction to the contributions in this volume, and finally, by way of conclusion, a discussion of the main results and the remaining problems.

In search of cultures of neurasthenia

It hardly needs saying that a comparative enterprise like the one discussed here requires at least some guidelines in order to make it work. In accordance with the title of the workshop, its central concern was the exploration of the mutual relationships between neurasthenia and society in the late-nineteenth and early-twentieth centuries. One of the main questions addressed the popularity of the neurasthenia concept, as compared to other concepts, in the different countries in the course of this period, and the reasons for this popularity or the lack of it. Another main question concerned the extent to which gender, class, and religion may have structured both

3

theory and practice with regard to neurasthenia in the various countries.

Special sessions were devoted to what were summarised as the professional view, the patient's view, and the public's view. The professional view comprised both medical theories and medical therapies for neurasthenia, including nervous diseases with similar symptoms. The patient's view comprised of patients' experiences and their therapeutical careers, with special attention to gender, age, marital and social/occupational status, and religion. Finally, the public's view related to how the neurasthenia concept was received, adapted and used in literature, politics, churches, and other societal and cultural settings, and what cultural impact it had more generally. Of course, it should be self-evident that there is no such thing as one professional view, or one patient's view, or one public's view. Each of these views should be conceived of in the plural, as they encompass many different views. The public's view is, moreover, a highly heterogeneous and fluid category.[10]

Themes that moreover figured fairly prominently, either in the (accounts of) historical cultures of neurasthenia or in their interpretation, were conceptions of the somatic and the psychic and their mutual relation; professional and lay appreciations of somatic versus psychic diagnoses; the changing professional status of neurology, psychiatry and psychology; and the construction of knowledge on their part, the development of a sexological domain, and the advance of psychotherapy and psychoanalysis. Another important, though somewhat less fully explored theme consisted of the connection between the character of the *fin-de-siècle* on the one hand, and the appropriation and popularity of neurasthenia on the other.

The three perspectives mentioned above are reflected in the contributions on Britain, Germany and the Netherlands. Each of these countries is first presented in an introductory chapter after which three chapters follow on respectively the professional, the patient's, and the public's view. Although these chapters are ordered per country, they may also, for comparative purposes, be read in thematical order. In the chapter on America and in the first chapter on France the three perspectives have been more or less combined, while in the concluding chapter on Pierre Janet's psychasthenia the professional view prevails.

•

The invention of neurasthenia

The volume opens with a contribution of Roy Porter on styles of nervous disorders in Britain in the eighteenth and nineteenth centuries. Of course, nervous maladies were by no means a new phenomenon before the neurasthenia diagnosis crossed the Atlantic. Britain even had its own English malady, an invention of the Scottish physician George Cheyne, dating from the 1730s. Like neurasthenia a century and a half later, the English malady was considered to be both an affliction of modern civilisation and, at least initially, a disease of the elite. However, whereas the English malady was primarily attributed to an overdose of luxury and laziness, American nervousness was primarily viewed as a disease of labour, an overburdening of the nerves. Porter also observes that the attribution of malfunctioning of the nervous system to lack of nerve force - according to Beard the primary cause of neurasthenia - had already been fairly current practice from the middle of the nineteenth century onwards. Nor were neurasthenia's symptoms considered to be all that new. Many British physicians were therefore inclined to judge that the neurasthenia diagnosis was just a new label for old nervous problems.

From neurasthenia's prehistory and early reception in Britain the focus moves in the next chapter to the early constructions of neurasthenia in America and what happened after. Tom Lutz is primarily interested in what the history of neurasthenia can reveal about the relation between culture and physiology if one tries to avoid anachronistic pitfalls, such as uncritically recreating the rift between somatic and psychic explanations, as they came into existence from Freud onwards. After a discussion of Beard's and Weir Mitchell's 'foundational' work on neurasthenia and its positive reception in America - the number of neurasthenics probably reached its peak between 1900 and 1910 – Lutz turns to what he calls the deconstruction of neurasthenia in the course of the 1920s and 1930s. The neurasthenia diagnosis was increasingly rejected as a blanket diagnosis, a cover for ignorance with regard to the 'real problem', namely a physical disorder or the beginning of a psychosis. In reaction to this criticism advocates of the neurasthenia diagnosis resorted to presenting neurasthenia as a mainly psychogenic disease. Lutz notes that this move resembled Freud's secession from physiological neurology, but that Freud had classified neurasthenia differently, namely as an organic, not a psychogenic disease. As Freud's influence in America had increased significantly by the

1920s, this meant a further blow to neurasthenia. However, in sanatoria and in Veterans' Hospitals the neurasthenia diagnosis remained in use much longer. This was also the case, even to this day, in China, Taiwan, and Japan, as Lutz shortly discusses in a final part, called Reconstructions. Because of its lack of stigma the diagnosis of neurasthenia, considered as a physiological rather than a psychological disease, could become fairly popular in these countries, as was initially the case in America and Europe. Interestingly, in present-day Western cultures neurasthenia is primarily associated with psychological disease, and as such considered to be stigmatised, not really curable, and therefore undesirable. Lutz concludes that both are manifestations of 'the overdetermined desire' to separate soma and psyche.

Britain

The next four chapters deal with Britain. In his introductory chapter Mathew Thomson demonstrates, in line with Roy Porter, that neurasthenia as a term may have been new, but the language of nerves and the somatic location of individual misery was by no means new. This is the reason why it is problematic to simply let neurasthenia's history begin with the introduction of the term. It is equally problematic to determine an end of neurasthenia: even if the term continued to be used, its meaning changed drastically. In Britain the diagnosis of neurasthenia remained in use until well after the First World War, but only after it had changed from a somatic into a psychic diagnosis. This change took place from the early-twentieth-century onwards, and would in the inter-war period result in the replacement of the language of nerves by the language of neuroses and psycho-neuroses, neurasthenia being reduced to just one psycho-neurotic symptom, namely abnormal fatigue.[11] However, ordinary general practitioners tended to stick to a vague and broad neurasthenia diagnosis until well after the First World War, while consumers tended to remain attracted to the older somatic explanatory model, though apparently accepting both somatic and psycho-therapeutic treatment.

Thomson queries the supposedly low profile of neurasthenia in Britain. Taking as a measure the circulation and republication of books and pamphlets on the subject, he is inclined to think that the practical interest in neurasthenia may well have been stronger than the modest number of publications and the critical treatment of the concept within the theoretical literature would seem to suggest. He also queries contemporary and later historiographical statements

6

with respect to the class and gender distribution of neurasthenia. British doctors may have written that neurasthenia could affect all classes, but in practice the better situated may well have been over-represented among those who were diagnosed as such and received treatment. A similar type of confusion reigns over gender: some doctors, and later historians, may have presented neurasthenia as a primarily male affair - the counterpart of female hysteria - but others disagreed, and the known examples of British diagnostic practice and treatment indeed show a fairly mixed picture.[12] Discussing the initial attractions of the neurasthenia diagnosis Thomson emphasises that the somatic explanation of a variety of conditions for which it was hard to find another organic origin, was welcomed by both doctors and patients, be it for different reasons. Doctors were pleased to be able to offer a diagnosis, patients did not want to labelled as mentally ill. Thomson further discusses the increasing use of psycho-therapeutic treatment, the growing influence of the state since the First World War, its impact on doctor–patient relations, and its indirect contribution – through insurance schemes for the shell-shocked – to the acceptance by both doctors and patients of a psychic explanation of neurasthenia.

Chandak Sengoopta discusses neurasthenia in British medical discourse more extensively, paying special attention to the roles of the neurasthenia concept in the professional controversies over medical specialisation. He first focuses on the new specialism of gynaecology, as represented by William Smout Playfair,[13] and the defence of generalism against the encroachment of specialisation, as undertaken by Sir Thomas Clifford Allbutt, both of them being leading British supporters of neurasthenia. Playfair attempted to position himself as the representative of a 'scientific' gynaecology by distancing himself from colleagues who were all too much inclined to interpret 'nervous' disorders in women as a uterine condition and treat them gynaecologically, and by promoting Weir Mitchell's rest cure instead. The general physician Allbutt was likewise opposed to standard gynaecological treatment of women's nervous disorders, but instead claimed that only general physicians possessed the wide knowledge that was required in such cases. Sengoopta describes the discussion organised by the British Medical Association in reaction to Allbutt's attack on gynaecology, and the resulting alliance between Allbutt and Playfair, culminating in their co-editing of a gynaecological handbook.

In the final part of his contribution Sengoopta moves on to neurasthenia's reception and appropriation within neurology and psychiatry. Never having been fervent supporters of the concept, British neurologists had by the second decade of the twentieth century completely lost interest, being preoccupied with organic disorders marked by structural lesions. They even left it to psychiatrists to treat the shell-shocked ex-servicemen, of whom supposedly some 100,000 were diagnosed as neurasthenic. Thus neurasthenia became a psychiatric rather than a neurological concern. As demonstrated by the career of the London alienist William Stoddart, some, but by no means all, British psychiatrists converted to Freudianism and psychoanalysis in the process. However, as the supposedly somatic foundation of neurasthenia was being removed and several different interpretations of neurasthenia were being offered by psychiatrists, neurasthenia's fate was sealed. The concept could no longer serve to unite the many different symptoms into one nosological entity. Nor could it any longer play a role in the controversies over medical specialism, for these had by then died down.

Hilary Marland concentrates on the experiences of British patients, in particular Playfair's all-female clientele, as revealed by Playfair himself in case notes and publications. Although the symptoms of his patients were quite similar, Playfair only diagnosed his well-to-do patients as neurasthenic, while he attributed the complaints of his poor patients at King's College Hospital, London, to long and hard work, sometimes in combination with childbearing. His standard treatment for the 'neurasthenic' women was the rest cure, which he had adopted at an early stage, in 1881. Marland provides interesting vistas of the regime these women were subjected to, and their relationship to Playfair, who took their condition seriously and inspired their trust. With respect to his poor hospital patients he only infrequently had recourse to surgical intervention, preferring less radical types of 'local uterine treatment', and offering these patients an opportunity to recuperate through rest and nutritious food. As Marland argues, Playfair's approaches in treating wealthy patients may well have had an impact on his hospital work.

Michael Neve completes the British quartet with a discussion of public perceptions of neurasthenia between 1880 and 1930, public meaning non-professional, lay. Observing that the history of the neurasthenia diagnosis is 'that of somaticism becoming increasingly supplemented by the language of psychological explanation and therapies from about the 1870s onwards',[14] Neve addresses the question to what extent this development was due to the patient's own involvement in the discussion and treatment of neurasthenia, as

8

manifested in his or her position and behaviour in the medical market-place. He also observes that the emergence of general practitioner and psychiatrist-based therapies at the end of the nineteenth century was first allied to a moderate form of feminism and then, especially in Britain, to diluted forms of psychotherapy and psychological medicine in which standard moral therapy ideals continued to play a part.

Neve approaches the question of the patient's involvement in a kaleidoscopic way. He first concentrates on what a number of printed British medical sources reveal about the problems of neurasthenic patients, their sexual problems included, on doctor/patient relationships and on various types of cures - suggestion played an important role. Next he analyses the huge growth of the commercial domain as evidenced by advertisements of medicines and remedies[15] – the vibrator making a wonderful case – and medical self-help books. It was a mainly middle and upper-middle-class public that was addressed. Neve then moves on to what he considers as a key context for aspects of the psychological developments at the end of the nineteenth century: the position of women, the women's movement and the matter of a possible sexual aetiology for neurasthenia. The well-known neurasthenia novel *A Dark Lantern* here serves as one of his sources. The line of feminist involvement with neurasthenia is drawn through to the 1920s and 1930s, with amongst others the example of Lady Chichester Hospital in Hove, Sussex, which specialized in the early treatment of nervous disorders, including neurasthenia, in poor women and children. Neve concludes that notwithstanding medical attempts to isolate, define or dispose of the concept, the general population used it in a much broader and less specific sense, located somehow between mental illness on the one side and serious physical injury or disease on the other. As such neurasthenia may well have been '*the* people's illness'.

Germany

The next four chapters focus on Germany from roughly the time of the Franco-Prussian War and the ensuing proclamation of the German Empire in 1871 to the First World War. It was a period of rapid industrialisation and other forms of modernisation, which had a distinct impact on the reception and appropriation of the neurasthenia diagnosis. In the introductory chapter Doris Kaufmann first sketches the general context in which neurasthenia gained and lost its importance in Germany, and then goes on to investigate the link between the German discourse on neurasthenia before the First

World War and the emergence of a 'sexual question'. As mentioned, Beard was translated into German at an early stage. Unlike what happened in Britain, Beard's neurasthenia concept was fully adopted in German psychiatry after 1880. German psychiatrists welcomed the concept because it covered a broad range of symptoms, because it implied a clear separation from mental disease, and because it provided an alternative for the diagnosis of hypochondria and hysteria, likewise classified as functional neuroses. Neurasthenia was considered to be mainly a disease of middle-class men and a few middle-class women, while hysteria was primarily associated with women and the lower-classes.

Mainly on the basis of contemporary medical literature, Kaufmann demonstrates that neurasthenia not only played a significant role in psychiatric discourse, but that it was also highly instrumental in promoting the discipline formation of psychiatry. This is thanks to the growing number of middle- and upper-class 'neurasthenic' patients who consulted specialists in nervous diseases. Kaufmann also makes mention of the emergence of a profitable 'neurasthenia-business' around numerous newly established private clinics and sanatoria for nervous diseases from the early-1880s onwards. By 1900 at least 500 private clinics were offering their services in Germany. Towards the end of the nineteenth century, moreover, clinics for working-class patients with neurasthenic problems were set up on the initiative of the neurologist Paul Möbius. As in other countries, psychological explanations of neurasthenia became increasingly important after 1900. However, in the 1910s the influential German psychiatrist Emil Kraepelin incorporated the symptoms of neurasthenia and hysteria into his description of psychosis, thus depriving both diseases of their separate status.[16] In the second part of her chapter, Kaufmann extensively discusses how neurasthenia provided a medical framework for sexual problems of male patients.[17] One of her conclusions is that neurasthenia promoted the emergence of a new psychiatric field of sexual knowledge and the widening of the psychiatric sphere into everyday life.

Volker Roelcke more fully discusses the medical discourses on neurasthenia in Germany until the First World War, including the theoretical and institutional consolidation of psychiatry as an academic discipline – and of neurology as a subspecialty – around 1910. Like Kaufmann, he demonstrates that the vicissitudes of the concept of neurasthenia were closely related to developments in psychiatry. He also observes that the 'career' of neurasthenia is

10

'indicative of the public demand for professional interpretation of individual discomforts and social concerns'.[18] As such discussions on neurasthenia formed an integral part of the broader debates on the effects of modern civilisation on health. Roelcke first pays attention to the intellectual and institutional resources for neurasthenia's reception and appropriation in the last decades of the nineteenth century. Important intellectual resources were the 'electrification' of the nervous system during the preceding decades, the combination of this idea with the idea of limited energy reservoirs in the body, and the availability of the category of 'neuropathic disposition' – resulting from both hereditary and environmental factors – as developed by Wilhelm Griesinger around the middle of the nineteenth century. Important institutional factors were the introduction of outpatients departments at university hospitals and the establishment of private clinics for nervous patients.

Roelcke thereafter sketches the development of the neurasthenia concept. Up to the early-1890s, the medical debate was primarily directed at the frequent occurrence of individual pathology and its connection with the electrophysiology of the nervous system. From the mid-1890s onwards the concept of neurasthenia converged with notions of heredity and degeneration, thus taking on the character of a collective pathology of the nation. As Beard had already observed, the concept of neurasthenia fell on particularly fertile ground in Germany. Initially it was representatives of the new field of neurology, like Wilhelm Erb and Paul Julius Möbius, who especially promoted neurasthenia. In a way similar to Beard, they stressed the external causation of neurasthenia: especially conditions of modern life such as urbanisation, railway traffic and steam power, telegraph and telephone, and also the competitive world of industry and commerce were thought to cause nervous problems. The most frequently advocated cure was electrotherapy, alongside other cures such as the therapeutic application of water, or a stay in the mountains or on the seaside. The rest cure, however, found little resonance in medical publications.[19]

Roelcke ends his chapter with a discussion of the increasing impact of notions of degeneration on the neurasthenia discourse, paying special attention to Emil Kraepelin in this respect. Advocating a somatic-biological perspective from which social causes were excluded, Kraepelin developed a new nosology in which he integrated the concept of degeneration. Already in the 1896 edition of his *Textbook* he no longer recognised neurasthenia as a distinct entity, now using the term 'disorders of exhaustion'. These disorders should in his view be countered or prevented by improving the physical strength of (potentially) affected individuals. As Kraepelin stated in 1908, degeneration was to a large extent caused by the damaging influence of alcohol and syphilis, and it was in its turn the cause of many problems of modern civilization, such as the increased frequency of insanity including 'functional neuroses' and the rapid spread of sexual 'aberrations'. In his view degeneration threatened ever greater parts of the nation. Of course, Kraepelin was by no means the only or the first one who vented such pessimistic ideas. Max Nordau and others had preceded him, at a time when the consequences of urbanization, industrialisation, and the rapidly increasing labour forces began to be interpreted in terms of a fundamental crisis of bourgeois culture. Kraepelin's contribution implied a major shift in the theoretical medical debates: neurasthenia had become a non-issue, whereas heredity and degeneration had become the central concerns. However, in psychiatric practice the concept of neurasthenia remained in use much longer.

This is where Joachim Radkau's highly personal chapter on the neurasthenic experience in imperial Germany comes in. Having studied a great number of patients' records from eight asylums or sanatoria all over Germany - including a public sanatorium for female patients of the lower-classes, opened in 1906 - Radkau presents the results of these forays.[20] Being one of the few authors in this volume who touches on possible connections between religion and neurasthenia,[21] he mentions that the Lutheran neurologist Möbius promoted the Catholic monastery as the best model for the public sanatoria (*Volksnervenheilstätten*). However, priestly status did not necessarily function as a prophylaxis against neurasthenia, for it appears that the hydrotherapeutic centre of Kneipp attracted many neurasthenic priests. Nor was the protestant clergy free from nervous problems. Radkau also points out that patients played an important role in the construction and further development of the neurasthenia concept. According to him it may well be that 'neurasthenia stems much more from the medical consultation room than from neurological theory.'[22] Patients consulted a doctor if their professional or sexual 'energy' and their 'nerves' were failing. Sexual frustrations figure most prominently in the patient's records: male patients especially frequently and quite openly spoke about their fear of having destroyed their nervous and sexual energy by masturbation. However, the overall sex ratio of neurasthenic patients, as represented in these patient's records, appears to be much less uneven, much less male dominated, than medical publications of the time suggested.

Interestingly, Radkau has found hardly any indication of anti-semitism in patients' records and medical commentaries.[23] The general feeling was rather, as he suggests, that nervousness was both a Jewish and a German disease.

The German patient's records show a shift in the concept of neurasthenia around 1900. While it had first stood for weakness, from then on it came to mean a malady of over-excitement. Radkau concludes that neurasthenia manifested itself in Germany, much more so than in England or France, as an acute and urgent mass phenomenon, and as a sign of the times. The connection with sexuality was stronger than in Britain, the connection with modern industrial stress stronger than in France.[24] Radkau observes that Germany bears most resemblance to the United States, albeit that American perceptions of neurasthenia tended to be much more optimistic than the German ones. He also suggests a close connection between the German 'neurasthenia boom' and particular political and cultural trends, such as the politics of social insurance,[25] the sanatorium movement, the spread of nature cures and other manifestations of life reform.

The last chapter on Germany deals with public perceptions of neurasthenia between 1880 and 1919. Heinz-Peter Schmiedebach approaches the subject by analysing articles and advertisements concerning neurasthenia as they were published in two widely-read, middle-class weekly magazines. Although the articles were written by doctors, they obviously addressed and influenced a lay public. Most of the advertisements were also meant for self-medication. Neurasthenia or nervousness was presented as a somatic condition which was primarily the product of modern times, over-excitement and the special requirements of brain-work. Hereditary conditions figured much less prominently than in medical publications at the time. The tone of the articles was rather optimistic, stimulating the readers to take some rest, or to apply other remedies. Apart from the numerous advertisements that dealt with 'premature male neurasthenia' (impotency), neurasthenia was not presented as a specifically male or female disease. Judging by the articles and adverts in these magazines, Schmiedebach suggests that neurasthenia was a very common and widespread disorder indeed. Neurasthenia was both a symbol of modern achievements and of the detrimental consequences of modernity. The advice was clear: slow down a bit.

•

The Netherlands

The next four chapters discuss the Dutch reception and appropriation of neurasthenia from the 1880s until World War I or even later. As in Germany the process of industrialisation took off fairly late, but on a much smaller scale. In his introduction Joost Vijselaar suggests that the distinct character of the reception and impact of neurasthenia in the Netherlands was connected to the fairly optimistic nature of the Dutch *fin-de-siècle*. He works this out for three domains in which neurasthenia manifested itself: politics, literature and medicine. In the political domain the concept of neurasthenia fell on fertile ground with liberal political commentators, who had already been complaining about the 'loss of nerve' of the Dutch population from the late 1870s onwards. Men especially had become 'unnerved' and 'effeminate'. Vijselaar sketches the political and social context of these concerns - the perceived threat to Dutch unity (and the liberal stronghold) by, amongst other things, the advent of denominational 'pillarisation' and the labour movement - and the program of moral regeneration they proposed. However, a younger generation that did not share the pessimism of these old-liberals would soon take over. In the arts, and especially in literature, a group of progressive radicals and 'young liberals' began to criticise bourgeois *mores* and lifestyle from the 1880s onwards. Inspired by French naturalism and contemporary medical ideas, the 'neurasthenic', the 'hysteric' and the '*dégénéré*' figured prominently in their novels. From the 1890s onwards this pessimistic naturalism made way for mysticism or a commitment to humanitarian or socialist reform. The cultural climate around 1900 radiated hope and optimism. By then the concept of neurasthenia had lost its political and moral 'usefulness'. As Vijselaar observes, the Dutch talk about neurasthenia was less pessimistic than the French debate, and degeneration a less important issue. It were rather moral concerns about character, education and sexual conventions that were stressed.

Medical circles were slower to pick up neurasthenia. The major Dutch treatise on neurasthenia by the later professor of psychiatry in Leiden, Gerbrandus Jelgersma, was published only in 1897,[26] four years after the first Dutch academic chair on psychiatry and neurology had been established. Compared to the relatively modest attention for neurasthenia in Dutch medical discussions, neurasthenia gained a certain significance in actual practice, as is for instance shown by the rising number of private institutions - medical sanatoria, specialised therapeutic institutions and nursing or rest

14

homes - for the care of neurasthenics from around 1890. The 'neurasthenia-business', as Vijselaar calls it, also functioned as a welcome alternative for well to do 'psychiatric' patients who were thus saved the stigma of insanity. The concept of neurasthenia appears to have been instrumental in expanding the psychiatric profession and in creating a new domain outside the asylum. Both in private practice and private institutions, doctors could experiment with all sorts of therapies, such as hydropathy, electrotherapy and psychotherapy in the form of hypnotism, early psychoanalysis and persuasive psychotherapy *à la* Dubois. Vijselaar moreover points to the recreational function of the neurasthenia-business, next to the therapeutic function. From 1910 onwards, medical interest in neurasthenia waned and the institutions for neurasthenics disappeared or they became primarily rest homes. As the somatic interpretation of neurasthenia as a disturbance of the nerves began to give way to psychological and psychoanalytical interpretations of what was then diagnosed as (psycho)neurosis, the private practice of the psychiatrist or the psychotherapist, mostly a psychoanalyst, may well have enjoyed an increasing demand on the part of the well-to-do.

In the next chapter Jessica Slijkhuis discusses the Dutch medical discourse with respect to neurasthenia, while concentrating on its most eminent advocate, Gerbrandus Jelgersma. Dutch doctors may not have been quick and diligent in publishing on neurasthenia, they could certainly read about it, if not in English or German, then in the Dutch translation of P.J. Möbius' book on nervousness which appeared in 1884. Around the turn of the century the medical interpretation of neurasthenia underwent a gradual shift from a somatic-physiological to a more psychological approach. Jelgersma can partly be seen as an exponent of this shift: having first adhered to a scientific oriented degenerationist approach, and designating neurasthenia's increase as one of the great social problems of his time, he later on propagated a psychodynamic approach to nervous diseases. Jelgersma also claimed that neurasthenia was more common among men than among women because men, excepting labourers, were more exposed to the strains of modern life. However, degenerationist theory attracted relatively few fervent adherents in Dutch medical circles, nor would a majority of Dutch psychiatrists become converts of Freud. Moreover, some physicians, notably Albert Willem van Renterghem and Frederik van Eeden, had already started with psychotherapy through hypnosis and suggestion *à la* Liébeault in the late 1880s.

In the following chapter Marijke Gijswijt-Hofstra attempts to reconstruct both the prevalence of neurasthenia in the Netherlands and the experiences of people suffering from neurasthenic complaints. Judging by statistics provided in medical publications and the establishment of institutions for neurasthenic patients, the Dutch medical profession appears to have been fairly slow in adopting the neurasthenia diagnosis. Nor did the diagnosis become particularly 'popular', at any rate not nearly as popular as in Germany, but its demise from about 1910 onwards was fairly protracted. It appears that it was mainly the educated and relatively well-off male members of society who were diagnosed as neurasthenic. Firsthand information on the experiences of the 'neurasthenics' themselves is fairly scarce. The article contains information on two professed neurasthenics who described their complaints and therapeutic career in letters or a diary: the author Lodewijk van Deyssel and Ernst Heldring, director of a big shipping company in Amsterdam. It further presents neurasthenic patients in the psychotherapeutic practice of Van Renterghem and Van Eeden, as they figure in their medical publications and in case notes by Van Eeden, and patients published on by other physicians or psychiatrists. The complaints of these patients were diverse, as were the circumstances from which their problems were supposed to have originated, for instance business problems, the strain of exams, family problems or self-imposed standards of superior creativity. Sexual problems or a sexual origin of other neurasthenic complaints were only seldom mentioned. The suffering of these patients tended to be protracted, and their therapeutical careers pluralist. The cures that eventually brought relief included, amongst others, hypnotic suggestion (Van Renterghem and Van Eeden's patients), a stay in the hills or the mountains, the Weir Mitchell cure and homoeopathy. Shopping around for cures like these may well have been the privilege of the well-to-do. People of modest means would not have been able to afford this.

In the last chapter on the Netherlands, Nelleke Bakker discusses a specific aspect of what could be called public perceptions of neurasthenia. This is the use of the psychiatric concept of neurasthenia and its more popular equivalents 'nervousness' and 'weak nerves' in relation to children and their upbringing during the first half of the twentieth century. She explains the 'second life' of neurasthenia in child-rearing advice, from immediately after 1900 until as late as the middle of the twentieth century, in terms of its use by child-rearing experts and their clients: teachers, parents and children. Initially Dutch educationalists were Germany-oriented. Interpretations of neurasthenia that emphasised hereditary determinism were much less popular than the ones that stressed the possibilities of prevention and cure by creating a positive environment, as advocated by Ludwig von Strümpell. However, at the time neurasthenia did not become a major concern of Dutch pedagogues. Child-rearing was mainly conceived of in terms of character formation. Children's insubordination, irritability, fear, eating or sleeping problems, bed-wetting or nail-biting were considered almost exclusively in moral terms. According to this interpretation these children were not ill, but suffered from a lack of self-control or will-power.

Nevertheless, the concept of neurasthenia continued to be used in the inter-war educational discourse. Bakker relates this development to the growing interest in school mental hygiene. Neurasthenic symptoms were considered to be the effect of the mental overburdening of school children. At around the same time the liberal educational discourse experienced a gradual shift from a moral interpretation of children's problematic behaviour to a psycho-medical interpretation of children's disorders. In the 1930s and 1940s Alfred Adler's individual psychology was the dominant theoretical approach in child-rearing literature. As Bakker observes, the concept of neurasthenia was gradually replaced by the less specific concept of nervousness to describe mentally unbalanced children, while at the same time the use of nervousness shifted from a neurological, physiological interpretation to a psychiatric interpretation in terms of family relations as pathogenic conditions. Orthodox Calvinists and Roman Catholics, being organised in their own 'polarised' organisations and having their own journals, took a bit longer than liberals to make the transition to a psycho-medical discourse on child-rearing. In these circles the concept of neurasthenia continued to be used, serving as a welcome medical concept for those experts who wanted to modernise the traditional authoritarian mode of child-rearing, and providing parents with freedom of guilt, for the child's suffering was not regarded as their fault. Neurasthenia also served to cover up a lack of intelligence or bad teaching in case a child failed at school. The diagnosis of neurasthenia moreover relieved children of being held responsible for their behaviour and being punished instead of receiving professional help.

•

France

The last two chapters are devoted to specific aspects of neurasthenia and its aftermath in France. Christopher Forth discusses the relationship between neurasthenia and conceptions of manhood in *fin-de-siècle* France. Was the diagnosis of neurasthenia indeed a safe way for men to be nervous without being associated with nervous, hysterical women, and thus compromising their sense of manhood? Moving between official medical discourses on neurasthenia and wider cultural understandings of what being a neurasthenic male meant in France at the time, Forth demonstrates that this became increasingly problematic from the 1890s onwards. He approaches the relationship between neurasthenia and masculinity by looking into the attitudes towards work and the problem of fatigue. Male nervous fatigue was an ambiguous phenomenon, both destructive and validating. Forth also deals with the problem of emotional and sexual control; it was considered unmanly to exhibit neurasthenic symptoms such as extreme susceptibility to external physical stimuli, the inability to exercise willpower and the collapse of personal boundaries. Forth also positions the increasingly negative attitudes towards male neurasthenia within the specific circumstances of France under the Third Republic. After the defeat in the Franco-Prussian War there was considerable concern about the state of French manhood, especially the martial and reproductive abilities of French men. These worries were reflected in medical discourses about degeneracy and national decline. In this context Jewish nervousness and the Dreyfus Affair also receive attention. In the final part on 'recapturing manhood' Forth relates that the beginning of the twentieth century brought an important shift, similar to the one observed by Janet Oppenheim for Britain. Neurasthenic men were now considered to be responsible for their own nervous problems. As reflected in adverts, popular health manuals and novels, men were expected to gain self-mastery, to get strong by engaging in sports, in short to be energetic and thus virile.

In the final chapter Sonu Shamdasani discusses the medical demise of neurasthenia in France as instigated by Pierre Janet by his launching of psychasthenia, together with a model of psychotherapy linked to a system of dynamic psychology, from the early-1890s onwards. As Shamdasani confirms, the birth of modern psychotherapy should by no means be solely ascribed to Freud. Janet had already developed and put into practice ideas similar to those of Freud, while Janet himself took part in a medical discourse that had already been developing concepts of functional nervous disorders and psychoneuroses, and that had also for some time been emphasising the importance of psychotherapy. After all, until 1902, when he got a post at the Collège de France, Janet had been working at the Salpêtrière hospital in Paris under Charcot, the French godfather of neurasthenia according to a contemporary colleague. Shamdasani shortly reports on neurasthenia's introduction and early reception in France, as mediated by Charcot, who refuted the American and elite character of the disease, while attributing it to organic lesions. Attention is also paid to the moral and hypnotic cures as developed by Hippolyte Bernheim and the Nancy school. It was mainly through Bernheim's work that psychotherapy both as a term and as practice was spread, including the notion that psychotherapy was the right treatment for most neuroses, incorporating 'acquired' as opposed to 'hereditary' neurasthenia. Charcot and colleagues, however, preferred forms of 'moral treatment', one of which being Weir Mitchell's rest cure.

Janet's main work on psychasthenia appeared in 1903. He presented psychasthenia as a major psychoneurosis, comprising 'simple' neurasthenia (in Charcot's sense), depression, phobias and obsessions. Its main characteristics consisted of what he called the sense of incompleteness, the loss of the function of the real and the physiological symptoms of nervous exhaustion. These disorders had a psychological origin. Shamdasani points out that the novel element in Janet's interpretation was that the psychological factor was supposed to act in a uniform, universal and law-like manner. The physical symptoms of psychasthenia and the corresponding symptoms of neurasthenia were the consequence of psychological problems, as Janet would have it. Attention is further paid to Janet's ideas on the treatment of psychasthenia – forms of 'moral treatment' – and, in a final part on 'the death of a disease', to the reception and decline of Janet's concept. Shamdasani concludes that the decline of psychasthenia was to a large extent due to the absence of a training institution of its own, for psychoanalysis did have its own training institutions and survived.

Cultures of neurasthenia compared: Results and remaining problems

The contributions in this volume confront us with a varied and complicated picture of neurasthenia's history or rather histories. The authors offer partly divergent, partly similar observations on the various countries. The question that remains is what actually were the

19

differences or similarities between the countries discussed here, and if these differences refer to per country specific circumstances. And also to what extent these variations should be attributed to either the particular scientific traditions – national or otherwise – the authors themselves work from, or the personal choices they have made. Moreover, as Colin Jones pointed out in his summing-up of the workshop, the comparative aspect also complicates things in other ways.[27] For was it not the implicit assumption that speaking about is speaking for England, or Germany, or the Netherlands? As if the matters discussed simply were and should be representative of a national tradition? But to what extent can one speak about neurasthenia in terms of national traditions or characteristics? Should we follow the idea of representativeness, or should we rather understand neurasthenia as an international movement or a below-national movement, for example along lines of region or denomination? Asking these questions is partly answering them, but no more than that.

The concept of neurasthenia

One of the problems is, of course, the concept of neurasthenia itself – being highly elusive and protean in nature. Neurasthenia seems to be about just everything, an umbrella term. It may be useful, as Colin Jones suggested, to also think about what it is not: it is not, say, a camel, nor an umbrella. This may seem a frivolous exercise. However, it is helpful to think of neurasthenia in this way. What then was included and what is not – what were its parameters? So much is clear: neurasthenia did not include the psychotic. It did initially, in Beard's time, include a whole range of physical and mental symptoms, but by no means new symptoms or even a new combination of symptoms. The label of neurasthenia itself was new, and, to a certain extent, was its explanation. This was not because of its somatic interpretation in terms of a lack of nerve force, or because it was seen as a disorder of modernity, but because of its specific, late nineteenth century interpretation in terms of the fast pace of urban life. In the course of time, depending on where and by whom it was used, the concept of neurasthenia acquired different meanings. Whereas in Beard's concept the notion of degeneration had not been included, degeneration became inextricably bound up with German and French medical discourses on neurasthenia from the 1890s onwards. In British and Dutch medical discourses this seems to have been much less the case. These divergent developments were, as several contributions in this volume indicate,[28] connected to broader socio-cultural and political developments in the respective countries during the *fin-de-siècle*.[29] In the German and French contexts the concern about national decline played an important role. In Germany, moreover, the fast pace of modernisation was a specific cause of concern.

Another change in neurasthenia's meaning, encompassing all these countries, took place from the early-twentieth-century onwards. Neurasthenia shifted from a somatic into a psychic diagnosis – not to be confused with therapy – eventually resulting in the replacement of the language of nerves by the language of neuroses and psycho-neuroses, neurasthenia being reduced to a single psycho-neurotic symptom, namely abnormal fatigue. This process was begun by neurologists and psychiatrists, or whatever they wished to call themselves.[30] They tended to be followed only later and more or less reluctantly by general practitioners and the sufferers themselves.[31] For them a broader and vaguer neurasthenia concept continued to be attractive. Moreover, patients may well have remained fairly reluctant to have their complaints diagnosed as mental, especially if a mental diagnosis entailed the risk of becoming associated with the insane. As Michael Neve suggests for the British context, the general population may well have interpreted neurasthenia as something in between mental illness on the one hand and physical injury or disease on the other. This theme needs to be pursued more fully, also for other countries, and through time.[32] Another shift, more or less related to the shift towards psychic interpretations of neurasthenia, and also taking place from around 1900, has been observed for all countries discussed here: having first been associated with weakness, neurasthenia now came to mean a malady of over-excitement. Indeed, a lack of willpower and self-mastery tended to be seen no longer as the result of nervous exhaustion, but as its cause.

Apart from these historical variations on the theme of neurasthenia, it also appears that historians themselves have developed different approaches to the concept. Some, especially German, historiographies, as Mathew Thomson observes in this volume, tend to use neurasthenia as a loose umbrella term for 'nervous' disorders, whereas others, especially British, use the term in a strictly particular sense. Whether this divergent historiographical use of the term reflects actual historical use remains to be seen. It may well be that in Germany and perhaps also in the Netherlands neurasthenia was more frequently used in a rather encompassing sense, referring to a broad condition of nervousness, for instance in the form of exhaustion, fatigue or depression, a condition that would later be called neurosis. Whereas in the United States and Britain neurasthenia could well have been more frequently used in a narrower sense, as a specific question of psychiatry. In Britain, moreover, the diagnosis of neurasthenia was controversial: medical circles were not inclined to consider it as a new disease, so why should they have needed the term? Of course, the former medical use of the term may not have corresponded with the non-medical use, which would probably have been fairly broad anyway.[33]

Neurasthenia may thus be considered as a form of knowledge that was produced, negotiated, contested and acknowledged. This volume provides partial information on how, where and by whom this was done. It was by no means only doctors who participated in this process. Patients, for instance, had their say as well. A suggestion for future research, offered by Colin Jones, is to look more closely at the topology of neurasthenia: where was neurasthenia at, where was it produced? To what extent was it an urban phenomenon, where, in which cities, faculties, newspapers, etc. do we find it? What was the print history of the term, and what was the print history of the translations?

Neurasthenia's 'popularity'

It is evident by now that the concept of neurasthenia came to mean many different things for the various parties involved. It is still less evident to what extent diagnoses of neurasthenia have in the course of time been actually applied. On the whole it has proved to be fairly difficult to find out about the actual incidence rates of the diagnosis, which, of course, is not the same as the actual incidence of the types of complaints that *could* have been diagnosed as such. Statistics, as published in medical publications or provided by therapeutical institutions, are scarce, and patients' records, if available, have seldom been systematically searched. Medical or other opinions about the prevalence of nervous complaints may well be lacking sufficient foundation and exaggerate one way or the other. Moreover, a more 'liberal' or a more 'strict' historiographical use of the term neurasthenia can result in yet other distortions, as may, according to Mathew Thomson, be the case with Germany's much higher incidence rates as compared with Britain. No more than tentative conclusions can therefore be offered at this stage. As it looks now, the diagnosis of neurasthenia gained most 'popularity' in Germany and least in Britain. The Netherlands are somewhere inbetween, but probably much nearer to Britain than to Germany. France may well prove to have a position nearer to Germany.

Of course, this is no more than a crude ranking. It should be complemented with data about class, gender and age of the sufferers. Statements about class and gender have been offered freely in medical publications on neurasthenia. They may or may not reflect the actual practice of diagnosing. If certain British physicians or a Charcot state that members of all classes were affected by neurasthenia, this should not be taken at face value. The same goes for gender: whether neurasthenia was presented as a disease of both sexes or as a primarily male disease, the distribution of actual diagnoses may have been different. Keeping this in mind, we may tentatively come to the following conclusions.

Initially neurasthenia was very much an affliction of the elite and the educated, not of the labouring-classes. This was the case in all countries discussed here. What started off as a more-or-less fashionable disease of the elites, later on became to a certain extent 'desocialised' or 'democratised', these being the terms that have been used in this volume. Whether or not this frightened off the elites, it appears that the diagnosis of neurasthenia has remained in use the longest amongst 'ordinary' sufferers and in general medical practice.[34] However, the extent to which members of the working-classes came to be diagnosed as neurasthenic is by no means clear. In Germany this process seems to have been well on its way before the turn of the century, after medical and accidence insurance schemes had, financially speaking, paved the way.[35] For Britain the situation is less clear: the available reports are contradictory, and only in the wake of World War I do we hear of shell-shocked soldiers being diagnosed as neurasthenic as a means of getting social insurance.[36] Judging from Playfair's hospital practice and the relative absence of information to the contrary,[37] we may assume that the diagnosis of neurasthenia was not as widely extended to the British working-class as was the case in Germany. In the Netherlands neurasthenia appears to have been primarily diagnosed amongst the upper and middle-classes, mainly the ones who could afford to finance their cure.

The gender distribution poses a similar problem. The German research provides a fairly mixed picture with both men and women represented, though male neurasthenic patients, many of them with sexual problems, constituted in all likelihood the majority. The British situation is fairly confusing, but it was certainly not that the majority of neurasthenic patients were women, as Elaine Showalter would have it.[38] Very much corresponding to Beard's view of neurasthenia as a primarily male affliction, Dutch research has so far produced an overwhelming majority of male neurasthenic patients as compared to only very few female patients. The French contributions in this volume point in the same direction of male majority. We may conclude that, notwithstanding these divergent and yet crude results, neurasthenia was not a large female condition.

It has been stated time and again that the diagnosis of neurasthenia was applied to men for what in women would have been called hysteria. Men were in this way saved the feminine label of hysteria. This may have been true for some, but by no means for all, men with nervous complaints, as Christopher Forth points out for the French context. Anyway, this does raise the important point of what the popular and also the elite patient's sense of neurasthenia was. To what extent, and by whom, was neurasthenia considered to be a masculine, gender-neutral, or a feminine disease? Would, for instance, feminist women have preferred the label of neurasthenia over that of hysteria if they suffered from nervous problems? Was neurasthenia partly considered as a way of rescuing people from being called hysterical, hypochondriacal, insane, etc.? One would indeed think so if one takes all those German and, to a lesser extent, Dutch institutions and nursing homes into account. One also wonders how far people, when they spoke about neurasthenia, had Beard in mind. In England there may have been some jealousy that the United States had come up with a new disease. But there was no such tension elsewhere.

Beard had anyhow faded to the background, when around 1900 German and in their wake Dutch pedagogues 'discovered' neurasthenia as an acceptable diagnosis for children with problematic behaviour, thereby replacing the repertoire of sin and guilt by a medical perspective. This line of research still needs to be pursued further, also for other countries.[39] As Colin Jones remarked, we here see an interesting example of neurasthenia as a professional strategy - in this case with respect to children - on the one hand, and the neurasthenia effect on the other, in this case alleviating guilt. The doctor's word had power, which was part of one's strategy. But it was also a strategy from the patient's or the parents' view. For, as we have seen, calling or having called oneself or their child neurasthenic could have its advantages. To return to the age issue: we could also do with more information about the age distribution of adults who were diagnosed as neurasthenic. The impression is that the age groups under forty to fifty were best represented: these were at any rate the groups who were expected to be energetic and productive, and failing to meet these standards meant that there was a problem.

Another, so far mostly neglected, approach to the actual distribution of neurasthenia would be the angle of religion.[40] Would it have made any difference from the point of view of prevention or susceptibility to have been Catholic, Protestant, Jewish or something else? And what difference would it have made to be Catholic, Protestant or Jewish in the one or the other country or region? Take for instance Catholics: did Dutch Catholics around 1900 have fewer nervous problems, or did they have a more wary attitude towards neurasthenia, or did they just lag somewhat behind with the organisation of their own 'polarised' institutions for nervous patients? These may all be reasons why only very few Catholic neurasthenic patients have so far been discovered in the Dutch context. In France, on the other hand, the majority of neurasthenic patients will have been Catholic. In this context a yet different angle would be the connection between neurasthenia and secularisation: neurasthenia may well have served as a new form of self-interpretation for people who wanted to situate and explain their being indisposed in non-religious terms in a secularising age. Neurasthenia offered a naturalistic explanation for ordinary, not really pathological trouble and affliction. Of course, secularisation may also have been a source of these problems.[41]

A last aspect of neurasthenia's incidence, which should receive more attention, is the question where these patients lived: where they indeed the urban dwellers for whom they were held by Beard, or did they also come from rural surroundings? Unfortunately the contributions in this volume offer very little information in this respect. German and also Dutch medical texts may have repeatedly ventilated Beard's view, but to what extent neurasthenia was in actual practice an urban phenomenon remains to be found out.

It hardly needs saying that there are also other ways of measuring neurasthenia's 'popularity' than by looking at the incidence of diagnoses. Although actual practice as it unfolds in patient–doctor consultations and negotiations is at the heart of the matter, there is more to it. For example the production of professional publications on neurasthenia, the production of medical advice literature, advertisements for remedies and cures, and, of course, the offered cures themselves. Not for nothing the term 'neurasthenia business' was used more than once during the workshop. Neurasthenia can indeed also be seen as business, and even as fashion production. One could even speak of a 'neurasthenia market', a market where medical advice, technology, remedies and cures were advertised and sold, thus creating and playing on the demand from (potential) patients. If not neurasthenia itself, then the cure was advocated as a desirable and possibly fashionable product. Spas, seaside and mountain resorts, and nursing homes, all combined the elements of medical treatment, rest and possibly even vacation, while sports too became increasingly important. All these aspects and the ways in which they were interconnected still deserve much attention.

Interpretations and connections

Neurasthenia's varying 'popularity' – in the course of time and in different regions, countries or groups – asks for explanations. Some have been offered in this volume, for instance the ones that point out the use or functions of neurasthenia for one or more of the parties involved. Patients were for instance saved a more stigmatising or unpleasant diagnosis and confinement in an asylum, and they could even try to make the best of it if they were wealthy enough to go to an attractive place for treatment. Doctors were pleased to have a label for a broad variety of vague complaints and to be able to offer some kind of treatment. Psychiatrists could make good use of neurasthenia for attracting a middle and upper-class clientele, which in its turn was highly instrumental in promoting the discipline formation of psychiatry. As it appears, this was most clearly the case in Germany. Quite a few medical boundary contests were fought out over neurasthenia, resulting in the further demarcation and filling-in of medical specialisations, for instance between neurology and psychiatry, and, in the British case, between gynaecology and general medical practice. As mentioned, neurasthenia also functioned as business. Apart from the doctors themselves, numerous others, such as nurses and other personnel in the many institutions or resorts where neurasthenic patients hoped to get cured, held a more or less important stake in the 'neurasthenia business'. It remains to be seen exactly how big this stake was in the different countries and how this fitted into already-existing therapeutical traditions.

Cultures of neurasthenia were very much intertwined with therapeutical developments, especially with regard to forms of psychotherapy and psychoanalysis. Although it should be added that neurasthenia was by no means the only affliction which was treated with psychotherapeutical methods. For instance, psychotherapy in the form of hypnosis and suggestion *à la* Liébeault was in the second half of the 1880s introduced into the Netherlands by the general practitioner Albert Willem van Renterghem, not with the intention only or even primarily to treat nervous patients. As it appears, Van Renterghem and his colleague Frederik van Eeden did indeed mainly attract nervous patients, including neurasthenics, but these types of patients were by no means the only ones. Suggestion became the keyword by which the doctor should inspire the patient to believe in his or her own healing powers. Later on both of them would also develop an interest in psychoanalysis. This example illustrates how complicated the connection between neurasthenia and forms of psychotherapy can be. It is also an example of what some time later would become fashionable: the private practice of the psychiatrist or the psychotherapist and especially the psychoanalyst. Several contributions to this volume touch on these and related themes.[42]

A final word about possible connections between the reception and the impact of neurasthenia on the one hand and the particular, more-or-less pessimistic, nature of the *fin-de-siècle* in different societies. It has been suggested that the relatively low profile of neurasthenia in the Netherlands may have been connected to the (supposedly) fairly optimistic nature of the Dutch *fin-de-siècle*. Similar remarks have been made about Germany and France in those cases, about the relationship between a greater preoccupation with neurasthenia and a more pessimistic nature of the *fin-de-siècle*. The problem is, of course, that these are fairly crude and also ambiguous types of statement. Even if we were to agree about what to understand by *fin-de-siècle* and how to assess its nature, then we would still be left with what could well turn out to be a chicken and egg problem, namely the nature of the connections between the two. Having said this, the temptation is great to pursue this path further. After all, neurasthenia's reception and appropriation in the various countries may have been very much a matter of its usefulness to the parties concerned, these parties in their turn were children of their time, sharing at least some of its concerns and hopes. Further reflections and research on these broader cultural contexts of neurasthenia would be very desirable. Or, to cite a former Dutch doctor: 'Be up and doing, and have guts'.[43]

Acknowledgements

My thanks to Roy Porter, August Gijswijt, Harry Oosterhuis and Joost Vijselaar for their help and comments.

Notes

1. Janet Oppenheim, '*Shattered Nerves': Doctors, Patients, and Depression in Victorian England* (New York & Oxford: Oxford University Press, 1991), 92–3. See also Roy Porter and Tom Lutz in this volume.
2. See Roy Porter and Mathew Thomson in this volume.

3. See Christopher Forth and Sonu Shamdasani in this volume.
4. Susan E. Abbey & Paul E. Garfinkel, 'Neurasthenia and Chronic Fatigue Syndrome: The Role of Culture in the Making of a Diagnosis', *American Journal of Psychiatry*, 148, 12 (1991), 1638–46.
5. See on America: F.G. Gosling, *Before Freud: Neurasthenia and the American Medical Community, 1870-1910* (Urbana, IL: University of Illinois Press, 1987); Tom Lutz, *American Nervousness, 1903: An Anecdotal History* (Ithaca, NY: Cornell University Press, 1991). See on Britain: Elaine Showalter, *The Female Malady: Women, Madness and English Culture, 1830-1980* (London: Virago Press, 1987); Janet Oppenheim, *op. cit.* (note 1). See on Germany: Joachim Radkau, *Das Zeitalter der Nervosität. Deutschland zwischen Bismarck und Hitler* (Munich: Hanser, 1998); Volker Roelcke, *Krankheit und Kulturkritik. Psychiatrische Gesellschaftsdeutungen im bürgerlichen Zeitalter 1790-1914* (Frankfurt/Main: Campus, 1999).
6. George F. Drinka, *The Birth of Neurosis: Myth, Malady, and the Victorians* (New York: Simon & Schuster, 1984). A. Rabinbach, *The Human Motor: Energy, Fatigue and the Origins of Modernity* (New York: Basic Books, 1990); Edward Shorter, *From Paralysis to Fatigue. A History of Psychosomatic Illness in the Modern Era* (New York, etc.: The Free Press, 1992).
7. Roy Porter, 'The Patient's View: Doing Medical History from Below', *Theory and Society*, 14 (1985), 175–198.
8. Lutz, *op. cit.* (note 5); Radkau, *op. cit.* (note 5).
9. With the addition of one further paper by Christopher Forth.
10. In his final comments at the workshop, Colin Jones raised the preliminary problem of how to establish what is public. Take for instance articles on neurasthenia in general magazines written by physicians: to what extent can these articles be considered to represent the public, non-professional sphere?
11. See also Chandak Sengoopta in this volume.
12. Similar observations have been made by Chandak Sengoopta and, for France, by Christopher Forth in this volume.
13. See on Playfair and his patients also Hilary Marland in this volume.
14. See Michael Neve in this volume, 139.
15. See Heinz-Peter Schmiedebach in this volume, 217.
16. See for a fuller discussion of Kraepelin's ideas Volker Roelcke in this volume, 175.
17. See on sexual problems of 'neurasthenics' also Joachim Radkau, Heinz-Peter Schmiedebach and Christopher Forth in this volume.
18. See Volker Roelcke in this volume, 175.
19. See, however, Edward Shorter, *A History of Psychiatry. From the Era*

of the Asylum to the Age of Prozac (New York, etc.: John Wiley & Sons, 1997), 133. Shorter states that 'by 1884 many private clinics had incorporated the "milk diet" (Mastkur), as some called it, or "Mitchell-Playfair Cure", into their palette of therapies for hysteria and neurasthenica.'

20. See also Radkau, *op. cit.* (note 5).
21. See also Marijke Gijswijt-Hofstra, Nelleke Bakker and Sonu Shamdasani in this volume.
22. See Joachim Radkau in this volume, 203.
23. See Christopher Forth in this volume on 'Jewish nervousness' in France, 327.
24. Radkau does not mention the Netherlands, but see the Dutch chapters in this volume, and the concluding part of this introduction.
25. See on this topic Heinz-Peter Schmiedebach, 'Post-traumatic Neurosis in Nineteenth-Century Germany: A Disease in Political, Juridical and Professional Context', *History of Psychiatry*, 10 (1999), 27–57.
26. See Jessica Slijkhuis in this volume for a fuller discussion of Jelgersma's ideas, 255.
27. With my thanks to Colin Jones who suggested that, rather than writing a conclusion to the volume himself, I could freely integrate elements of his summing-up in this introduction.
28. See for instance Michael Neve, Doris Kaufmann, Volker Roelcke, Joost Vijselaar, Marijke Gijswijt-Hofstra and Christopher Forth in this volume.
29. See also Daniel Pick, *Faces of Degeneration: A European Disorder, c.1848-c.1918* (Cambridge etc.: Cambridge University Press, 1989).
30. See also the recent publication on Krafft-Ebing by Harry Oosterhuis, *Stepchildren of Nature. Krafft-Ebing, Psychiatry, and the Making of Sexual Identity* (Chicago & London: The University of Chicago Press, 2000).
31. Of course, the appropriation of neurasthenia as a psychic instead of a somatic diagnosis should be distinguished from the appropriation of certain types of therapy. Sufferers, for example, may well have been clinging to a somatic diagnosis while welcoming psychotherapy at the same time. They may thus have indirectly furthered the shift towards a psychic diagnosis of neurasthenia. See also Henri F. Ellenberger, *The Discovery of the Unconscious. The History and Evolution of DynamicPsychiatry* (New York: Basic Books, 1970).
32. See also Tom Lutz in this volume, 49.
33. See also Michael Neve on this point, 139.

34. Nelleke Bakker moreover points in this volume to the 'second life' of the diagnosis of neurasthenia in Dutch child-rearing advice. It remains to be seen to what extent other countries knew similar developments, 307.

35. Schmiedebach, *op. cit.* (note 25).

36. See Mathew Thomson in this volume, 75.

37. Thomas Savill, for instance, treated neurasthenic working-class patients in the 1880s and 1890s. See Mathew Thomson in this volume.

38. Showalter, *op. cit.* (note 5). See also Mathew Thomson in this volume.

39. It is interesting to see that at around the same time when children with problematic behaviour were alleviated of guilt, nervous adults began to be admonished to exhibit self-mastery and will-power, thus being held responsible for their own recovery if not for their illness in the first place.

40. See Joachim Radkau, Nelleke Bakker and Christopher Forth in this volume.

41. This suggestion was offered by Joost Vijselaar.

42. See for example Mathew Thomson, Chandak Sengoopta, Michael Neve, Doris Kaufmann, Joost Vijselaar, Marijke Gijswijt-Hofstra and Sonu Shamdasani in this volume.

43. H. van der Hoeveen, 'Neurasthenie', *Nederlandsch maandschrift voor geneeskunde*, 10 (new series 2) (1921), 35–36: 44. See also Gijswijt-Hofstra in this volume.

1

Nervousness,
Eighteenth and Nineteenth Century Style:
From Luxury to Labour

Roy Porter

> How can we be cheerful when our nerves are shattered?
> **Peacock, Nightmare Abbey**[1]

> Phenomena which cannot otherwise be accounted for are commonly
> attributed to nervousness; - but to what is nervousness attributable?
> The world may rest on Atlas, but on what does Atlas rest?
> **James Manby Gully**[2]

This paper opens by exploring the framing of 'nervous disorders' in
eighteenth century England; it then proceeds to analyse nineteenth
century developments in general, focuses down on neurasthenia in
the USA and UK, and concludes by highlighting continuities and
discontinuities.

Enlightenment nervousness

As early as the 1660s, Thomas Willis, to whom we owe the term
'neurologie', was maintaining that study of the nervous system
revealed 'the hidden causes of diseases and symptoms';[3] and in
succeeding generations, physicians of a iatromechanical bent
addressed the traditional humoral discourse of melancholy, as
definitively elaborated by Robert Burton, reconfiguring it as a
nervous disease. The Edinburgh professor William Cullen
established neurosis as a pathological entity and made the nervous
system central to physiology and pathology.[4] Though the nature
of the nerve fibres remained contested (were they wires or hollow
tubes, did they conduct electrical impulses or some aetherial
fluid?), their role in connecting body and brain gave
neuroanatomy a prima facie prominence in the elucidation of
maladies of mood and behaviour.

In the Georgian era, such popular labels as the spleen and the vapours, hysteria and hypochondriasis were thereby provided with a neurological substrate. 'Nervous' maladies became privileged in polite society, as tokens of their victims' cultivation, and 'nervousness' turned into a badge of honour, a mark of superior sensibility. 'Upwards of thirty years ago', declared James McKittrick Adair in his *Essays on Fashionable Disorders* (1790),

> a treatise on nervous diseases was published by my quondam learned and ingenious preceptor Dr Whytt, professor of physic, at Edinburgh. Before the publication of this book, people of fashion had not the least idea that they had nerves; but a fashionable apothecary of my acquaintance, having cast his eye over the book, and having been often puzzled by the enquiries of his patients concerning the nature and causes of their complaints, derived from thence a hint - 'Madam, you are nervous!' The solution was quite satisfactory, the term because fashionable, and spleen, vapours and hyp were forgotten.[5]

The 'nervousness' diagnosis itself enjoyed a rise and fall in fashion. 'My complaints', complained Colonel Ellison in 1744, 'are what the Modern Physicians term nervous, a cant word the Gentlemen of the Faculty are pleased to make use of when a distemper proves obstinate and does not yield to their medicines'.[6]

In the 1730s, George Cheyne judged that a third of all disorders were nervous.[7] Seventy years later, Thomas Trotter thought they constituted 'two thirds of the whole, with which civilised society is afflicted'.[8] Like fashion itself, disease evidently obeyed the 'trickle down' effect: 'we shall find, that nervous ailments are no longer confined to the better ranks in life', fretted Trotter, 'but rapidly extending to the poorer classes'.[9]

The identification of nervousness as the key to modern malaises was boldly made early by George Cheyne, the Scottish physician whose impeccable Enlightenment credentials included endorsement of the iatromechanistic teachings of the Leiden-Edinburgh school and eminence as a Newtonian populariser. Did the wealth of nations secure the health of nations? Far from it, he concluded. For as England rose to riches, her people were sinking in health, succumbing to that clutch of chronic and constitutional conditions he dubbed 'The English Malady.'[10]

Cheyne spelt out familiar primitivist tropes: 'when Mankind was simple, plain, honest and frugal, there were few or no diseases. Temperance, Exercise, Hunting, Labour, and Industry kept the Juices

Sweet and the Solids brac'd'.[11] As early as the Ancients, however, the rot had set in. It was conventional to praise the Greeks for inventing medicine. But had they not been driven to it by the proliferation of sickness caused by their softened, sedentary, urban lifestyle?

> The ancient Greeks, while they lived in their Simplicity and Virtue were Healthy, Strong and Valiant: But afterwards, in Proportion as they advanced in Learning, and the Knowledge of the Sciences, and distinguished themselves from other Nations by their Politeness and Refinement, they sunk into Effeminacy, Luxury, and Diseases, and began to study Physick, to remedy those Evils which their Luxury and Laziness had brought upon them.[12]

Thus Enlightenment - the Greek Enlightenment - had proved the forcing-house of disease. Thereafter it was downhill all the way. Prosperous England was suffering in particular: 'Since our Wealth has increas'd, and our Navigation has been extended, we have ransack'd all the Parts of the Globe to bring together its whole Stock of Materials for Riot, Luxury, and to provoke Excess'.[13] Various components of the nation's commercial and social success were now conspiring to exacerbate sickness:

> The Moisture of our Air, the Variableness of our Weather, (from our Situation amidst the Ocean) the Rankness and Fertility of our Soil, the Richness and Heaviness of our Food, the Wealth and Abundance of the Inhabitants (from their universal Trade) the Inactivity and Sedentary Occupations of the better Sort (amongst whom this Evil mostly rages) and the Humour of living in great, populous and consequently unhealthy Towns, have brought forth a Class and Set of Distempers, with atrocious and frightful Symptoms, scarce known to our Ancestors, and never rising to such fatal Heights, nor afflicting such Numbers in any other known Nation.[14]

As the kingdom grew 'luxurious, rich and wanton', distempers mushroomed.[15] Fashionable living was deleterious, with its late rising, later nights, artificial lighting and heating, tight-lacing, and worst of all, sophisticated cuisines culled from all corners of the globe, prizing dishes rich, salted, sauced, pickled, smoked and highly-seasoned, all washed down with fortified liquors and ardent spirits.[16] High living in high society carried high health risks.

To complement his history of disease, Cheyne also pointed up a sociology. Agricultural labourers were the contemporary equivalents of savages, physically-robust 'No Thinkers': 'Fools, weak or stupid Persons, heavy and dull Souls, are seldom much troubled with

Vapours or Lowness of Spirits'.[17] By contrast, top people sacrificed their health and equanimity to the calls of business, pleasure, ease and fashion. Particularly vulnerable were the *literati*:

> Now since this present Age has made Efforts to go beyond former Times, in all the Arts of Ingenuity, Invention, Study, Learning, and all the contemplative and sedentary Professions (I speak only here of our own Nation, our own Times, and of the better Sort, whose chief Employments and Studies these are) the Organs of these Faculties being thereby worn and spoil'd, must affect and deaden the whole System, and lay a Foundation for the Diseases of Lowness and Weakness.[18]

Doubtless with his own 'case' in mind – gourmandising at one point blew him up to 450lbs – Cheyne noted that 'Great Wits are generally great Epicures, at least, Men of Taste'.[19] If the stimuli of the bottle and the table were needed, if one was to shine, no wonder the nerves became debilitated and damaged.

Sickness, held Cheyne, made terrible inroads into the sensibilities of those fine spirits blessed, or cursed, with exquisite feelings and a hyperactive brains. Such highly-strung people were spinning downwards on a dizzying spiral. Fleeing 'Anxiety and Concern', they sought diversion in dissipation - 'Assemblies, Musick Meetings, Plays, Cards, and Dice', which jeopardised their health.[20] The irony (or cosmic justice), in short, was that it was the Quality who were chiefly doomed to suffer.[21]

Since Cheyne's formulation of the 'English Malady' as a constitutionally crippling yet choice disorder has been widely analysed of late,[22] I shall now draw attention to just three facets of it. First, he was emphatic that civilisation bred self-inflicted sickness: 'these monstrous and extreme Tortures, are entirely the Growth of our own Madness and Folly, and the Product of our own wretched Inventions'.[23] Second, he insisted, the fact that he embraced such a view did not make him a primitivist, a railer, or a Rousseauvian *avant la lettre*. Critics of his advocacy of dietary reform - moderation for all and vegetarianism for some - were utterly wrong to accuse him of being 'at Bottom a mere Leveller, and for destroying Order, Ranks and Property'.[24] For - my third point - Cheyne was not for rejecting, but for refining, civilisation. He wanted to sublimate the grossness of affluence into something altogether more aetherial and elevated. To the end of achieving this lightness of being, he formulated a new sociology (an aesthetic of elite living), a new psychology (heightened sensibility, indeed, taste) and predicated them upon a new physiology, which discarded classical humoralism in favour of the iatro-mechanist and medically materialist idiom of the nerves as the key to 'the Human Machin'.[25]

Health, explained the English Malady, hinged not upon humoral equipoise but upon nervous tone. Nerves were designed to carry impulses rapidly and efficiently throughout the body. Being so delicate, their channels were readily clogged by swill from overloaded guts, rendering them 'glewy' and sluggish. In particular, acidities produced irritations, provoking ulcers, inflammations and other obstructions. Weakened, relaxed nerves would in time lead to diarrhoeas, phlegm, dropsy, diabetes, scrofula and other chronic malaises.

Fine physical health, it followed, depended upon keeping these vital nerves springy and tonic. All the more so as the beau monde 'have a great Degree of Sensibility; are quick Thinkers, feel Pleasure or Pain the most readily, and are of most lively Imagination'.[26] Psycho-physiology thus supported the 'common Division of Mankind into Quick Thinkers, Slow Thinkers and No Thinkers'; 'Persons of slender and weak Nerves are generally of the first Class: the Activity, Mobility and Delicacy of their intellectual Organs make them so'. Indeed, nervous affliction 'never happens or can happen, to any but those of the liveliest and quickest natural Parts, whose Faculties are the brightest and most spiritual, and whose Genius is most keen and penetrating, and primarily where there is the most delicate Sensation and Pain'.[27] Highly-strung people living on their nerves were thus disproportionately prone to debility.

Cheyne's blaming of mood disorders on the nerves gave expression to an astute strategy of patient management, not least because it dissociated English malady sufferers from any imputation either of downright lunacy on the one hand, or of self-indulgent malingering on the other. Catering for wealthy and influential patients, and aware that couching a diagnosis in tactful terms was not only an essential but a delicate business (John Radcliffe was reputed to have been dismissed from Queen Anne's service after telling her Majesty she was suffering from the 'vapours'), enlightened physicians made great play of the organic origins of mysterious maladies and ambiguous ailments.

The diplomacy of diagnostic negotiation was pondered by Cheyne: physicians were commonly put on the spot by 'nervous cases', because such conditions were easily dismissed by the 'vulgar' as tell-tale marks of 'peevishness' or, when ladies were afflicted, of 'fantasticalness' or 'coquetry'.[28] Somatic categories, by contrast were music to patients' ears, craving as they did diagnoses which confirmed the reality of their disorders. Foolish people might suppose that the extended family of disorders which included hysteria and the spleen were 'nothing but the effect of Fancy, and a delusive Imagination'; such charges were ill-founded, however, because 'the consequent Sufferings are without doubt real and unfeigned'.[29] Even so, hitting upon *le mot juste* required great tact. 'Often when I have been consulted in a Case ... and found it to be what is commonly call'd Nervous', Cheyne mused:

> I have been in the utmost Difficulty, when desir'd to define or name the Distemper, for fear of affronting them or fixing a Reproach on a Family or Person.... If I said it was Vapours, Hysterick or Hypochondriacal Disorders, they thought me mad or Fantastical.[30]

His contemporary, Richard Blackmore, chewed over similar difficulties. 'This Disease, called Vapours in Women, and the Spleen in Men, is what neither Sex are pleased to own', he emphasised,

> for a doctor cannot ordinarily make his Court worse, than by suggesting to such patients the true Nature and Name of their Distemper.... One great Reason why these patients are unwilling their Disease should go by its right Name, is, I imagine, this, that the Spleen and Vapours are, by those that never felt their Symptoms, looked upon as an imaginary and fantastick sickness of the Brain, filled with odd and irregular Ideas.... This Distemper, by a great Mistake, becoming thus an Object of Derision and Contempt: the persons who feel it are unwilling to own a Disease that will expose them to Dishonour and Reproach.[31]

Any such imputations of shamming would be scotched, insisted Dr Nicholas Robinson, once it was made clear that such disorders were not 'imaginary Whims and Fancies, but real Affections of the Mind, arising from the real, mechanical Affections of Matter and Motion'; for 'neither the Fancy, nor Imagination, nor even Reason itself...can feign...a Disease that has no Foundation in Nature'.[32] After all, stressed that vocal medical Newtonian, one could not 'conceive the Idea of an Indisposition, that has no Existence in the Body'.[33]

In explicating hysteria and hypochondria, nerve doctors did not seek altogether to deny the contribution of the mind. But their wish to be identified as modern, scientific physicians treating superior people disposed iatromechanists to insist upon the primacy of physical stimuli, principally the nerves, as part of a strategy designed to win the confidence of both their professional peers and their patients. Establishing the credentials of nervous disorders would enhance the status of medicine itself, while enlightened nerve doctors were ostentatiously sympathetic to the tribulations of their clients. In the many case-histories detailed in the final section of *The English Malady*, Cheyne made much of the real woes of sufferers burdened with misery, depression, taedium vitae, hysteria and so forth - not least, his very own case.

The nineteenth century

Nervous breakdown, depression, collapse, exhaustion, prostration, agitation and irritability - all these were central life-experiences to Darwin, Huxley, Florence Nightingale and scores of other eminent Victorians. Their doctors had to confront a constellation of symptoms: fatigue, insomnia, emptiness, weeping, impotence, obsessive fears, headache, backache, neuralgia, dyspepsia, excruciating headaches, and so forth.[34] 'In the most remarkable of these cases', according to Henry Holland, discussing nervous collapse,

> all the voluntary movements of walking, speaking, eating, etc., were
> in a sort of abeyance - the mind inert, as if unable to force itself into
> any effort of thought or feeling - the circulation exceedingly feeble -
> and great torpor of all the natural functions.[35]

As in the Enlightenment writings just discussed, nineteenth-century discourses of shattered nerves standardly rooted all such symptoms in the body, though it was widely acknowledged that 'functional nervous disorder' and similar labels might be convenient diagnostic cloaks for medical ignorance: Clifford Allbutt, Regius Professor of Medicine at Cambridge, thus lamented that 'the so-called diseases of the nervous system' were 'a vast, vague, and most heterogeneous body, two-thirds of which may not primarily consist of diseases of nervous matter at all'.[36]

Various theoretical models were tendered for those thus stressed-out. Till mid-century, nervous collapse was mainly attributed to 'spinal irritation'. At a later stage explanations hinging on nervous energy moved stage centre, with malfunctionings of the nervous system being attributed to lack of 'nerve force'. Drawing upon high-prestige experimental physics, it became commonplace to liken the grey matter of the brain, regarded as the source of nervous energy, to a faradic battery generating electrical current, with the nerve fibres acting as wires, conducting power throughout the body.[37]

Articulated around mid-century, the second law of thermodynamics furthermore posited that the quantum of energy available in the Universe was gradually and inexorably decreasing. This entropy theory was incorporated in medicine in such assertions as Henry Maudsley's dictum that the 'energy of a human body [is] a definite and not inexhaustible quantity'.[38] Reserves of nervous energy were finite, Victorian doctors warned: over-exertion, mental or physical, would sap an individual's supply, leaving a depleted nervous system incapable of activity. Just as an epileptic fit might be explained in terms of excessive build-up and then discharge of nervous energy, so the symptoms of depression, fatigue, melancholia and nervous breakdown could be attributed to the ebbing of the same force. Utter paralysis might follow, indicating that so-called weakness of will had a nervous foundation.

Such borrowings from energy physics were intimately linked, semantically and symbolically, to dominant economic metaphors. Within the idiom of a nervous economy, the language of 'depression' bridged the economic and the neurological, whether it was thought of as reduced capital expenditure in an economic depression, the fall of atmospheric pressure in a meteorological depression, or a draining of nervous energy. In Victorian writings which abound in phrases like 'taxing nervous resources' and 'wasting nervous reserves', nerve force was widely represented as a deposit which could be wisely invested for the future, spent prudently, or splashed out recklessly, precipitating bankruptcy. 'Money now is almost exclusively made at the expense of the wear-and-tear of nerve', commented the Harley Street nerve doctor, Alfred Schofield, 'and it is a matter of ever-increasing economical importance to keep the money-making machine, the brain and the mind, at the highest productive pitch - in short, in a state of perfect health'.[39] Given the Victorian esteem for the Protestant work-ethic, the prospects of nervous breakdown or physiological bankruptcy - demand exceeding supply, or one's mental bank-balance being catastrophically overdrawn - were particularly daunting.

Brought on by pressure, exertion, anxiety and tribulation, mental strain was widely viewed as the cause of decreased nerve energy and fatigue.[40] When the distinguished Scottish geologist, religious leader and newspaper editor Hugh Miller committed suicide, it was precisely such a theoretical model which was invoked by way of exoneration: Miller was said to have become fatally overwrought as a result of overwork and anxiety.[41] Late in the century, theories of nervous collapse were increasingly integrated into hereditarian and degenerationist frameworks. Schofield, for instance, insisted that an array of functional nervous disorders, including hysteria, neurasthenia and migraine, were 'all strongly hereditary'.[42]

Neurasthenia and nervous collapse

British medical writings on nervous complaints were a motley mix before the new diagnostic category of 'neurasthenia' held out the promise of creating coherence out of chaos, and conferring new medical legitimacy upon the protean symptoms of depression.[43] A pathological construct meaning nerve weakness or debility of the nervous system, neurasthenia was floated from 1869 by George Miller Beard, a New York neurologist and electrotherapist.[44] It was a concept which owed something to the Brunonian idea that disease was divisible into two categories, sthenia and asthenia - that is, respectively, an excess of stimulation, and an incapacity to react to stimulus.[45]

Beard painted a panorama of the physical and mental symptoms of neurasthenia: anxiety, despair, phobias, fretfulness, insomnia, nightmares, inattention, extreme fatigue, migraine, palpitations, indigestion, impotence, neuralgia, and many more. If the list seemed interminable, he was at least more precise when it came to questions of social aetiology. Neurasthenia was a disorder of modernity, and it was, as was blazoned forth by the title of his chief book, primarily a matter of American Nervousness, for 'gilded age' United States was a land of unparalleled social mobility, bursting with dynamic entrepreneurs and ambitious achievers, whose high-tension, non-stop tempo of life was rightly, for Beard, a matter of national pride: 'American nervousness is the product of American civilisation'.[46] This 'distinguished malady'[47] moreover surfaced almost exclusively among the educated middle and upper-classes – those intellectuals, professionals and businessmen who took up most intensively the challenge of modern urban life.[48] Only 'our nervous century' could breed neurasthenia, he wrote, for contemporary civilisation alone, especially in its American manifestation, had produced the unique combination of elements so deleterious to nerve force: 'steam power, the periodical press, the telegraph, the sciences, and the mental activity of women'.[49] With the erosion of religious faith, top people, moreover, were adrift in a sea of doubt. Competition, insecurity and ceaseless striving made for an exhausting schedule, as Americans battled to make good and prove themselves in a market place whose law was the survival of the fittest. Such a demanding milieu made the sapping of nervous energy inevitable.

In Beard's medical model, insufficient nerve force offered a comprehensive explanation for every neurasthenic symptom. For men and women temperamentally or constitutionally doomed to deficient output of nerve force, or for those whose lifestyle and imprudent habits squandered otherwise adequate supplies, any additional strain – from business cares, domestic trouble, excessive mental labour or anything else – would hurtle the wretched victim into a neurasthenic tailspin. The brain, the digestive organs and the reproductive system, Beard explained, were all centres for the body's nervous reflex action. Depletion of nerve force through excess demands upon any one of these nuclei would send irritation and exhaustion pulsing through the body, with physical symptoms appearing in what might seem the most implausible places.

Beard's neurasthenic formulation was to be given its distinctive therapeutics by Silas Weir Mitchell. In highly successful works like *Wear and Tear, or Hints for the Overworked* (1871) and *Fat and Blood: and How to Make Them* (1877), he elaborated the rest cure, which prized seclusion, enforced bed-rest, electrical treatments, a milk diet, and passive exercise through massage. This schedule of treatment, Mitchell insisted, represented an organic remedy for a somatic condition.[50]

The neurasthenia diagnosis crossed the Atlantic. Like their American counterparts, British medical writers insisted that it was, if 'protean',[51] a real 'functional' disorder of the nervous system,[52] rather than a disorder of the imagination or a species of insanity. They likewise insisted that its chief causes were 'overstrain' and 'overwork',[53] if placing more blame than the Americans on high-pressure educational 'brainwork', especially amongst women.[54] The spiritually destabilising effects of the progress of science and technology were also often cited.[55] It was widely categorised as a disorder of the more 'civilised races'.[56]

Though highly popular in America, the neurasthenia diagnosis won, however, rather a mixed reception amongst British neurologists and clinicians. It had a handful of renowned supporters, notably Clifford Allbutt in Cambridge and the obstetrician William Playfair at King's College Hospital in London. The concept was welcomed as a useful addition to medical terminology by others as well, including the aptly-named Thomas Stretch Dowse, author of *On Brain and Nerve Exhaustion: "Neurasthenia"* (1880).[57] Many, however, judged it a case of old wine in new bottles, the familiar malady of shattered nerves tricked out in new clothes. The entry in Tuke's *Dictionary of Psychological Medicine* thus traced its pedigree back to the sixteenth century,[58] while Sir Andrew Clark of the London Hospital similarly observed that its symptom cluster had 'been more or less fully recognised and described by every competent observer and writer from the days of Cheyne and Whytt until now'. Neurasthenia 'is not a novelty', insisted Leonard Guthrie: 'under other names it has always flourished'.[59]

While certain late Victorian and Edwardian medical men thus approved the handle of 'neurasthenia' because it imposed coherence on a pot pourri of disparate symptoms, or bestowed an air of precision on a protean affliction, others were thus not so impressed or ready to forego the old diagnostic categories of spinal irritation or hysteria. Hopes of forging diagnostic clarity had thus foundered in terminological controversy.

Rather as with Trotter's gloss on Georgian nervousness, quoted above, or Charcot's strategy with hysteria, efforts were made further to validate the condition by insisting on its prevalence and universality. According to Cyril Bennett, it was 'as common in the slums of the East End as in the mansions of the West',[60] while Leonard Guthrie proclaimed, 'it is not confined to any class or any district.... It may be met with in the castle and in the cottage, in the highlands or in city slums'.[61] Neurasthenia's apparent predilection for superior sorts was, it was suggested, an artefact of the class orientation of the clienteles of superior physicians.[62] But such a strategy was liable to backfire, since what had initially made neurasthenia putatively so attractive as a pathographic profile was its social exclusivity. And when its claimed neurophysiological foundations were not validated, neurasthenia became increasingly vulnerable to the charge that it was, after all, merely a terminological fig-leaf to cloak ignorance in cases of what was essentially (merely) a psychological condition.

At that point, as Simon Wessely has noted, it became easy for hostile medical critics to trash it as a fantasy or to expose the so-called neurasthenic as a fraud, the ignominious demise of the diagnosis being transferred to taint the patients themselves. It was said that, at the Johns Hopkins Hospital, 'the neurasthenic patient is treated by physicians... with ridicule or a contemptuous summing up of his case in the phrase "there is nothing the matter, he is only nervous"'. The American Smith Jelliffe described neurasthenics as 'purely mental cases. Laziness, indifference, weakness of mind and supersensitiveness characterise them all. They are... ill because of lack of moral courage'. Such patients, according to Guthrie Rankin, were 'the terror of the busy physician ... occupied by their symptoms beyond reason', traipsing from physician to physician where they 'write down their sensations in long memoranda which they hasten to read and to explain'. It all sounds like a dress-rehearsal for the stigmatising of ME sufferers today.[63]

Not surprisingly by around the time of the First World War, neurasthenia was losing its place in the diagnostic armoury in the West, though interestingly it still enjoys a lease of life in China and Japan, where it serves 'as a more respectable somatic mantle to cover mental illnesses and psychological and social problems that otherwise raise embarrassing issues of moral culpability and social stigma'.[64]

Comparisons and contrasts:
How new was neurasthenia?

Strong similarities link nervous disorders as carved out by the Enlightenment and by Beard's neurasthenia. Both were diseases of civilisation, both mapped maladies of affect and behaviour onto organic sites in the nervous system. Behind both lay the desire to obviate the stigma of psychiatric illness. In Britain both were, initially at least, launched as eligible conditions, disorders of the officer class rather than the ranks.

Nervous depression eighteenth- and nineteenth-century styles differed in one key respect, however. Sufferers from the English malady were said to have succumbed to profound anxiety because they were engaged in the performance of glamorous, if taxing, parts on the Spectatorial stage of fashionable society; the disorder was thus the product of affluence, politeness and excess. A century later, neurasthenics were said to develop exhaustion and depression because they constituted an ambitious elite living in the fast-lane in an economic system whose law was struggle. The English malady was a refinement of the old pathology of luxury; American nervousness was a disease of labour. The malaise of the *bon ton* had given way to the disorder of the businessman.[65]

Notes

1. David Garnett (ed.), *The Novels of Thomas Love Peacock* (London: Rupert Hart-Davis, 1948), 413.
2. James Manby Gully, *An Exposition of the Symptoms, Essential Nature and Treatment of Neuropathy, or Nervousness* (London: Churchill, 1837), vii.
3. Cited in Janet Oppenheim, *'Shattered Nerves': Doctors, Patients and Depression in Victorian England* (Oxford: Oxford University Press, 1991), 105. For background, see G. S. Rousseau, 'Nerves, Spirits

and Fibres: Towards Defining the Origins of Sensibility ; with a Postscript', *The Blue Guitar*, ii (1976), 125–53; *idem*, 'Science and the Discovery of the Imagination in Enlightenment England', *Eighteenth-Century Studies*, iii (1969-70), 108–35; *idem*, 'Psychology', in G. S. Rousseau and Roy Porter (eds), *The Ferment of Knowledge* (Cambridge, Cambridge University Press, 1980), 143–210; J. Spillane, *The Doctrine of the Nerves* (London: Oxford University Press, 1981); C. J. Lawrence, 'The Nervous System and Society in the Scottish Enlightenment' in B. Barnes and S. Shapin (eds), *Natural Order: Historical Studies of Scientific Culture* (London: Sage Publications, 1979), 19–40; *idem*, 'Medicine as Culture: Edinburgh and the Scottish Enlightenment' (University of London PhD Thesis, 1984); R. French, *Robert Whytt, the Soul and Medicine* (London: Wellcome Institute for the History of Medicine, 1969).

4. C. J. Lawrence, 'The Nervous System and Society in the Scottish Enlightenment', in Barry Barnes and Steven Shapin (eds), *Natural Order: Historical Studies of Scientific Culture* (London: Sage Publications, 1979), 19–40.

5. J. McKittrick Adair, *Essays on Fashionable Disorders* (London: Bateman, 1790), 1.

6. E. Hughes, *North Country Life in the Eighteenth Century*, 2 vols (London: Oxford University Press, 1965-69), i, 95.

7. George Cheyne, *The English Malady; or, A Treatise of Nervous Diseases* (London: G. Strahan, 1733). For Cheyne's life see Anita Guerrini, *Enlightenment and Obesity: Natural Philosophy, Medicine and Culture in Eighteenth-Century Britain: George Cheyne and Some Contemporaries* (University of Oklahoma Press, 2000). Cheyne's other works offer similar outlooks: see *An Essay on Regimen* (London: C. Rivington, 1740); idem, *The Natural Method of Cureing* (London: G. Strahan, 1742); *idem, The Method of Cureing Diseases of the Body and the Disorders of the Mind* (London: G. Strahan, 1742).

8. Roy Porter, 'Addicted to Modernity: Nervousness in the Early Consumer Society', in J. Melling and J. Barry (eds), *Culture in History* (Exeter: Exeter Studies in History, 1992), 180–241. Thomas Trotter, *A View of the Nervous Temperament* (London: Longman, Hurst, Rees & Orme, 1807), xvi, xvii; see also 'Introduction' by Roy Porter to Thomas Trotter, *An Essay on Drunkenness* (London: Routledge Reprint, 1988).

9. Trotter, *View of the Nervous Temperament*, xvii.

10. O. Doughty, 'The English Malady of the Eighteenth Century', *Review of English Studies*, ii (1929), 257–69; J. F. Sena, 'The English Malady: The Idea of Melancholy from 1700 to 1760' (Princeton

University PhD Thesis, 1967). It would be good to know how far
the affluent bourgeois Netherlands of the 'golden age' produced an
equivalent: Simon Schama, *The Embarrassment of Riches: An
Interpretation of Dutch Culture in the Golden Age* (New York: Knopf,
1987; London: Fontana, 1988).

11. Cheyne, *English Malady, op. cit.* (note 7) 66.
12. *Ibid.,* 56.
13. *Ibid.,* 174, 49.
14. *Ibid.,* Preface, i-ii.
15. *Ibid.,* 174.
16. *Ibid.,* 174.
17. *Ibid.,* 52.
18. *Ibid.,* 54.
19. *Ibid.,* 54.
20. *Ibid.,* 181, 52.
21. *Ibid.,* 188.
22. See, for instance, G. S. Rousseau, 'Mysticism and Millennialism:
    "Immortal Dr Cheyne"', in R. H. Popkin (ed.), *Millenarianism and
    Messianism in English Literature and Thought 1650-1800* (Leiden:
    E.J. Brill, 1988), 81–126; David E. Shuttleton, '"My Own Crazy
    Carcase": The Life and Works of Dr George Cheyne, 1672-1743'
    (Ph.D. thesis, University of Edinburgh, 1992); *idem,* 'Methodism
    and Dr George Cheyne's "More Enlightening Principles"', in Roy
    Porter (ed.), *Medicine and the Enlightenment* (Amsterdam: Rodopi,
    1994), 317–35; and the 'Introduction' by Roy Porter to G. Cheyne,
    The English Malady (London: Routledge Reprint, 1989).
23. Cheyne, *English Malady, op. cit.* (note 7), 34.
24. *Ibid.,* iii.
25. *Ibid.,* 14. As Joost Vijselaar has pointed out in an admirable
    commentary on my paper, nervous disorders were treated with a
    variety of therapeutic interventions. Cheyne liked strong drugs;
    electrotherapies later came into vogue, and indeed massaging,
    presaging Weir Mitchell.
26. Cheyne, *English Malady, op. cit.* (note 7), 105.
27. *Ibid,* 60.
28. Quoted in L. Feder, *Madness in Literature* (Princeton: Princeton
    University Press, 1980), 170.
29. Quoted in Richard Hunter and Ida Macalpine, *Three Hundred Years
    of Psychiatry, 1535-1860* (London: Oxford University Press, 1963),
    353.
30. Quoted in Richard Hunter and Ida Macalpine, *Three Hundred Years
    of Psychiatry, 1535-1860* (London: Oxford University Press, 1963),

353.

31. Sir Richard Blackmore, *A Treatise of the Spleen and Vapours* (London: Pemberton, 1725), quoted in Richard Hunter and Ida Macalpine, *Three Hundred Years of Psychiatry, 1535-1860* (London: Oxford University Press, 1863), 320.

32. Nicholas Robinson, *A New System of the Spleen* (London, 1729), quoted in Richard Hunter and Ida Macalpine, *Three Hundred Years of Psychiatry, 1535-1860* (London: Oxford University Press, 1983), 344.

33. *Ibid.*

34. See Ralph Browne, *Neurasthenia and its Treatment by Hypodermic Transfusions* (London: Churchill, 1894), 33.

35. Henry Holland, *Chapters on Mental Physiology*, 2nd ed. (London: Longman, 1838), 314–5.

36. Janet Oppenheim, *'Shattered Nerves': Doctors, Patients and Depression in Victorian England* (Oxford: Oxford University Press, 1991), 9.

37. *Ibid.*, 81; Thomas D. Savill, *Lectures on Neurasthenia* (London: Gleisher, 1906), 68.

38. Henry Maudsley, 'Sex in Mind and in Education', *Fortnightly Review*, ns, xv (1874), 467. Trevor Turner, 'Henry Maudsley: Psychiatrist, Philosopher and Entrepreneur', in W. F. Bynum, R. Porter and M. Shepherd (eds), *Anatomy of Madness* (London, Routledge, 1988), iii, 151–89; Anson Rabinbach, 'The Body without Fatigue: A Nineteenth Century Utopia', in S. Drescher, D. Sabean and A. Sharlin (eds), *Political Symbolism in Modern Europe: Essays in Honor of George L. Mosse* (London: Transaction Books, 1982), 42–62; idem, 'The European Science of Work: The Economy of the Body at the End of the Nineteenth Century', in Steven L. Kaplan and C. J. Koepp (eds), *Work in France: Representations, Meaning, Organization and Practice* (Ithaca, N.Y.: Cornell University Press, 1986), 415–513; *idem, The Human Motor: Energy, Fatigue, and the Origins of Modernity* (New York: Basic Books, 1990).

39. Alfred T. Schofield, *Nerves in Disorder: A Plea for Rational Treatment* (London: Hodder and Stoughton, 1903), 4.

40. Stanley W. Jackson, *Melancholia and Depression from Hippocratic Times to Modern Times* (New Haven: Yale University Press, 1986).

41. Roy Porter, 'Miller's Madness', in Michael Shortland (ed.), *Hugh Miller and the Controversies of Victorian Science* (Oxford: Oxford University Press, 1996), 285–309.

42. Alfred T. Schofield, *Nerves in Disorder: A Plea for Rational Treatment* (London: Hodder and Stoughton, 1903), 4.

43. For historical accounts, see Tom Lutz, 'Neurasthenia and Fatigue

Syndromes', in German E. Berrios and Roy Porter (eds), *A History of Clinical Psychiatry. The Origin and History of Psychiatric Disorders* (London: Athlone, 1995), 533-544; Edward Shorter, *From Paralysis to Fatigue. A History of Psychosomatic Illness in the Modern Era* (New York: Free Press, 1992).

44. Beard did not, however, coin the term. His two main works are *A Practical Treatise on Nervous Exhaustion (Neurasthenia): Its Symptoms, Nature, Sequences, Treatment* (New York: W. Wood, 1880) and *American Nervousness: Its Causes and Consequences* (New York: Putnam, 1881). See F. Gosling, *Before Freud: Neurasthenia and the American Medical Community, 1870-1910* (Chicago: University of Illinois Press, 1987); Tom Lutz, *American Nervousness, 1903: An Anecdotal History* (Ithaca: Cornell University Press, 1991); Charles Rosenberg, 'The Place of George M. Beard in Nineteenth Century Psychiatry', *Bulletin of the History of Medicine,* xxxvi (1962), 245–59; Simon Wessely, 'Neurasthenia and Fatigue Syndromes', clinical section, in German E. Berrios and Roy Porter (eds), *A History of Clinical Psychiatry. The Origin and History of Psychiatric Disorders* (London: Athlone, 1995), 509–32; Tom Lutz, 'Neurasthenia and Fatigue Syndromes', social section, in *ibid.,* 533–44.

45. W. F. Bynum and Roy Porter (eds), *Brunonianism in Britain and Europe* (London: Medical History, Supplement 8, 1989).

46. George M. Beard, *A Practical Treatise on Nervous Exhaustion (Neurasthenia)* (New York: William Wood, 1880), 3. Beard made much of the fact that, at long last, in neurasthenia, America had its own special and authentic disease. It was not just a disease of civilisation, but a disease of American civilisation; 9.

47. 'Neurasthenia is rather considered a mark of distinction than a weakness': Emile Durkheim, quoted in Arthur Kleinman, *Social Origins of Distress and Disease: Depression, Neurasthenia, and Pain in Modern China* (New Haven, Conn.: Yale University Press, 1986), 19.

48. George M. Beard, *American Nervousness* (New York: Putnam's, 1881), 176; *idem, A Practical Treatise on Nervous Exhaustion* (Neurasthenia) (New York: Wood, 1880), 3.

49. *Idem, American Nervousness,* vi.

50. Kenneth Levin, 'S. Weir Mitchell: Investigation and Insights into Neurasthenia and Hysteria', *Transactions and Studies of the College of Physicians, Philadelphia,* xxxviii (1971), 168–73; Tom Lutz, *American Nervousness, 1903: An Anecdotal History* (Ithaca: Cornell University Press, 1991); *idem,* 'Neurasthenia and Fatigue Syndromes', in German E. Berrios and Roy Porter (eds), *A History of*

Clinical Psychiatry. The Origin and History of Psychiatric Disorders (London: Athlone, 1995), 533–544; Ernest Earnest, *S. Weir Mitchell, Novelist and Physician* (Philadelphia: University of Pennsylvania Press, 1950); S. Weir Mitchell, *Fat and Blood: An Essay on the Treatment of Certain Forms of Neurasthenia and Hysteria* (Philadelphia: Lippincott, 1877); *idem, Lectures on the Diseases of the Nervous System, Especially in Women* (Philadelphia: Lea, 1881); *idem, Doctor and Patient* (Philadelphia: Lippincott, 1888).

51. J. B. Hurry, *The Vicious Circles of Neurasthenia and their Treatment* (London: Churchill, 1915), xiii.

52. Thomas D. Savill, *Lectures on Neurasthenia* (London: Gleisher, 1906), 17. Savill was physician to the West-End Hospital for Diseases of the Nervous System.

53. Cyril Bennett, *The Modern Malady: Or, Sufferers from Nerves* (London: Edward Arnold, 1890), 132; J. Mitchell Clarke, *Hysteria and Neurasthenia* (London: John Lane at the Bodley Head, 1905), 171, 179. Clarke was Professor of Pathology at University College, Bristol.

54. Ivo Geikie Cobb, *A Manual of Neurasthenia* (London: Baillière, Tindall and Cox, 1920), 27; Cyril Bennett, *The Modern Malady: Or, Sufferers from Nerves* (London: Edward Arnold, 1890), 103; see also 144 and 170, which refers to women's 'highly-strung nervous systems'. Thomas D. Savill, *Lectures on Neurasthenia* (London: Gleisher, 1906), 60, 61.

55. Cyril Bennett, *The Modern Malady: Or, Sufferers from Nerves* (London: Edward Arnold, 1890), 126.

56. J. Mitchell Clarke, *Hysteria and Neurasthenia* (London: John Lane at the Bodley Head, 1905), 175. For a standard litany of complaints against towns, newspapers, railways, etc. see Thomas D. Savill, *Lectures on Neurasthenia* (London: Gleisher, 1906), 111.

57. Janet Oppenheim, *op. cit.* (note 3), 332.

58. Daniel Hack Tuke (ed.), *Dictionary of Psychological Medicine* (London: Churchill, 1892), ii, 840–1.

59. Sir Andrew Clark, 'Some Observations Concerning What is Called Neurasthenia', *Lancet,* i (1886), 1; Leonard George Guthrie, *Functional Nervous Disorders in Childhood* (London: Frowde, 1907), 17.

60. Cyril Bennett, *op. cit.,* (note 55), v.

61. Leonard George Guthrie, *Functional Nervous Disorders in Childhood* (London: Frowde, 1907), 17.

62. Ivo Geikie Cobb, *A Manual of Neurasthenia* (London: Baillière, Tindall and Cox, 1920), 27.

63. Simon Wessely, 'Neurasthenia and Fatigue Syndromes', clinical
    section, in German E. Berrios and Roy Porter (eds), *A History of
    Clinical Psychiatry. The Origin and History of Psychiatric Disorders*
    (London: Athlone, 1995), 509–32: 523.

64. Arthur Kleinman, *Social Origins of Distress and Disease: Depression,
    Neurasthenia and Pain in Modern China* (New Haven: Yale
    University Press, 1986), 15.

65. This conclusion holds, I believe, if we draw a simple contrast
    between two 'ideal types': Cheyne's English malady and Beard's
    American nervousness. The contrast is, however, excessively stark.
    Around 1800, and writing from commercial Bristol, Thomas
    Beddoes in particular was already construing nervous disorders as the
    product of business worries and money mania:

    > Among the faces that appear at high 'Change, mark those that
    > bespeak the cares attendant upon wealth already accumulated; and
    > those others, where an added air of wildness characterises the
    > speculator, too much in haste to wait for the reward of regular
    > industry, and burning to get rich by the lucky hit. Some of these
    > men will grow mad enough to be watched at home or sent to a
    > lunatic asylum, where they will be haunted by the fear of coming
    > upon the parish.

    Thomas Beddoes, *Hygëia: or Essays Moral and Medical, on the Causes
    Affecting the Personal State of our Middling and Affluent Classes*
    (Bristol: J. Mills, 1802-3), 3 x 77; Roy Porter, *Doctor of Society:
    Thomas Beddoes and the Sick Trade in Late Enlightenment England*
    (London: Routledge, 1991), 61f. The South Sea bubble was said to
    have produced a one-off crop of nervous cases and suicides: John
    Midriff, *Observations of the Spleen and Vapours: Containing
    Remarkable Cases of Persons of Both Sexes, and All Ranks, from the
    Aspiring Director to the Humble Bubbler, Who Have Been Miserably
    Afflicted with Those Melancholy Disorders since the Fall of South-Sea
    and Other Publick Stocks* (London: Roberts, 1721).
    It will have been noticed that this paper omits to discuss the
    gendering of nervous disorders. There is a reason for this: in both
    the eighteenth and the nineteenth centuries hysteria was the prime
    vehicle of female nervous disorders. The English malady and
    neurasthenia were mainly imagined as male. It was often said that
    neurasthenia was to men what hysteria is to women, and it appears
    that more men were so diagnosed: J. S. Haller, 'Neurasthenia: the
    Medical Profession and the "New Woman" of Late Nineteenth
    Century', *New York State Journal of Medicine*, xv (1971), 473–82;

Nervousness, Eighteenth and Nineteenth Century Style

Katharina Rowold (ed. and intro.), *Gender and Science. Late Nineteenth-Century Debates on the Female Mind and Body* (Bristol: Thoemmes Press, 1996).

2

Varieties of Medical Experience:
Doctors and Patients, Psyche and Soma in America

Tom Lutz

'It is no longer the height of good form,' Wade Wright announced in dismissing neurasthenia in *Mental Hygiene* in 1921, 'to enjoy poor health.'[1] Using one of the staple figures of neurasthenia's medical competitors, Wade suggests that neurasthenia was a fashionable disease, that it was not suffered so much as 'enjoyed,' that it was class-based bad science more than it was a real disease, that it was cultural, finally, more than it was physiological. Many historians, if less dismissively than Wade, equally definitively, have seen in the disease a cultural formation more than a medical one, myself included, and turn-of-the-century physicians sometimes helped provide evidence.[2] 'This distinguished malady' is the way George M. Beard, MD, described it and he bragged that 'not Greece, nor Rome, nor Spain, nor the Netherlands, in the days of their glory, possessed such maladies.' Almost forty years after Beard's first papers, William Marrs, MD, in *Confessions of a Neurasthenic*, claimed that the best thing about the disease is that it allowed one to 'move in neurasthenic circles,' as if the disease was a form of social attainment.[3] One can safely assume that this kind of talk helped, through the negotiations between doctors and patients, swell the ranks of the diagnosed, and point more patients toward specialists. If we assume that the frequency of diagnosis ran roughly parallel to the publication of case studies in the major journals, then the number of neurasthenics in America increased in every decade until it peaked in 1900-1910. That decade saw the peak of medical discussion of the disease, including a flurry of criticism, most of which centred on the idea that neurasthenia was insufficiently rigorous as a diagnostic category.

These criticisms have continued to this day, but they have often been beside the point in America after the 1920s and 1930s, when, thanks in large part to such criticism, the disease was largely dismantled. In subdividing neurasthenia into two halves, one physiological and the other psychic in origin, Freud and his followers also helped bring about its temporary demise and, more broadly, helped create a psychiatric culture that T.M. Luhrmann has recently analysed as dominated, over the last century, by precisely this split.[4] What F.G. Gosling correctly, if somewhat anachronistically, called the 'holistic' view of the theorists of neurasthenia devolved into a fundamentally riven culture with physiologically-based and psychically-based theories of psychology and psychiatry continually, and as Luhrmann shows often deleteriously, unable to speak to each other.[5] Those historians most closely tied to the history of psychoanalysis have thus seen the disease primarily as either a precursor of Freudianism or a form of medical error, mistaking psychological problems for physical ones, while some historians hostile to psychoanalysis nonetheless maintain the same sense of neurasthenia's purely ideological character.[6] Those in the physiological camp who would banish the couch completely in favour of the CAT scan and chemicals assume that the study of both consciousness and culture are equally superfluous.[7] Rather than a history of error, however, I want to suggest that what neurasthenia can offer historians is more than just a ripe field for understanding the relation between medicine and cultural fashions, but a paradigmatic site for re-examining the very relation between culture and physiology in ways that do not recreate the rift that divides the disciplines we are attempting to study.

Early constructions

The two most important physicians in the rise of neurasthenia were Beard and S. Weir Mitchell. Beard's first official contribution appeared in 1869 in *The Boston Medical and Surgical Journal*, in which he states that although the 'morbid condition or state expressed by this term has long been recognised, and to a certain degree understood, but the special name neurasthenia is now, I believe, for the first time presented to the profession.'[8] The term had, in fact, been introduced earlier, and was, for instance, listed in Dunglison's *Medical Lexicon* in 1851, and 1869 also saw the use of the term in an article by E.H. Van Deusen in the *American Journal of Insanity*.[9] But it is Beard's work that helped put neurasthenia on the medical and cultural map, and it is his work, and then Mitchell's, that were taken as foundational by most subsequent writers.

Neurasthenia is to the nervous system, Beard argues, what anemia is to the vascular system. Both may be the effects of acute or chronic diseases, such as 'wasting fevers, exhausting wounds, parturition, protracted confinement, dyspepsia, phthisis, morbus Brightii and so forth.'[10] And both may cause chronic and acute diseases, including 'dyspepsia, headaches, paralysis, insomnia, anaesthesia, neuralgia, rheumatic gout, spermatorrhea in the male and menstrual irregularities in the female.'[11] And anemia and neurasthenia can cause each other. These co-morbidities, the various and interchangeable physiological causes and effects (a constant in Beard's thinking), had framing social causes: Beard argues that both anaemia and neurasthenia are 'most frequently met with in civilised, intellectual communities. They are part of the compensation for our progress and refinement.'[12] But the cure was not social. Just as anaemia was treated by tonics for the blood, so should neurasthenia be treated, according to Beard, by tonics for the nerves – especially electricity.

The pathology of neurasthenia, Beard acknowledges, is not known, and must be reasoned 'from logical probability.' In a move analogous to Freud's in breaking neurasthenia off from the 'actual neuroses,'[13] Beard suggested that diagnosis needed to be 'obtained partly by the positive symptoms, and partly by exclusion.' If the positive symptoms are present, and the patient 'at the same time gives no evidence of anaemia or of any organic disease, we have reason to suspect that the central nervous system is mainly at fault, and that we are dealing with a typical case of neurasthenia.' The central nervous system problems he had in mind are purely physiological. As Beard wrote:

> My own view is that the central nervous system becomes dephosphorised, or perhaps, loses somewhat of its solid constituents; probably also undergoes slight, undetectable, morbid changes in its chemical structure, and as a consequence, becomes more or less impoverished in the quantity and quality of its nervous force.[14]

For evidence, he cites the experimental studies on the central nervous system reported by Reynolds, Bois-Reymond, L'Hertier, and Maudsley. He admits that his conclusions are speculative, but feels that they will 'in time be substantially confirmed by microscopical and chemical examinations of those patients who die in a neurasthenic condition.'[15] In a typical case study ten years later, Beard discusses a clergyman who, he claims, suffered from neurasthenia because he had an inherited nervous diathesis (what Freud would later call a 'predisposition,' but one that was primarily physical rather than psychological), a strenuous and stressful job (Freud's 'specific cause'), had recently suffered heat prostration (Freud's 'contributory cause'), and was 'excited' by the 'mental annoyance' of having to write sermons (Freud's 'exciting cause').[16]

But by 1881, with the publication of *American Nervousness*, Beard's emphasis had moved from the physiological, genetic, and otherwise personal explanations to more specifically include cultural ones, and he listed his famous five causes of the epidemic of neurasthenia: 'steam power, the periodical press, the telegraph, the sciences, and the mental activity of women.'[17] These different causes were expressly additive, by what Beard called an 'algebraic formula,' and he gives the equation:

> civilisation in general + American civilisation in particular (young and rapidly growing nation, with civil, religious, and social liberty) + exhausting climate (extremes of heat and cold, and dryness) + the nervous diathesis (itself a result of previously named factors) + overwork or overworry, or excessive indulgence of appetites or passions = an attack of neurasthenia or nervous exhaustion.[18]

Beard's preferred cure was the application of electric current to replenish the nerve force, and along with A.D. Rockwell he published several works on the use of electricity as a therapy. In one case study, for instance, the full report of cure is that he applied 'interrupted galvanic current in the inner angle of the eye with the negative pole, the positive being placed at the back of the neck, or on the temples. Immediate relief followed a single application.'[19] But he thought it should be combined with the 'concentration of all possible tonic influence on the nervous system – air, sunlight, water, food, rest, diversion, muscular exercise, and the internal administration of those remedies, such as strychnine, phosphorus, arsenic, &c., which directly affect the central nervous system.'[20] By 1876, according to Charles Dana, Beard would add suggestion to his list; whether or not this was because, as Dana would write, he realised one day that he had cured a patient with electricity even though his battery was dead, he came to believe that 'effects which have been brought about through the emotions had been as permanent as those realised through the agency of medicines or electricity.'[21] As Gosling notes, however, Beard was more interested in diagnosis than cure, often stating that neurasthenia was 'relatively easy to manage, if not cure.'[22]

S. Weir Mitchell, by contrast, would concentrate most of his writing on cure, and he especially recommended two therapies from Beard's list: rest and food. Mitchell was a graduate of Jefferson Medical College and studied physiology in Paris with the pioneering experimentalist Claude Bernard. In the period before the establishment of university physiological laboratories in the US Mitchell founded his own private laboratory in Philadelphia and is often regarded as the outstanding American physiologist of his day. The co-founder of the American Physiological Society and its second president (after declining the position for the first term), his experimental work dealt with gunshot wounds, snake venom, the function of the cerebellum, the knee jerk, and the physiology and pathology of nerves. Mitchell's *Fat and Blood and How to Make Them* (1878) uses a series of statistical epidemiological surveys to set the stage, starting with Adolphe Quetelet's *Sur l'homme et le developpement de ses facultés, essai d'une physique sociale* (1835), which first introduced what is now known as the body mass index (BMI).[23] He discusses the measurements reported by Dr. Henry Bowditch (president of the AMA, founder of the American Public Health Association, and along with Mitchell of the American Physiological Society) in *Growth of Children* (1894), the public health research in John Stanton Gould's *A Report on Health and Diet* (1852), and J.H. Baxter's 1875 GPO survey of physiological statistics. When he reviews the medical literature on the relation between fat and the number of red corpuscles in blood, he has to admit that physiologists do not yet know the exact relations between optimal blood counts and the production of fat, but he cites studies that help suggest that the two are complexly interrelated. He concludes this introduction by insisting that although the main job of the physician when encountering a neurasthenic is to bring her or him to optimal levels of corpuscles and corpulence, to do this the physician must also alter the patient's social and moral situation, and it is only this combination of interpersonal readjustment and physiological repair that works.

> If I succeed in first altering the moral atmosphere which has been to the patient like the very breathing of evil, and if I can add largely to the weight and fill the vessels with red blood, I am usually sure of giving relief.[24]

Mitchell goes on, in *Fat and Blood*, to describe his treatment regimen of diet, rest, massage, and electricity. He sums up what he calls 'numerous clinical studies,' in which he tried different combinations of these four therapies, and says, again without offering any actual numbers, that electricity was the least significant variable.[25] He describes his elaborate feeding schedules, including milk, beef soups, iron supplements, supplements to prevent constipation, and eventually full meals. He recounts over two dozen cases, reporting on temperature changes after massage and electrical treatments and in some detail about weight gain. The men and women gain between 18 and 51 pounds over the course of several weeks. Following standard procedure in medical reports of this kind, the case studies are given in a short paragraph or two, and no statistical data is given about his patient population as a whole. (Gosling and Ray found a total of 307 case studies reported by physicians in American medical journals between 1870 and 1910, but none of these gained the iconic status of Freud's more famous case studies, and indeed none were reported in much detail.[26])

In 1904 Mitchell gave a retrospective lecture on the rest cure, which by that time had become famous and had been adopted by many other physicians. He opens by explaining what he sees as his relation to scientific method:

> You all know full well that the art of cure rests upon a number of sciences, and that what we do in medicine, we cannot always explain, and that our methods are far from having the accuracy involved in the term scientific. Very often, however, it is found that what comes to us through accident or popular use and proves of value, is defensible in the end by scientific explanatory research.[27]

In the case of the rest cure, his first evidence was the cases of acute exhaustion among soldiers in the Civil War, and since he had little to offer them than rest and nutriment, he had his first glimpse of their value by accident. In a case of locomotor ataxia in 1872, a man broke each of his legs in succession, and the subsequent enforced rest moderated his condition. And when his first serious case of neurasthenia proper did not respond to the available treatments, he noticed that the patient (who he describes in his earlier work as well) felt marginally better when she rested and when she got moderate exercise, but too much of either made her worse. He hit on the 'pregnant' idea of using massage as a form of passive exercise, and thus using 'rest in bed without the injurious effects of unassisted rest.'28 The patient gained forty pounds in two months and had remained well ever since. The cure was thus somewhat accidentally discovered, but 'justified by the later scientific studies of Lauder Brunton, myself and others' on the therapeutic value of massage. 'It is one of the most scientific,' he concludes with no more evidence, 'of remedial methods.'[29] It is clear that his sense of the scientific validity of the disease was sealed, however, by its adoption by William Playfair, MD, in London, and its gradual acceptance by others in the British Medical Association.

Mitchell's *Doctor and Patient* (1887) is the kind of thing to give fuel to those who find him more a Victorian moralist than a scientific analyst.[30] He declaims on topics as diverse as the education of young women, sexual morality, racial difference, marriage relations, literary excellence, and the separate and converging responsibilities of labour and capital. Mitchell was in the position to make such pronouncements not just because of the prestige of his expertise, but because the theories of neurasthenia were imbued at every level by cultural beliefs and norms. His audience either lived or envied some version of the ideal American, late-Victorian, elite, WASP lifestyle, the underlying assumptions of which governed the theory of neurasthenia; that women were more sensitive than men, Anglo-Saxons more aware of their surroundings than Asians, Protestants more refined than Catholics, brainworkers more fastidious than workers, and whites more intelligent than blacks all helped explain why WASP brainworkers suffered from the disease more than any other group. Since one of the causes of women's illnesses was their rejection of traditional roles in favour of college or social work, Mitchell had an obligation to explain to women the health benefits of household management and child-rearing. And since men could lose their nerve strength through an unmanly overindulgence in such things as aesthetic experience (it was Mitchell, himself a novelist, who claimed that the literary monthlies had become so feminised that they would soon begin to menstruate), physicians had a responsibility to proselytise for strenuous, old-fashioned masculinity. But this book is straightforwardly presented as a set of 'lay sermons,' not as a contribution to medicine. And if laying down such laws was, as the earlier case studies make clear, part of the physician's responsibility in effecting a personal or societal cure, it was not the same as scientific understanding, which, Mitchell believed, preceded and legitimated his sermonising.

Deconstructions

The defences of neurasthenia by other physicians at the turn of the century, like Freud's defences of his methods around the same time, remained very similar to those of Mitchell and Beard in that they admitted the inconclusiveness of scientific findings while bolstering theoretical reasoning with available studies. In some cases, the arguments were more 'holistic' than defensive. The improbably named I.N. Love, MD, writing about neurasthenia in the *Journal of the American Medical Association* in 1894, for instance, argued that 'There are many things in man which the test tube and the microscope cannot discover, and in our work as bacteriological delvers and in our desire to be superlatively scientific, we should not lose sight of the fact.'[31] But as the practice of neurology became more specialised in the first decades of the twentieth century, its subspecialties more narrowly defined and disciplined, cultural explanation and cultural criticism became seen as tainted by unscientific moralising, and physicians began to do their damnedest to avoid them. Sinclair Lewis's novel *Arrowsmith* (1925), for which he did research with Paul de Kruif, most clearly represents the disdain scientists and honest doctors had for public sermonising. In the novel, the clownish pitch-man Dr. Pickerbaugh expounds on the moral value of not spitting in the streets and the saintliness of hygiene, but at the price of appearing foolish, dishonest, and unscientific. Pickerbaugh is not a practicing physician but a public health official, and only the few neurologists who allied themselves with this newest medical speciality (in its newly-founded journals such as *Mental Hygiene*, started in 1916) continued to argue the morality of medical news. Wright's condemnation of neurasthenia in that journal, then, needs to be seen as the critique of a direct competitor not just for the scientific field but for its diverse social functions and cultural prestige as well.

In fact, all the various schools of psychotherapy retained to some extent the earlier neurologists' emphasis on advice-giving, as easily seen in Freud's tracts of the 1920s and 1930s on the history and future of civilisation, art, and religion. John B. Watson, famous as the father of behaviourism and of pop psychology, and who maintained serious physiological interests, wrote an immensely popular child-rearing manual that promised a better world through scientific parenting and otherwise offered what despite his caveats can only be seen as moral advice. Many lesser-known psychologists felt comfortable propounding moral and cultural theory, such as Harvard's Leonard T. Troland, who maintained that philosophical ethics was well within the realm of psychological experimentation and theory. Psychologists of the 1920s thereby acquired the authority on cultural issues formerly enjoyed by the neurologists, with all its aura of scientificity. As Frederick Lewis Allen remembered at the end of the decade, 'Of all the sciences . . . psychology was king. . . . [O]ne had only to read the newspapers to be told that psychology held the key to the problems of waywardness, divorce, and crime.'[32]

At the same time, the neurologists were refigured as myopic, nerdball scientists out of touch with daily life. In 1920, J. W. McConnell, MD, in trying to explain why many general practitioners avoided neurology altogether, invoked the current stereotype:

Neurology is regarded as an unknown land, the exploration of which should only be attempted by high brow individuals who wear heavy spectacles, have stooped shoulders, and who consider the greatest pleasure in life to be the changing of fluids on the specimens in their laboratories.[33]

The psychologist had moved from being an egghead researcher to being a revered scientific expert offering advice about everyday life and the neurologist had gone the opposite route.

As any schematic analysis does, of course, this greatly oversimplifies a diverse and disparate field. William James argued for an applied psychology in the 1890s and there was a vocal and influential contingent of academic psychologists in the 1920s who believed that applied psychology was charlatanry, since the science of psychology was not advanced enough to be applied. And likewise, there were nerve specialists in the 1890s working in laboratories who considered Mitchell *et al.* to be unscientific quacks catering to popular prejudice, just as there were still nerve specialists in the 1920s prescribing milk, tonics and vacations for a hefty fee. But the overall ground had shifted significantly, and by 1920, although books continued to pour off the presses giving outlines of neurasthenia and related illnesses and recipes for cure, they were regularly derided by the major scientific journals. In a review of Edwin Ash's *The Problem of Nervous Breakdown* (1920) in *Mental Hygiene*, for instance, M. W. Raynor pooh-poohed what he saw as an extreme 'conservatism,' claiming that the time for such repetitions of Mitchellesque lore (Ash had three chapters on the rest cure) was long past. The marks of Ash's lack of scientificity were his inattention to 'the biological viewpoint' and his ignorance of the latest psychological findings.[34] Ralph Truitt, in the same issue, claimed that while W. Charles Loosmore's *Nerves and the Man* (1921) was perhaps uplifting and useful to some patients, it was nonetheless completely unscientific and therefore had nothing to do with medicine proper.[35] And most medical articles on the disease were even less forgiving.

The first and most serious charge against neurasthenia was that it was simply a cover for ignorance. Although this charge was made implicitly by unbelieving neurologists in the nineteenth century, and explicitly as early as 1904 by Charles Dana (in the very journal in which Beard had introduced the term), it was not until the 1920s that it became a general chorus. In the *New York Medical Journal* in 1920, J. W. McConnell claimed that 'neurasthenia as a blanket diagnosis for early tuberculosis, chronic appendicitis, or the querulous depressed stage of general paresis has not been at all uncommon.'36 W. C. Ashworth, though he went on to defend the term in the August 1921 *Virginia Medical Monthly,* argued that 'neurasthenia is a sort of blanket term to cover our ignorance of some functional nervous disorder which we find difficult to diagnose without careful and painstaking examination.'[37] In the *U.S. Veteran's Bureau Medical Bulletin* in 1926, M. D. Clayton asked the medical question 'When is the Diagnosis of Neurasthenia Justified?' and concluded that the answer was never. 'This one diagnosis has been allotted greater use and greater abuse than any other diagnosis known,' he wrote, claiming that neurasthenia was diagnosed when the real problem was a physical disorder or the early development of a definite psychosis. 'It is my opinion that the diagnosis of neurasthenia has served its purpose, outlived its usefulness,' Clayton concluded, 'and could at this time be left out of the nomenclature.'[38] Denunciation of the term's semiotic vagrancy became over time a formulaic opening to essays on neurasthenia, whatever the writer's final conclusions about how the term should be correctly used or about whether it should be discarded. Peter Bassoe, writing in the *Wisconsin Medical Journal* at the end of the decade offered what amounted to an obituary for the term:

Nowadays, among up-to-date physicians a diagnosis of neurasthenia is usually not well received. . . for the term as now used does not stand for anything definite either as to etiology, pathology, or prognosis. A good many men prefer to discard the term altogether, some because they think the original conception is wrong, others because they feel that the term has been so much abused that it is hopeless to restore it to stand for something definite. . . . When neurasthenia began to be considered a disease entity it deteriorated into a convenient wastebasket and encouraged superficiality and laziness. . . . To sum up, the term neurasthenia is a mile stone in the history of medicine, which at first marked progress but now impedes it . . . as its use leads to neglect of necessary inquiry into the inner life and the environment of the individual patient.[39]

Not all neurologists were ready to do away with the term altogether, and even Bassoe, in response to criticism backed down, if only slightly:

Any physician who uses that term should get a little bad taste in his mouth every time he uses it and not think he has done anything brilliant when he calls a case one of neurasthenia. It is not like a diagnosis of a heart lesion. It must be understood that it is just a general descriptive term that includes a great many dissimilar cases which have certain features in common. If we use it in that spirit, then we shall go on and improve ourselves.[40]

This conclusion, that neurasthenia was a description of a complex of symptoms that might indicate a number of different diseases, was the middle road to its temporary abandonment. Medical writers who adopted this middle road did so by claiming it as not a disease, but as a 'reaction.' Clarence C. May, writing in the *New Orleans Medical and Surgical Journal* in 1925 agreed that 'nervousness is not a separate and distinct disease entity with clearly defined symptoms and easily elicited causes in each instance or a uniformly outlined course. It is not, in itself, disease of the brain or body; nor is it exhaustion, poisoning, fatigue or weakness of the nerves.' Instead, May argued, neurasthenia 'is a type of reaction to physical and mental maladjustment, subtle, extensive, far-reaching and often disastrous in its effects, though almost invariably preventable and curable.'[41] Some writers were less successful than others at walking this rhetorical tightrope. C. F. Neu in the *Medical Record* seemed to worm his way into a corner and settle there, however uncomfortably:

> The term neurasthenia should be restricted to an enfeeblement or fatigue neurosis, a primary fatigue neurosis, its cardinal characteristics being an inordinate sense of physical or mental fatigue, or both, a difficulty of concentration, of attention and application to work, a sense of pressure in the head, and irritibility of the spine, various paresthesias, and more or less disturbance of function of the various visceral organs, all being more or less closely related to psychogenic factors.[42]

This is, 'more or less,' a narrowing of the category, but with plenty of clauses and modifiers to keep it wide.

The move to isolate neurasthenia in psychogenic factors that Neu and others made imitates the Freudian secession from physiological neurology, but Freud himself had come to an opposite conclusion about neurasthenia some years earlier. In an 1895 paper, 'On the Grounds for Detaching a Particular Syndrome from Neurasthenia under the Description "Anxiety Neurosis,"' Freud set up shop by making a distinction between 'psycho-neuroses' and 'actual neuroses,' the former being psychogenic and amenable to psychoanalysis, the latter being organic and the province of neurologists.[43] The latter, including neurasthenia, were not psychogenic and therefore not treatable by psychotherapy. Freud was interested in carving away some of the territory that the epidemic of neurasthenia still engulfed. Rather than challenging the medical establishment's authority over 'actual' diseases, Freud simply asserted the value of his analytic therapy for a small subset of 'psychoneuroses.'

By the 1920s Freud's influence was, however lacking in orthodoxy, nonetheless omnipresent in American intellectual and professional circles. The journal that had been most friendly to theorists of neurasthenia during the preceding decades, the *Journal of Nervous and Mental Diseases*, was edited from 1902 to 1945 by Smith Ely Jelliffe, who along with William A. White, president of the American Psychopathology Association, produced major new systems of classification for diseases of the nervous system that made room for Freudian thinking (Jelliffe was also the editor of *Psychoanalytic Review* from 1913 to 1945). White wrote in the journal in 1922 that 'Freud's contribution may very properly be considered of as great importance to psychopathology as Darwin's was to biology.'[44] *The Journal of Nervous and Mental Diseases* helped lead the campaign for the abandonment of neurasthenia in its articles and reviews. Pierre Prengowski's *Les maladies neurasthéniques* was dismissed by its reviewer because 'neurasthenic disorders are a bit out of fashion at the present day' and in an article on 'Influenza and Melancholy,' Karl Menninger felt free to ridicule a colleague's use of the term thusly: 'The neurasthenic (sic!) state persisted...'[45] To vitiate the category of neurasthenia made its apparent sufferers available to other diagnoses. As one doctor put it, 'the neurasthenic, and his neurotic associates, are at the threshold of a more fair consideration,' and this consideration involved new disease entities, of which neurasthenic symptoms were secondary signs.[46] In a comparison of psychiatry in 1895 and 1915, Lawson G. Lowery argued in the same journal that diagnostic terms in 1895 were 'merely clinically descriptive, with little basis of pathology or etiology'; by 1915, diagnostic terms were 'in part etiologic, in part prognostic, and in part clinically descriptive.'[47] In the pages of the *Journal of Nervous and Mental Diseases* these new, more dynamic diagnostic terms tended to leave no room for neurasthenia as a disease entity.

To a certain extent, then, the theoretical rejections of neurasthenia as elaborated in the late teens and early twenties simply accounted for changes already underway. In a 1917 article in the *Journal of the American Medical Association* Theodore Diller analysed his own caseload and that at the New York Neurological Institute.

'Twenty-five years ago practically all the neuroses or psychoneuroses were classified as hysteria or neurasthenia,' Diller reported, but by 1894, these two categories accounted for some 21% of his caseload.[48] By 1916, this figure had shrunk to 12%. The Neurological Institute reported 430 cases of neurasthenia in 1916 out of a total caseload of 8,103, or just over 5%. When Charlotte Perkins Gilman experienced mental disorder after childbirth in 1885 not she, her husband, or her doctors had any hesitation in recognising a case of neurasthenia.[49] But by 1911, postpartum disorders were rarely diagnosed as neurasthenia; in 'A Study of Psychoses Occurring in Relation to Childbirth,' Elizabeth Kilpatrick and Harry M. Tiebout categorised 72 cases of mental disorder associated with childbirth between 1911 and 1923 as 50% manic-depressive, 32% deleria, 14% dementia praecox, and 4% psychoneuroses.[50] One study of 1000 cases of arthritis noted that 'fatigue, mental lethargy, headache, and migraine ... practically the whole complex of neurasthenia' was the most common 'clinical disturbance' related to arthritis, but that nonetheless the organic, metabolic processes involved with the arthritis should be the prime concern for physicians, not the secondary symptoms.[51]

Many physicians in the 1920s, on the other hand, assumed that what had happened over the last two decades was the standard, ongoing process of renaming with more specificity the same disease entities that previous physicians had seen – it was a simple case of the march of scientific progress.[52] If the study of nervous disease had 'long been handicapped by the confusion of symptoms and diseases,'[53] then fine-tuning the nomenclature could provide an end to confusion. This implied that changing disease categories represented a process of simple translation. Charles Dana, in a 1923 article commemorating Beard as 'the father of neurasthenia,' casually refers to neurasthenia as 'what we now call psychoneuroses,' suggesting that little had changed with the change of names.[54] This way of thinking could cut both ways, of course, for if little had changed, little advance could be claimed. 'To label a patient neurasthenic is no diagnosis at all,' Tom A. Williams wrote in the 1921 *Medical Record,* but by the same token, 'to say manic depressive ... is no therapeutic help' either.[55]

Other professionals took over some of what practitioners like Mitchell had offered. Faith-healers like Aimee Semple McPherson ('Oh, you who are down in the Shadowland of sickness and despair ... there is health in His wings for you'), homeopaths, chiropractors, and hydropaths continued to peddle their wares. With the discovery of vitamins in the teens a school of scientific nutritionists arose to promise relief from fatigue, worry, autointoxication and other ills. The physical culture movement continued to offer services that reversed the relation of soma to psyche promoted by the psychogenesists. And relief from psychological and nervous ailments was promised in advertisements for hundreds of products, from yeast, breakfast cereals and other food products to detergents, appliances, automobiles, tours, spas, and, of course, nostrums and other over-the-counter medicines. Official spokespeople like Morris Fishbein, the president of the American Medical Association, wrote denunciations of the most profitable of what he called quackeries.[56] Ernest Jones echoes the AMA in his defence of psychoanalysis in a volume edited by White and Jeliffe in 1913, and making clear that he thinks of psychoanalysis and medicine as allies in the fight against charlatanry; he claims that the new study of neuroses is in fact 'destined to enhance the general importance of medicine.'[57] And after claiming that 'not more than 1 per cent of the cases usually called neurasthenic are really of this nature,' Jones divides the spoils between psychoses, which should be treated by psychiatrists, and neuroses, which should be handled by psychoanalysts.[58] He grants psychiatrists their continuing majority share of asylum business by agreeing that they are the only practitioners capable of treating the two-thirds of asylum cases that are psychoses. But what this argument about the relative provinces of the two specialities elides is perhaps the most far-reaching consequence of the disappearance of neurasthenia. Neurasthenia had become the main diagnostic category used by general practitioners for the many emotional, psychological or nervous disturbances they were called upon to treat. As it was replaced by more specialised diagnoses, neurasthenia was delegitimised and finally demedicalised, and the specialists effectively disposed of the general practitioner as a professional rival.

Even Jones's apparent acquiescence in his fellow specialists is only partially sincere. In a move typical of the imperialism of these competing paradigms, Jones claims priority for the insights of psychoanalytic study as necessary aids to 'the elucidation of the previously unintelligible tangle of mental processes present . . . in insanity,' and he goes further: 'No one who is destitute of this knowledge [of psychoanalytic findings] can hope to unravel the more complicated problems of insanity'; this knowledge 'is capable of throwing an astonishing amount of light on the psychology of both the normal and the abnormal,... on the development of genius ... and of the criminal, ... on the significance of art, religion, and philosophy, and on character formation in the normal as well as the eccentric.'[59] And so while he helps establish the split between the physiological and psychological sciences, he in fact claims more explanatory power for his own side.

Some of the older neurologists clearly saw this as usurpation of their ground. Sir James Crichton-Browne, a leading British writer on neurasthenia, acknowledged in the *Lancet* in 1920 what he called 'our debt to psychoanalysis for having induced us to take a more psychical and less material view of insanity,' but he claimed that this was finally not new, and that insofar as it was, it tended to let practitioners slight the somatic.[60] Successful psychotherapy still needed to be accompanied by other changes in the environment, Crichton-Browne argued, and hence voyages and rest cures were still important therapies. And psychoanalysis was also, Crichton-Browne argued, closely akin to the moral treatments of mid-century, and therefore not so much an advance as a retreat from some of his and Mitchell's methods.

Crichton-Browne was not the only one arguing for an adherence to the old label. Two kinds of institutions continued to use the diagnosis regularly. As might be expected, the sanatoria with a thriving business in treating nervousness continued to go with the proven thing. Many continued to advertise in the same journals that now derided their methods, and sanatorium directors wrote occasional articles salvaging this or that notion. W. C. Ashworth, Medical Director of the Glenwood Park Sanatorium in Greensboro, North Carolina, argued in 1921 that the real heyday was yet to come: 'In the progress of the medical sciences, the provision in the schools and hospitals for the study and treatment of neurasthenia is only beginning to receive proper attention in this country.'[61] All he offered, however, was a repeat of the turn-of-the-century line: the problem was a 'bankrupted nervous system', the treatment consisted of 'rest and isolation, massage, electricity, hydrotherapy, forced feeding, and the use of appropriate drugs.'[62] The other institutions that promoted the diagnosis were Veterans' Hospitals. L. W. Day, of the Perry Point, Maryland Veterans' Hospital asked, 'Which authority is right? Are constitutional psychopathic inferiority and neurasthenia the same, or are we confounding the one with the other?'[63] The most important difference between the two for patients, Day explains, is that neurasthenia is 'compensable,' covered as a veteran's benefit, while the other is not. Thus to diagnose a poor patient as having one of the new disease entities would be in effect to deny them treatment. As a result, in some Veterans' clinics even late in the 1920s, neurasthenia accounted for the majority of all psychopathological diagnoses. At the Minneapolis clinic, for instance, there were 1295 diagnoses of neurasthenia among 2100 neuropsychiatric cases.[64]

As the use of neurasthenia in Veterans' hospitals suggests, the original connection between the 'highly civilised' elites and the disease had largely broken down by the 1920s, leading to the fairly logical conclusion that its elite status was essential to its meaning for doctors, patients, and the public. Nonetheless, as Gosling and Ray have shown, neurasthenia was never in fact simply an elite disease. In their study of the 232 case studies published in the medical literature between 1885 and 1910, 167 identified patients by gender and class, and of these 107 (56 male, 51 female) were middle- (or professional) class, and 60 (37 male, 23 female) were lower-class.[65] The theory of over-civilisation, in other words, did not seem to be supported by the patient population, but remained part of the theory nonetheless. And Gosling and Ray also note that physicians' understandings of the disease was affected by the patient's status; 'working-class men were half as likely to be found neurasthenic due to overwork and twice as likely to be considered neurasthenic due to sexual excess or substance abuse than middle-class men.'[66] The cures undertaken were in part determined by these status differences and in part by the specialty of the physician.

By the twenties, there were other competitors in the field as well. Endocrinology seemed to hold out the promise of a new set of physiological bases for what were increasingly being called emotional disturbances rather than mental disturbances. And glandular explanations threatened to wreak havoc with attempts to isolate any disturbances as clearly psychogenic, the final claim of psychoanalysts and psychologists. And at the same time endocrinological explanations could serve as a buffer between those disease categories which were 'organic' in the old sense, meaning that there were lesions somewhere, and those that were purely psychic or psychological. Jelliffe identified three levels of activity in the nervous system: the vegetative or physiochemical, which included the endocrines and 'visceral neurology'; the sensorimotor, which is what used to be considered neurology proper, based in the central nervous system; and the psychic or symbolic, the 'highest, most complex' level of activity which included cognition and the relation of the individual to the environment, especially the social environment.'[67] At this highest level only, of course, did moralistic therapies for individuals and societies make sense. As these three levels coexisted in mutually interdependent relations, the universe of nervous activity was necessarily the province of all (and only) specialists; and the highest of these, each of these groups argued to themselves, were themselves. The separation of psyche and soma, central to these specialisations' self-definition even when they talked about the necessary connections, grew more and more rigid.

Reconstructions

What then, does this tell us about the rift between somatic and psychic explanations? To answer this one should look further afield for a moment, to the experience of neurasthenia in other cultures. Neurasthenia has continued to be an active diagnostic category in several countries in Asia since its introduction earlier in the century (1900s in Japan, 1920s in China). In a national epidemiological study in China in 1982, 59% of all patients with some form of neurosis were diagnosed as neurasthenic.[68] Later studies that attempted to rediagnose these cases using more recent diagnostic entities found that 42 to 52% of cases fit no other category as clearly.[69] In Taiwan, the prevalence of neurasthenia is much lower; at National Taiwan University Hospital, only 63 patients received the diagnosis between 1980 and 1990, accounting for only 0.2% of psychiatric outpatients. But the entity is used much more widely in discussing disorders with patients, as it is 'much easier to accept by patients without stigma, prejudice, fear, guilt feeling, and ambivalence attached to the disorder for which they are seeking medical help.'[70] In Japan, this lack of stigma results in official as well as unofficial diagnoses. Shizuo Machizawa, chief of psychiatry at the Japanese National Institute of Mental Health, found that 70% of Japanese psychiatrists declined to tell their patients that they were schizophrenic, 20% using a 'euphemistic diagnosis,' often neurasthenia.[71] Tsung-Yi Lin claims that the same is true in Taiwan, where neurasthenia's status as a physiological rather than psychological disease, combined with its ongoing association with brainworkers and thus greater prestige, make it a less stigmatised diagnosis than psychoneuroses or psychoses. Lin also notes that as Western-trained doctors (like himself) gradually used the diagnosis less over time, it experienced 'a rapid rise of popularity among the traditional Chinese doctors and the lay public.'[72]

According to Ware and Weiss, this process of the 'legitimation of otherwise stigmatised symptoms' is common to neurasthenia and a series of similar syndromes, such as *nervios* in Latin America, dhat syndrome in India, *hwa byung* in Korea, and *shinkeishitsu* in Japan.[73]

In other words the function these diagnoses have for patients is not in any direct or necessary relation to the function the same distinctions have for practitioners as they fine-tune their diagnostic categories and fix the boundaries of their specialities. For Ware and Weiss this points towards the 'social construction of psychiatric knowledge,' but we might see it as well as public resistance to the psychiatric severing of soma and psyche.[74]

In the West, such resistance can be seen in the patient activism surrounding one of neurasthenia's acknowledged successor syndromes, Chronic Fatigue Syndrome (CFS). A fairly large literature on the relation between neurasthenia and CFS is complicated by the contributions of researchers working for pharmaceutical companies which clearly desire to cast as wide a net as possible in the marketplace (much of which in the last few decades is documented by Kutchins and Kirk's *Making Us Crazy*[75]). This argument seems less cynical than it might otherwise if one considers the PRIME-MD (Spitzer *et al.*, 1994), a 26-question psychiatric questionnaire, developed by physicians with funding by (and copyrighted by) Pfizer, one of the largest manufacturers of psychiatric drugs in the U.S., or the SPHERE (Hadzi-Pavolic *et al.*, 1997) checklist of 36 questions developed by their competitor Bristol-Myers-Squibb.[76] SPHERE works by asking patients whether, in the last few weeks, they have experienced:

1. Headaches?
2. Feeling irritable or cranky?
3. Poor memory?
4. Pains in your arms and legs?
5. Feeling nervous or tense?
6. Muscle pain after activity?
7. Waking up tired?
8. Rapidly changing moods?
9. Fainting spells?
10. Nausea?
11. Arms and legs feeling heavy?
12. Feeling unhappy & depressed?
13. Gas or bloating?
14. Fevers?
15. Back pain?
16. Needing to sleep longer?
17. Prolonged tiredness after activity?
18. Sore throats?

19. Numb or tingling sensations?
20. Feeling constantly under strain?
21. Joint pain?
22. Weak muscles?
23. Feeling frustrated?
24. Diarrhoea or constipation?
25. Poor sleep?
26. Getting annoyed easily?
27. Everything getting on top of you?
28. Dizziness?
29. Feeling tired after rest or relaxation?
30. Poor concentration?
31. Tired muscles after activity?
32. Feeling lost for words?

The patient that answers 'yes' to any of these questions is a candidate for further psychiatric testing and treatment. Broad enough that no sentient being could go a week without being able to answer at least one of these affirmatively, SPHERE commingles somatic symptoms like back, joint, or throat pain with everyday occurrences like frustration or annoyance in a list that despite its amazing breadth could describe the 32 effects of one ill-spent night in a pub.

Simon Wessely and others have argued that CFS and Myalgic Encephalomyelitis (ME) have in the past been diagnosed as neurasthenia, which Wessely calls 'the disease that did not disappear,' and that neurasthenia would 'readily suffice' as a diagnosis for ME and some other syndromes now.[77] These calls for a revival of the diagnosis have received severe and warranted criticisms from CFS activists and others, who claim that doing so would jump the scientific gun. They worry that labelling CFS as neurasthenia gives it the onus of a psychiatric, rather than, as they see it, a viral or otherwise physiological illness. In *The Illness Narratives*, Arthur Kleinman describes the case history of a lady in New York who never recovered from a severe case of mononucleosis (an infectious blood disease) and who had developed what most doctors would call ME or chronic fatigue syndrome. He ascribes all her symptoms to psychiatric causes such as depression and anxiety, suggests that she is a classic case of neurasthenia and recommends psychotherapy as the best treatment. In a speech before the 1999 Sydney conference on Chronic Fatigue and related illnesses, patient-activist Ted Shaw scoffed at Kleinman's easy translation of categories, and feared that the labelling of CFS as neurasthenia, and neurasthenia as a psychiatric illness, would hinder research into the physiological basis of the disease.[78] What Shaw counselled was more activism on the part of CFS sufferers, a kind of proactive social construction to combat the professional construction of the neurasthenia revivalists. It is no accident that one of the voices calling for the revival of neurasthenia as a diagnosis in the West is Ian Hickie, MD, one of the three authors of SPHERE.

The fact that neurasthenia is regarded as a protection against psychiatric diagnoses in some cultures and a dangerous slide into a psychogenic diagnosis in others is the mark of its ability, as a diagnosis, to bridge this fundamental divide. It may very well be that neurasthenia in late-nineteenth-century America helped naturalise the psychologisation of certain kinds of suffering, but this was against the background of the growing prestige of physiological research. But what is interesting in today's anti-neurasthenic arguments is that, although they are concerned with the stigma attached to psychiatric diagnoses, their main complaint is that the diagnosis makes finding a real cure impossible. The patient activists believe that CFS and related diseases have viral, bacterial, and possibly other physiological causes, and so assume that these organic causes would need to be addressed. Recent papers have discussed mycoplasma, rickettsias, chlamydia, RNaseL dysfunction, channelopathy, stealth viruses, solvent exposure, and psoas muscle deterioration, among other things, as causes of CFS.[79] The hope is that one or more of these avenues of research will result in the development of therapies that will alleviate the symptoms, at least, of patients with this constellation of fatigue disorders. Since cognitive and behavioral therapies obviously cannot deal with the viral or other causative agents and many drugs would simply mask symptoms, these are considered non-therapies by the CFS activists. These latter present their arguments, then, as explicit counterweights to market construction: against the imperialist forces of the DSM-IV crowd, they propose the need for more scientific research – they argue, in other words for the scientific construction of disease over and against market constructions and professional constructions. So if in some Asian cases neurasthenia allows cure by combating social constructions of psychoneuroses, in the West neurasthenia is attacked for the opposite reason. In both cases, at stake is the question of the relation of soma to psyche in the disease, or the overdetermined desire to separate them.

Notes

1. Wade Wright, 'Industrial Hygiene', *Mental Hygiene*, 5 (July 1921), 497–98: 497.
2. Suzanne Poirier, 'The Weir Mitchell Rest Cure: Doctors and Patients', *Women's Studies*, 10 (1983), 15–40; Barbara Sicherman, 'The Uses of Diagnosis: Doctors, Patients, and Neurasthenia', *Journal of the History of Medicine and Allied Sciences*, 32 (1977), 33–54: 36; Charles E. Rosenberg, *No Other Gods: On Science and American Social Thought* (Baltimore: Johns Hopkins, 1976); Ann Douglas, 'The Fashionable Diseases: Women's Complaints and Their Treatment in Nineteenth-Century America', *Journal of Interdisciplinary History*, 4 (1973), 25–52; T.J. Jackson Lears, *No Place of Grace: Antimodernism and the Transformation of American Culture, 1880-1920* (New York, Pantheon, 1981); George F. Drinka, *The Birth of Neurosis: Myth, Malady, and the Victorians* (New York: Simon & Schuster, 1984); Tom Lutz, *American Nervousness, 1903: An Anecdotal History* (Ithaca, NY: Cornell University Press, 1991).
3. William Taylor Marrs, *Confessions of a Neurasthenic* (Philadelphia: FA Davis, 1908).
4. T. M. Luhrmann, *Of Two Minds: The Growing Disorder in American Psychiatry* (New York: Knopf, 2000).
5. F. G. Gosling, *Before Freud: Neurasthenia and the American Medical Community, 1870-1910* (Urbana, IL: University of Illinois Press, 1987).
6. See Gosling, *op. cit.* (note 5); Peter Gay, *The Bourgeois Experience, Victoria to Freud.* Volume II *The Tender Passion* (New York: Oxford University Press, 1986); Henri F. Ellenberger, *The Discovery of the Unconscious: The History and Evolution of Dynamic Psychiatry* (New York: Basic Books, 1970); Edward Shorter, *A History of Psychiatry: From the Era of the Asylum to the Age of Prozac* (New York: John Wiley & Sons, 1997).
7. Cf. F.M. Corrigan, 'Neurasthenic Fatigue, Chemical Sensitivity and GABAa Receptor Toxins', *Medical Hypotheses*, 43 (1994), 195–200; David S. Bell, 'Taking Chronic Fatigue Syndrome Seriously' [Letter], *American Journal of Psychiatry*, 149 (1992), 1753.
8. George M. Beard, 'Neurasthenia, or Nervous Exhaustion', *Boston Medical and Surgical Journal*, ns 3 (1869), 217–21.
9. Robley Dunglison, *Medical Lexicon: A Dictionary of Medical Science* (Philadelphia: Blanchard and Lea, 1851); E.H. Van Deusen, 'Observations on a Form of Nervous Prostration (Neurasthenia), Culminating in Insanity', *American Journal of Insanity*, 25 (1869),

445–61.

10. G. Beard, 'Neurasthenia', *op. cit.* (note 8), 217.

11. *Ibid.*

12. *Ibid.*

13. Sigmund Freud, 'A Reply to Criticisms of Anxiety Neurosis', in *A General Selection from The Works of Sigmund Freud*, eds Rickman and Brenner (New York: Doubleday, 1957).

14. G. Beard, 'Neurasthenia', *op. cit.* (note 8), 218.

15. *Ibid.*

16. S. Freud, 'Reply'; G. Beard, 'Nervous Exhaustion (Neurasthenia) with Cases of Sexual Exhaustion', *Maryland Medical Journal*, 6 (1880), 289–97: 294.

17. G. Beard, *American Nervousness: Its Causes and Consequences* (New York: Putnam's, 1881), 96.

18. G. Beard, *ibid.*, 176.

19. G. Beard, 'Nervous Exhaustion', *op. cit.* (note 16), 294.

20. G. Beard, *American Nervousness*, *op. cit.* (note 17), 219.

21. Charles L. Dana, 'The Partial Passing of Neurasthenia', *Boston Medical and Surgical Journal*, 60 (1904), 339–4.

22. F. Gosling, *op. cit.* (note 5), 86.

23. S.W. Mitchell, *Fat and Blood and How to Make Them* (Philadelphia: Lippincott, 1878).

24. Mitchell, *ibid.*, 46.

25. Mitchell, *ibid.*, 72.

26. F.G. Gosling and Joyce M. Ray, 'The Right to Be Sick: American Physicians and Nervous Patients, 1885-1910', *Journal of Social History*, 20 (1986), 251–67: 264–7.

27. S. Mitchell, 'The Evolution of the Rest Cure', Journal of Nervous and Mental Diseases, 31 (1904), 368–73: 370.

28. *Ibid.*, 371.

29. *Ibid.*, 373.

30. S. Mitchell, *Doctor and Patient* (Philadelphia: Lippincott, 1887).

31. I.N. Love, 'Neurasthenia', *Journal of the American Medical Association*, 22 (1894), 539–44: 540.

32. Frederick Lewis Allen, *Only Yesterday: An Informal History of the Nineteen-Twenties* ([1931] New York: Harper & Row, 1964), 165.

33. J.W. McConnell, 'The Relation of Neurology to the Practice of General Medicine', *New York Medical Journal*, 111 (May 29, 1920), 944–46: 944.

34. M.W. Raynor, Review of Edwin Ash's *The Problem of Nervous Breakdown* (1920), *Mental Hygiene*, 5 (July 1921), 638.

35. Ralph P. Truitt, Review of W. Charles Loosmore's *Nerves and the*

Man, *Mental Hygiene*, 5 (July 1921), 655.

36. J. W. McConnell, 'The Relation of Neurology to the Practice of General Medicine', *New York Medical Journal*, 111 (May 29, 1920), 944.

37. W.C. Ashworth, 'Neurasthenia', *Virginia Medical Monthly*, 48 (Aug 1921), 247–54: 247.

38. M.D. Clayton, 'When is the Diagnosis of Neurasthenia Justified?', *U.S. Veteran's Bureau Medical Bulletin*, 2 (January 1925), 61–64: 61, 64.

39. Peter Bassoe, 'The Origin, Rise and Decline of the Neurasthenia Concept', *Wisconsin Medical Journal*, 27 (January 1928), 11–14: 11.

40. *Op. cit.*, (note 15); for criticism see B.B. Rowley, [Reply], Wisconsin *Medical Journal*, 27 (January 1928), 14.

41. Clarence C. May, 'Nervousness', *New Orleans Medical and Surgical Journal*, 77 (February 1925), 307–309: 307.

42. C.F. Neu, 'Treatment and Management of the Neurasthenic Individual', *Medical Record*, 97 (Feb 28, 1920), 341–45: 341.

43. Sigmund Freud, 'On the Grounds for Detaching a Particular Syndrome from Neurasthenia under the Description 'Anxiety Neurosis', *Standard Edition of the Complete Psychological Works of Sigmund Freud*, ed. J. Strachey (London: Hogarth Press, 1953), 3: 87–139.

44. William A. White, 'Existing Tendencies, Recent Developments and Correlations in the Field of Psychopathology', *Journal of Nervous and Mental Disease*, 56 (1922), 1–15: 1.

45. Review of Pierre Prengowski's *Les maladies neurastheniques*, *Journal of Nervous and Mental Disease*, 69 (1929), 353; Karl Menninger, 'Influenza and Melancholy', *Journal of Nervous and Mental Disease*, 53 (April 1921), 257–81: 263.

46. Frank R. Fry, 'The Neurasthenic at the Threshold', *Journal of the American Medical Association*, 69 (22 September 1917), 955–6: 956.

47. Lawson G. Lowery, 'Notes on the Psychiatry of 1895 and 1915', *Journal of Nervous and Mental Disease*, 54 (August 1921), 97–106: 97, 106.

48. Theodore Diller, 'The Psychoneuroses: How Shall We Look at Them Today?', *Journal of the American Medical Association*, 69 (22 September 1917), 956–58: 957.

49. See Lutz, *op. cit.* (note 2), 224–231.

50. Elizabeth Kilpatrick and Harry M. Tiebout, 'A Study of Psychoses Occurring in Relation to Childbirth', *American Journal of Psychiatry*, 6 (July 1926), 145–60.

51. Ralph Pemberton, 'The Nature of Certain Functional Nervous

Disturbances and Their Treatment Along Metabolic Lines', *Archives of Neurology and Psychiatry*, 9 (February 1923), 208–17.

52. This has been true for historians as well. The only major interpretation of the end of neurasthenia has been advanced by Gosling in *Before Freud*. Although Gosling recognises increasing specialisation and European influences as contributing factors, his main conclusions are that neurasthenia was abandoned because 'doctors became more knowledgeable about the characteristics of nervousness' and 'perceived important dissimilarities among so-called neurasthenics,' and because 'the difficulty of achieving permanent cures in cases of neurasthenia led to dissatisfaction with diagnosis as well as with therapeutics' (164). What this doesn't explain, of course, is why, after almost a half century, these differences and difficulties became perceived not as puzzles to be solved but as proof that the paradigm should be abandoned. See also Janet Oppenheim, *'Shattered Nerves': Doctors, Patients, and Depression in Victorian England* (New York: Oxford University Press, 1991), which treats 'neurasthenia' and 'depression' as different names for the same phenomenon, and Peter Gay, *op. cit.* (note 6).

53. K. Menninger, *op. cit.* (note 45), 257.

54. Charles Dana, 'Dr. George M. Beard: A Sketch of His Life and Character, With Some Personal Reminiscences', *Archives of Neurology and Psychiatry*, 10 (October 1923), 427–35: 433.

55. Tom A. Williams, 'The Genesis of Some So-Called Neurasthenic States', *Medical Record*, 99 (1921), 681–83: **681–82**.

56. Morris Fishbein, *Medical Follies* (New York: Boni & Liveright, 1925). See Paul Starr, *The Social Transformation of American Medicine* (New York: Basic Books, 1982), for the history and function of this form of competitiveness by physicians. Psychoanalysts have repeated many of the techniques for attaining internal cohesion and external legitimation as did medical doctors. See especially the introduction and chapters three and six. See also Harvey Green, *Fit for America* (New York: Pantheon, 1986) and Lutz, *op. cit.* (note 2).

57. William A. White and Smith Ely Jelliffe (eds), *The Modern Treatment of Nervous and Mental Diseases*, Vol. 1 (Philadelphia: Lea and Febiger, 1913), 335.

58. *Ibid.*, 342.

59. *Ibid.*, 335.

60. James Crichton-Browne, 'Notes on Psychoanalysis and Psychotherapy', *Lancet*, 198 (June 5 and 12, 1920), 1248–9, 1296–7: **1248**.

61. W. Ashworth, *op. cit.* (note 37), 249.
62. *Ibid.*
63. L. W. Day, 'A Study of the Last One Hundred Cases of Neurasthenia discharged from United States Veterans' Hospital, Perry Point, Maryland', *US Veteran's Bureau Medical Bulletin*, 3 (June 1927), 559–73: 559.
64. Ralph E. Davis, 'The Mechanism of Neurasthenia among Ex-service Men', *ibid*, 549–59: 550.
65. F. Gosling and J. Ray, 'Right to Be Sick', *op. cit.* (note 5), 253.
66. *Ibid.*, 255.
67. Smith Ely Jelliffe and William A. White, 'Principles Underlying the Classification of Diseases of the Nervous System', *Journal of the American Medical Association*, 66 (11 March 1916), 781–83: 782. In the 1920s, with the rapid growth of endocrinology, researchers continued to worry about the relation of hormones to psychological and psychiatric phenomena. Robert Rea made a typical move by stressing the importance of hormonal activity while asking without answering the question of whether it was 'causal, coordinate, or incidental.' This conspicuous indeterminacy effectively neutralized the competing explanation.
68. Yan He Qin, 'The Necessity of Retaining the Diagnostic Concept of Neurasthenia', *Culture, Medicine, and Psychiatry*, 13 (1989), 139–45.
69. Yan He Qin, 'Neurasthenia in China', *Psychiatric Annals*, 22 (1992), 188–9.
70. Eng-Kung Yeh, 'Neurasthenia in Taiwan: A Diagnostic Entity or Destigmatized Paradigm of Mental Disorders?', *Psychiatric Annals*, 22 (1992), 192–3.
71. Shizou Machizawa, *ibid.*, 190–1.
72. Tsung-Yi Lin, 'Neurasthenia Revisited: Its Place in Modern Psychiatry', *Psychiatric Annals*, 22 (1992), 173–87: **181**.
73. Norma C. Ware and Mitchell G. Weiss, 'Neurasthenia and the Social Construction of Psychiatric Knowledge', *Transcultural Psychiatric Research Review*, 31 (1994), 101–24: **101**.
74. *Ibid.*, 101.
75. Herb Kutchins and Stuart Kirk, *Making Us Crazy: DSM: The Psychiatric Bible and the Creation of Mental Disorders* (New York: The Free Press, 1997).
76. R. Spitzer, *et al.* 'Utility of a New Procedure for Diagnosing Mental Disorders in Primary Care: The PRIME- MD 1000 Study', *Journal of the American Medical Association*, 272 (1994), 1749–56; D. Hadzi-Pavolic, I. Hickie, and C. Ricci, 'The SPHERE Somatic and Psychological Report', *Technical Report TR-97-002*, School of

Psychiatry, University of NSW and Academic Department of
Psychiatry at St George Hospital, 12 April 1997.

77. Simon Wessely, 'Neurasthenia and Fatigue Syndromes: Clinical
    Section', in German E. Berrios and Roy Porter (eds), *The History of
    Clinical Psychiatry: The Origin and History of Psychiatric Disorders*
    (London: Athlone, 1995), 509–32; Arthur Kleinman, *The Illness
    Narratives: Suffering, Healing & the Human Condition* (New York:
    Basic Books, 1988); I. Hickie, D. Hadzi-Pavlovic, and C. Ricci,
    'Reviving the diagnosis of neurasthenia [editorial]', *Psychological
    Medicine*, 27 (1997), 989–94.

78. Ted Shaw, 'Patient Information Day Speech', 1999 Sydney ME/CFS
    Conference, http://www.ahmf.org/Conf99_2.htm

79. A. Chaudhuri and P. Behan, 'Chronic Fatigue Syndrome is an
    Acquired Neurological Channelopathy', *Human Psychopharmacology
    Clinical Experiment*, 14 (1999), 7–17; W.J. Martin, L.C. Zeng, K.
    Ahmed, and M. Roy, 'Cytomegalovirus-Related Sequences in an
    Atypical Cytopathic Virus Repeatedly Isolated from a Patient with
    the Chronic Fatigue Syndrome', *American Journal of Pathology*, 145
    (1994), 441–52; V. Roca, 'Transient Acquired Immunodeficiency
    During Rickettsial Disease' [Letter], *Archives of Internal Medicine*,
    144 (1984), 198–99.

3

Neurasthenia in Britain:
An Overview

Mathew Thomson

The problem of a beginning

A language of 'nerves', a popular bodily economy of nervous energy, an expanding medical culture of nerve management, and a belief that civilisation produced nervousness were all in place in Britain long before Beard coined of the term 'neurasthenia'.[1] There is a careful and particular history to be told of how Beard's concept and the treatment regime associated with it, such as the 'Rest Cure' of Silas Weir Mitchell, fitted into this existing climate and were received and translated to suit another culture as they spread across the Atlantic. However, in a broader sense, the history of neurasthenia may be better conceptualised as beginning well before the birth of the category itself. Indeed, there is a case for arguing that the concept and its somatic location of individual misery acted as a kind of holding operation for a medical model which both long predated it and was already in the early stages of decline.

It is perhaps significant that the subject of British neurasthenia has attracted little specific attention from historians, particularly set against studies of the United States and, more recently, Germany.[2] The main authority on Britain locates the subject fairly seemlessly and as a minor episode within the nineteenth-century culture of 'shattered nerves'.[3] There is an extensive literature on the history of insanity and asylums in the Britain of this period, but this scarcely mentions neurasthenia. Is this low profile simply a reflection of the relative neglect of a history which reaches beyond confinement and madness? Or does it accurately mirror the comparative unimportance of the category in the British context? Reasons can readily be suggested to account for its higher profile elsewhere. For instance, it is hardly surprising that a condition which was framed as peculiarly that of the most modern nation in the world should take off in that country, the United States, with a certain sense of national pride. In

Germany, the relatively advanced development of out-patient care and research in psychiatry, at a time when British counterparts were generally as bound as their patients by the walls of the asylum, may have encouraged more interest in borderline conditions like neurasthenia. However, the higher profile may also reflect a greater tendency in these other historiographies to use neurasthenia as a loose umbrella term for 'nervous' disorders, rather than in a strictly particular sense; and in this respect, Britain may be less exceptional than is at first suggested by a survey of the historiography.

One can gain a crude impression of the relative importance of neurasthenia as a particular category by surveying books and pamphlets circulating in Britain during the period. Only thirty six titles included the term. Eleven of these were published after the First World War: an event which is usually seen as marking the end of the concept's heyday.[4] Nine were foreign works.[5] A similar proportion were handbooks directed at a lay audience, written in a popular style, often but not always by unqualified practitioners, and sometimes conveying an unorthodox message.[6] A few recounted patients' experiences.[7] Only a handful of orthodox British doctors wrote on the subject, and when they did it was usually in a second-hand way as a guide to practitioners and often as part of broader accounts covering a range of nervous disorders. There is certainly no sense that the concept was to the fore in orthodox medical debate. On the other hand, a number of these surveys of the literature were regularly republished. For instance, Thomas Stretch Dowse's fairly slim and derivative paper on the subject, first read before the Medical Society of London in 1880, went into four further editions before the end of the century. Such a pattern of publication might be seen as a product of the paucity of publications in the field, but it may also suggest that there was an undercurrent of demand for practical information on neurasthenia among general practitioners, despite its rather marginal position within medical theory.[8] Significantly, one of the most substantial and successful of these volumes, written by Thomas Dixon Savill, was not published until as late as 1899: three decades after Beard and after years of criticism of the vague nature of the neurasthenia diagnosis within the medical literature. Three further editions would follow in quick succession. Again, this raises the possibility that practical interest may have been considerably stronger and more persistent than suggested by the relative neglect and dismissal of the concept within the theoretical literature.[9] In the immediate aftermath of the First World War there was a brief surge of interest provoked by shell shock and another of these general accounts appeared though this time in only a single edition.[10] Thereafter, such orthodox surveys disappeared altogether; the post-war publications were almost all towards the popular end of the market.

Attractions of neurasthenia

It has been argued that one of the great attractions of the neurasthenia diagnosis was that it provided classificatory order and unity to an existing confusion of nervous disorders.[11] However this overarching ambition was also, paradoxically, one of its main weaknesses. In 1897 even one of its greatest British advocates acknowledged that: 'For a long time the word neurasthenia was absolutely denounced by some physicians on the ground that its meaning was vague, unscientific and unsound, and that to use it was a blot upon the canons of science'. He claimed that such 'balderdash has had its day'.[12] But, in truth, it remained a vague and contested category, even more prone than it had ever been to criticism, fracture, and rejection.

More convincing, therefore, as an attraction of the diagnosis in the last decades of the century is that it offered a somatic location - the nerves - for a vast range of conditions which had no other obvious organic origin, from lethargy to insomnia, depression, headache, and bodily aches and pains, and thereby successfully satisfied the needs of doctors and patients within the medical marketplace: 'validating both the doctor's ministrations and the patient's suffering'.[13] Crucial here is the relationship of private medical practitioner and consumer. Doctors were desperate for explanation, on the one hand; a growing population of wealthy and leisured patients were ready and able to create a market, on the other. The somatic location of these ailments suited all concerned: there was no sense that the proper role of medicine extended beyond ministering to the body; and to suggest that the conditions were partly in the mind would have been to cast in doubt the reality of suffering at best and to have questioned will power, honesty and even sanity at worst - neither acceptable to clients who held the purse strings. Neurasthenia's location in the condition of the nervous system as a whole was attractive in practice to doctors because, in diet, rest and drugs, they were already armed with a panoply of readily accessible, seemingly therapeutic strategies which could be prescribed in infinite and seemingly expert combination. It is also important to note that such regimes of intense, individualised, patient-management enabled doctors to integrate what was in effect a psychological approach in all but name and thus without the negative connotations of a self-willed illness.[14] Indeed, in the American context it has been suggested that the success of the neurasthenia diagnosis lay in this covert opening up of an acceptable space for the development of psychotherapeutic medicine and an escape from the cul-de-sac of asylum-based psychiatry.[15] To a certain extent, and within the context of an increasingly explicit materialist emphasis in medical culture, this may also be a useful way to think about medical practice in the British situation.[16]

Epidemiology

One obvious approach to any comparative history of illness is epidemiological. However, such scrutiny reveals how little we really know, and perhaps can ever know, about such an impressionistic condition as neurasthenia. Historians are in no position to calculate rates of neurasthenia in the way that they might physical diseases and even mental illness. On the basis that neurasthenia was so successfully serving the interests of producer and consumer, Oppenheim speculates that it probably encouraged an increase in the number of nervous cases in the final third of the century.[17] However, beyond such guesswork, with so much imprecision in the use of the term, and with an unknown volume of medical treatment hidden in the realms of the private sphere and spilling over into the realms of the quack and the self-help book, it is difficult to see how even the most ardent of empiricists could attempt to map an epidemiology with any real confidence. We are largely left to draw cautious conclusions based on contemporary opinion and the shifting production of published ideas. The very logic of neurasthenia as a disease of civilisation - the result of urbanisation, the increased pace of life, and the demands of 'brain work'- encouraged contemporaries to claim an increase in prevalence as if this was common knowledge.[18] However, precision and reliable data rarely accompanied such views. One early-twentieth-century specialist claimed that neurasthenia was six times more common than hysteria;[19] but how trustworthy is this estimate when it is stretched beyond his own fashionable practice; and does this solve the problem when we are unable to estimate with confidence the number of hysterics, or even be sure that the two diagnoses were not to some extent interchangeable?

It is even difficult to be confident about the basic class and gender composition of the neurasthenic population. In the United States, Beard had framed neurasthenia as having a particular association with the wealthy classes; the archetypal sufferer was infamously the businessman exhausted by the hustle and bustle of modern life. British doctors, on the other hand, often went out of their way to assert that the condition could affect all classes.[20] Despite this, both the logic of the consumerist argument and the preponderance and greater introspection of middle-class, compared to working-class memoir material, have perpetuated the stereotype originally set up by Beard.[21] And as Hilary Marland's case study of William Smout Playfair and Anne Digby's work on General Practice suggest, because of the importance of class in determining the style of the doctor–patient encounter and deterring time-intensive neurasthenic case histories at the bottom of the social scale, there may be something to this view in practice.[22]

There is further confusion when it comes to gender. It is tempting to see neurasthenia as the male alternative to hysteria: one which lacked the suggestion of malingering associated with the predominantly female condition;[23] and one which positioned male breakdown as the result of hard work - nothing to be ashamed of - rather than a body unable to cope with its sexual burden.[24] Some statistics and opinion from the period supports this. For instance, in the 1880s and 1890s Thomas Savill, treating mainly working-class patients, found that 61% of the neurasthenics were men, while 97% of the hysterical cases were women.[25] As late as 1920, Cobb also regarded the condition as slightly more common among men.[26] However, a number of doctors also emphasised that strains attributed to the female reproductive system could lead to neurasthenia.[27] Moreover, the Rest Cure for neurasthenia has come to be closely associated with women, particularly through the experiences of prominent patients like Virginia Woolf and Charlotte Perkins Gilman; even if in reality men also appear to have been readily sent on such courses.[28] Lending a degree of support to this stereotype, in the first decade of the twentieth century Dr Alfred Schofield reported that 228 of 350 cases treated by him were women; noting, moreover, that this was perhaps a higher proportion of men than might have been expected.[29] In her influential The Female Malady, however, cultural historian Elaine Showalter went substantially further to assert that the majority of neurasthenic patients in the United States were women and that in Britain it was mainly associated with young women.[30] Historians, we might conclude, like contemporaries, have made what sense they have wanted out of the protean condition.

•

From body to mind

It is generally agreed that the waning of neurasthenia (and more generally the location of a broad range of ills in the physical condition of nervous system as a whole) can be explained by a fundamental shift in medical paradigms in the early-twentieth-century. The origin of physical symptoms was now to be found in the mental problems which arose from the individual's struggle to adjust to a changing environment. Bearing in mind the comparative conservatism of British medicine, it is perhaps unsurprising that such a transition was in practice more protracted and tentative than suggested by the concept of a 'paradigm shift'. And this is confirmed when analysis extends to the ordinary general practitioner, unorthodox medicine, and popular attitudes.

By the turn of the century, there was growing criticism of the efficacy and safety of the drugs that had been the mainstay of nineteenth-century treatment of neurasthenia.[31] The search for a demonstrable and specific organic origin which could be targeted by medicine continued, but was proving similarly disappointing.[32] Instead, some doctors turned towards an emerging literature which more explicitly recognised the psycho-therapeutic role of the doctor, the power of the subconscious mind over the body, and the malleability of this mind to suggestion.[33] This had potentially radical implications for the diagnosis and treatment of neurasthenia. By the inter-war period, therefore, the language of 'nerves' and 'neurasthenia' was making way for that of 'neuroses' and 'psycho-neuroses' which assumed a primarily mental origin, the organic implications of the latter term now notably notwithstanding.[34] In his 1923 study of the 'neuroses', T.A. Ross still used the term 'neurasthenia' but it was now a synonym for 'anxiety neurosis' and that 'series of symptoms, which arise from faulty adaptation to the strains and stresses of life.'[35] Thereafter, 'neurasthenia' would persist in British medical language, but in an increasingly narrow sense: now no more than one psycho-neurotic symptom - abnormal fatigue - among many, rather than the grand umbrella category of its youth.[36]

An embrace of psychotherapy and a redefinition of neurasthenic states in increasingly mental rather than somatic terms did not take place overnight.[37] There was some trenchant initial resistance to the new psychology, within the British medical profession.[38] A desire of some to offset the challenge of the 'ever-growing hordes of quacks' claiming the psychotherapeutic territory as their own tended to be cancelled out by a more general fear of guilt through association.[39]

And even though there were regular calls for medicine to take seriously the importance of mind as well as body in all questions of health and illness, progress was held back by the marginal position of psychology within the medical curriculum.[40] Some elite clinicians supported the study of psychology as the key to a more holistic style of medicine.[41] However, the ordinary general practitioner remained largely ignorant of psychological theory, regarding it as the terrain of psychiatric specialists though rarely having the insight or confidence to refer cases.[42] For these busy doctors, neurasthenia may have remained a convenient label - perhaps along with another bottle of medicine - for a vast range of unexplainable conditions and hundreds of apparently intractable patients.[43] With its amorphous character, neurasthenia proved adaptable to the changing climate of opinion. The idea that mental and somatic factors both played a part had after all always been implicitly if not explicitly accepted. Moreover, acknowledging that mental worry might precipitate bodily ills left such ills no less real for this; and it left the possibility that the same was true in reverse. And since treatment to alleviate these conditions might be attempted at any point of this 'vicious circle' it did not invalidate the doctor's traditional therapeutic strategies.[44] In exasperation at this persistence, one psycho-therapeutically inclined doctor in 1930, found himself forced to complain about the 'dumping ground of neurasthenia'.[45] But as late as the 1950s general practitioners were still to be found utilising the unreliable and vague diagnosis.[46]

At a popular level, advertisements in the press testify to the persistence of a nerve-centred discourse and therapeutics, with tonics such as 'Wincarnis', 'Hall's Wines', and 'Sanotogen' claiming to ameliorate a broad range of nervous conditions. These included 'neurasthenia', and there was even a product called 'Antineurasthin'. On the other hand, this was by no means the most common nerve ailment by the interwar period. Instead, conditions like 'neuralgia' and 'neuritis' came to the fore suggesting that even at a popular level 'neurasthenia' was becoming old-fashioned or seemingly too vague.[47] T.A. Ross reported that one forty-eight-year-old woman, having been in and out of rest cures for a decade before arriving for treatment at the psycho-therapeutically-orientated Cassel Hospital in 1921, 'regarded herself as storage battery. No one had let her stay long enough on the charger, and everybody had allowed a larger discharge to be drawn off from her than her battery could stand.' And as he noted: 'this view is a very common one among patients.'[48] But the general public were also increasingly influenced by the new 'climate of opinion' in which maintaining mental energy was a question of satisfying drives and instincts, avoiding resulting conflicts, and off-setting anxiety.[49] Like H.G. Wells' Sir Richmond Hardy, they might therefore combine a language of 'neurasthenia', 'fatigue', and 'flagging' with a 'popularised psycho-analysis': 'one strains and flags, and then the lower stuff in one, the subconscious stuff, takes control.'[50] In fact, although the preponderance of lay guides to neurasthenia at first sight suggests a persistence of somaticism, these texts were also invariably open to psychotherapy, sometimes pioneeringly so. An individualist self-help culture readily accepted the idea that individuals could conquer ailments like neurasthenia through self mastery of brain and body. It has recently been suggested that in the United States neurasthenia was replaced by 'nervous breakdown': a culture which merged the nervous-energy and psycho-therapeutic models.[51] Even if the neat packaging of this argument is rejected (and in Britain, at least, the term 'nervous breakdown' already appeared regularly in nineteenth-century writing), it does again highlight that we may need to think about the persistence of neurasthenia in its broader sense, albeit alongside emerging psycho-dynamic conceptions of mental health and illness, long after its official 'end'.

The great strength of neurasthenia in the late-nineteenth century had been that it satisfied the interests of both doctors and medical consumers. Shorter and Oppenheim both suggest that the increasingly explicit acceptance by doctors of mental origins to somatic conditions began to change this equation. Consumers, on the other hand, tended to remain more attracted to the older explanatory model which was readily understood, absolved them of individual responsibility, asserted the somatic reality of their suffering, and shaped a treatment regime which in its somatic therapies and also in its less overt psycho-therapeutic dimensions satisfied many of their physical and emotional needs.[52] It has been suggested that this may also help to explain the longer persistence of somatic models within popular culture and the 're-emergence' in the form of new illnesses such as 'ME' and Chronic Fatigue Syndrome in the late-twentieth century.[53] Overlooking for the moment the qualifications suggested above to a dichotomy of psychologically-inclined doctors and somatically- resilient patients, the logic of this position is that the end of neurasthenia depended upon a shift in power between doctor and patient. Why were doctors now able and willing to break the neurasthenic contract against the will of their patients?

The state

In beginning to answer this question, it seems sensible to address the era's most seismic development for doctor–patient relations: the increasing influence of the state. In doing so, it is worth reiterating that Oppenheim's picture of the nineteenth-century neurasthenic contract is based on the relationship between private doctor and medical consumer. In such circumstances, it is hardly surprising that patients' interests tended to be served. Without this type of pecuniary incentive, as they increasingly found themselves in the twentieth century, doctors may have been more likely to question the somatic basis of conditions which had no obvious or specific organic origin.

In dealing with compensation claims for neurasthenia arising from 'railway spine' or industrial injury under the Workmen's Compensation Act of 1897, doctors could find themselves employed to police malingering in the interest of insurance companies or the state. By the inter-war period five to six per cent of the working population were making successful claims annually.[54] Even doctors who were not so employed often came to recognise that neurasthenia would often persist as long as the issue of compensation remained to be resolved.[55] General practitioners also had less incentive to embark on a possibly endless assault on the symptoms of neurasthenia if the patients were not paying - it was said that nine out of ten applying for medical relief at out-patient departments were neurasthenics.[56] The busy general practitioner was liable to come to see seemingly incurable and interminable neurasthenics as more trouble than they were worth – 'known in every consulting room... the terror of the busy physician'.[57] There was a similar exasperation with 'bottle of medicine loving patients' from Stephen Taylor, at the time a junior doctor dealing with 'poor teaching cases' in a London hospital, leading him to coin the term the 'suburban neurosis' for what half a century earlier had been classic neurasthenia.[58] Treatment of such cases almost inevitably involved a cat and mouse game which was always prone to become increasingly inquisitorial.

The shell-shock issue of the First World War would bring the issue of malingering to the fore in spectacular fashion, with doctors employed to act in the interests of the state and country.[59] However these doctors were also torn by the fact that the shell-shocked, albeit lacking the power of the consumer, were putting their lives on the line and as such assumed a different kind of status, especially in the case of officers who were more prone than the other ranks to be removed from the front line with a diagnosis of neurasthenia.[60] As a result, it proved difficult to hold back neurasthenia in the form of shell-shock;[61] particularly, since in providing a reasonably harmless outlet for tension, exhaustion and collapse of morale, it was in a sense 'functional' for the military as well as the soldiers involved.[62] Nevertheless, the shift from a private medical market to an albeit temporary wartime situation of state control had radically transformed the relationship between doctor and patient and made it much easier to conceptualise neurasthenia in psychological terms.[63] By the end of the war it was recognised that it might be very difficult to cure shell-shock if this was to result in the removal of a war pension. Many ex-soldiers who succumbed to neurasthenia in the post-war years, now diagnosed in terms of anxiety, and became unemployed as a result would be unable to obtain a war pension, and would fall back on charitable aid from groups like the Ex-Services Welfare Society.[64]

In the inter-war period, with the spread of panel doctors under the National Insurance Scheme and an increasing proportion of the unemployed forced to seek relief, the doctor as state employee was once more placed in the role of policing malingering. Again, in such circumstances there was no longer the interest of the consumer to hold back the view that physical ills were often the result of psychological causes. Some doctors became openly critical of what they saw as a burgeoning culture of 'compensation neurosis'.[65] One influential study suggested that a third of those claiming incapacity to work were the result of psychoneuroses, though only a small proportion of these cases were in fact labelled as such.[66] If they had been, they might no longer have been covered by national insurance on the grounds that treatment demanded a specialist skill beyond the capacity of the panel doctor.[67] A 'nervous' diagnosis by contrast remained more ambiguous.[68] For inter-war governments and for a Ministry of Health under George Newman concerned to deflect criticism about responsibility for ill health, particularly as a result of unemployment, benefit levels, and poor diet, the idea that psychology rather than economic well-being was the root cause had a natural appeal.[69] However, doctors did not necessarily act in the interests of the state. With the effect of poverty and emotional misery often visibly apparent in this era of economic insecurity, they may have been understandably reluctant to adopt a psychological diagnosis that only added to this dire situation by jeopardising their patients' chances of obtaining relief through the National Insurance scheme. As H.V. Dicks, Physician to the Institute of Medical Psychology in London recognised, for all its theoretical redundancy, the neurasthenia diagnosis served a useful purpose as a generic term for any psychological condition apart from insanity because it left the self-esteem of the patient intact and 'fortunately the approved societies [who administered the insurance scheme] are not yet so advanced in psychopathology as to quarrel with it.'[70] The ideal solution would have been to treat what was becoming recognised as a huge reservoir of psychoneurotic problems among the population as early as possible and thus with real hope of cure in the national interests, however with psychotherapeutic resources so limited and treatment time-consuming this was never a realistic prospect.[71]

The state's influence on the neurasthenia diagnosis also resulted from its concern about what has loosely been termed 'national efficiency'. In 1870, the still largely non-interventionist British state assumed a radical extension of responsibility: elementary education of children. In doing so, it was faced by the question of whether all children had the necessary brain power to be educable. Concern arose that the very system, through 'cramming' and its effect on weak young minds, could result in neurasthenia.[72] And a process of marking off, and eventually segregating, a section of the population as mentally defective was given impetus.[73] This, together with alarming evidence about the silting up of mental asylums, prisons, and poor law institutions with adult mental defectives, contributed significantly to turn-of-the-century degenerationist anxieties. In this climate, it may well have become harder than before to maintain neurasthenia as a condition of distinction and fashion. If there really was an increasing number of neurasthenics, could this be a further sign of a decline in the national stock? Was neurasthenia, like mental deficiency, the result of a morbid inheritance or at least one unable to cope with modern conditions? There were clearly some who did adopt this sort of position. Sir Havelock Charles, President of the Medical Board at the India Office, for instance, argued that the country was 'breeding a race of neuropaths', their condition made worse by the competitive examination system, who were unfit to maintain Imperial rule and invariably collapsed from neurasthenia in the climate of India.[74]

Once the state, and an ever-growing host of professional and voluntary bodies competing to serve its interests, had assumed a concern about national health, it was likely that neurasthenia would come to be seen in collectivist terms as a problem and a drain on potential national resources. For instance, in the aftermath of the national mobilisation of the First World War, concern about fatigue shifted its locus from the individual, neurasthenic body to the organisation and efficiency of the workplace and the working day.[75] The neurasthenic worker in these depression years was more characteristically regarded as the victim of insecurity and absence of work than of that classic neurasthenic symptom of business 'hustle and bustle'.[76] All this can have done little for the allure of the condition. By the inter-war period, mental hygienists were claiming that conditions like neurasthenia were a huge financial burden on the nation, both in terms of working days lost and the cost of care.[77] The state was called upon to increase its vigilance in detecting likely cases. Prevention was presented as more efficient than cure. And there was an incentive to find a quick mode of cure: lengthy, and to some minds self-indulgent, psycho-analysis was out; but so too was pandering to patients' beliefs in the somatic basis of their conditions; blunt persuasion (used more commonly and with more immediate results than the more celebrated 'talking cure' in the Great War, it should be noted), was to be in.[78] In sum, the state's growing concern about mental health had shifted attention to the working-class and had significantly modified the environment in which patients would encounter doctors. It was less likely as a result that sufferers would now either choose or be able to negotiate a diagnosis of neurasthenia as had their more affluent forebears.

The patient's paradigm changes?

Thus far, an examination of the decline of the neurasthenia diagnosis has followed Shorter in accepting that the doctors had more to gain than the patients from a shift away from the somaticism of neurasthenia. But was this always the case? Do we need to consider more seriously the positive attractions to a lay audience of the shift of paradigms? It is worth pointing out at this juncture that there is an interesting qualification to Shorter's argument. He notes that before psychotherapy was 'highjacked by psychoanalysis' and the patient thereby denied a belief in the somatic basis of suffering, there was an initial psychotherapeutic era in which techniques like suggestion and persuasion were used productively while continuing to allow patients to believe that they were receiving organic therapy.[79] There is surely no reason to believe that such a mix of the organic with the psychological might not have been more attractive to patients than earlier therapeutic regimes, particularly if they were therapeutically effective. In this respect, it is worth noting that in Britain it was quacks, 'psycho-cults', and mystics who were the initial driving force behind the emergence of a psychotherapeutic culture: a fact which surely does point towards the potential popular appeal of such therapy. Moreover, these popular movements usually did mix together the psychological with the somatic (and the spiritual) in an eclectic but holistic mix. As far as they were concerned, there were a number of limitations to a merely somatic approach to a condition like neurasthenia. First, there was a lack of confidence in the efficacy of medicine and its drug-centred approach, exposed by failure in addressing conditions ranging from cancer to neurasthenia, to insanity. Secondly, it appears that these movements catered to a need and desire for therapeutic action, self-help and commodification of health and lifestyle which was not satisfied by the orthodox medical culture of the era (and this continued to be the case even after psychotherapy became part of orthodoxy). And finally, it seems that among a significant population there was a desire for something more that a materialist medicine; psychotherapeutic approaches, linked as they so often were to beliefs about finding a spirituality through the discovery of the whole self, catered to this disenchantment. It is also important to point out that such an argument about the potential popular attractions of a shift beyond the somatic paradigm of neurasthenia can be extended into the realm of orthodox medicine in the inter-war period. For although this medicine remained slow and cautious to accept psychotherapy, partly because of this it tended to integrate it holistically alongside somatic (and at times even spiritual, or at the very least 'humanistic') approaches. Moreover, there is evidence to suggest that forcing patients to acknowledge the psychological basis of conditions like neurasthenia - a stance which did not necessitate denying the reality of their suffering - could be attractive, effective and empowering.[80]

Conclusions

The end of neurasthenia in Britain may be a story of both sides – not only doctors, but also to some extent the patients – finding this diagnosis increasingly unsatisfactory, albeit for rather different reasons. It has also been suggested that such a history can benefit from going beyond mere analysis of changing ideas to consider the importance of their location in an evolving doctor-patient relationship. And it may be revealing to explore variations between different levels of medical practice. However, it is important to point out that this essay has attempted to problematise a clear narrative trajectory of 'beginning to end'; perhaps an inevitability with such a malleable diagnostic category which could so readily offer different things to different groups. Thus, the roots of a demise can be found at the very start and in the heyday of neurasthenia; and apart from

Mathew Thomson

the terminology itself, it may make little sense to think of a beginning which begins with 'neurasthenia'. At the other end of the spectrum, the end would prove to be a protracted and uneven process: in Britain, 'neurasthenia' in fact had a significant history and continuing attractions for some time after the First World War.

Notes

1. See for instance Roy Porter's chapter in this volume.
2. For instance, on the United States: Tom Lutz, *American Nervousness, 1903: An Anecdotal History* (Ithaca: Cornell University Press, 1991); Edward Shorter, *A History of Psychiatry: From the Era of the Asylum to the Era of Prozac* (New York & Chichester: Wiley, 1997). And on Germany: Joachim Radkau, *Das Zeitalter der Nervosität. Deutschland zwischen Bismarck und Hitler* (Munich & Vienna: Carl Hanser Verlag, 1998); Volker Roelcke, *Krankheit und Kulturkritik: Psychiatrische Gesellschaftsdeutungen im bürgerlichen Zeitalter (1790-1914)* (Frankfurt/M: Campus, 1999).
3. Janet Oppenheim, *Shattered Nerves: Doctors, Patients and Depression in Victorian England* (Oxford: Oxford University Press, 1991).
4. A different picture might emerge from a survey of articles in periodicals. It has been estimated that over 300 articles appeared on the subject in American medical journals: M. Barke, R. Fribush & P. Stearns (eds.), 'Nervous Breakdown in 20th-Century American Life', *Social History*, 33 (2000), 565–84: 567.
5. For instance: Paul Hartenberg, *Treatment of Neurasthenia*, translated by Ernest Playfair (Oxford Medical Publications, 1914). Adrien Achille Proust & Gilbert Ballet, *The Treatment of Neurasthenia*, translated by Peter Campbell Smith (London: Henry Kimpton, 1902); Dr Rumler, *The Causes, Nature and Cure of Neurasthenia in General and of the Nervous Disorders of the Generative System in Particular* (Geneva: The Author, 1901), 15th edition.
6. For instance: Edwin Lancelot Hopewell Ash, *Mind and Health: the Mental Factor and Suggestion in Treatment with Special Reference to Neurasthenia and Other Common Nervous Disorders* (London: H.J. Glaisher, 1910); J.M. Graham, *Neurasthenia: its Nature, Origin and Cure* (London: The Psychologist, 1936); James Russell Sneddon, *Self-Treatment for Neurasthenia by Nature Cure Methods* (London: Health for All Publishing Company, 1951); 'A Specialist', *From Terror to Triumph: How to Fight and Conquer Neurasthenia, Insomnia, and Other Nervous Disorders* (Epsom: E.G. Pullinger, 1932); Roger Vittoz, *Treatment of Neurasthenia by Means of Brain Control* translated by H.B. Brooke (London: Longmans, 1911; 2nd edn. 1913).

7. Doris Mary Armitage, *A Challenge to Neurasthenia* (London: Williams & Norgate, 1929,1931,1935); Wilfred Northfield, *Conquest of Nerves: The Inspiring Record of a Personal Triumph over Neurasthenia* (London: Fenland Press, 1933); Joseph Snowball Milne, *Neurasthenia, Shell Shock and the New Life* (Newcastle-on-Tyne: Robinson & Co., 1918).

8. Thomas Stretch Dowse, *On Brain and Nerve Exhaustion: 'Neurasthenia', Its Nature and Treatment* (London: Ballière, Tindall, 1880, 1887,1892,1894).

9. Thomas Dixon Savill, *Clinical Lectures on Neurasthenia* (London: Henry J. Glaisher, 1899, 1902, 1908).

10. Hamilton Clelland Marr, Psychoses of the War, including Neurasthenia and Shell Shock (Oxford Medical Publications, 1919); Ivo Geikie Cobb, *A Manual of Neurasthenia - Nervous Exhaustion* (London: Ballière & Co., 1920)

11 Oppenheim, *op. cit.* (note 3), 96, 109.

12. Thomas Stretch Dowse, *The Pocket Therapist* (Bristol: J. Wright & Co., 1897), 108.

13. Oppenheim, *op. cit.* (note 3), 97.

14. Though there is always in practice such a psychological component to the doctor-patient encounter, neurasthenia was located within a medical culture which was becoming more stridently somaticist, albeit at a theoretical rather than necessarily practical level: Charles Rosenberg, 'Body and Mind in Nineteenth-Century Medicine: Some Clinical Origins of the Neurosis Construct', in C. Rosenberg (ed.), *Explaining Epidemics* (Cambridge: Cambridge University Press, 1992), 74–89.

15. B. Sicherman, 'The Uses of Diagnosis: Doctors, Patients and Neurasthenia', *Journal of the History of Medicine,* 32 (1977), 33–54.

16. See for instance: Dennis de Bardt Hovell, *On Some Further Conditions of Neurasthenia: A Psychological Study* (London: J.& A. Churchill, 1887).

17. Oppenheim, *op. cit.* (note 3), 99.

18. See for instance the continued support for Beard's position: J. Michell Clarke, Hysteria and Neurasthenia (London: John Lane, The Bodley Head, 1905), 171.

19. Edward Shorter, *From Paralysis to Fatigue, A History of Psychosomatic Illness in the Modern Era,* (New York: Free Press, 1992), 222.

20. For instance: Cobb, *A Manual of Neurasthenia, op. cit.* (note 10), 26; Clarke, *op. cit.* (note 18), 175.

21. Oppenheim, *op. cit.* (note 3), 105–8.

22. Marland, this volume; Anne Digby, *The Evolution of British General*

Practice, 1850-1948 (Oxford: Oxford University Press, 1997), 209–11.

23 Oppenheim, *op. cit.* (note 3) 144.

24. *Ibid*, 152-3.

25. Shorter, From Paralysis to Fatigue, op. cit. (note 19) 224. See also Guthrie Rankin, 'Neurasthenia: the Wear and Tear of Life', *British Medical Journal* (BMJ) (2 May 1903), i, 1017–20.

26. Cobb, *op. cit.* (note 10), 23.

27. Oppenheim, *op. cit.* (note 3), 188. See Sengoopta and Marland in this volume.

28. Oppenheim, *op. cit.* (note 3), 107–8, 212–3.

29. Alfred T. Schofield, *The Management of a Nerve Patient* (London: J.A. Churchill, 1906), 106.

30. Elaine Showalter, *The Female Malady: Women, Madness and English Culture, 1830-1980* (London: Virago, 1987), 137

31. Oppenheim, *op. cit.* (note 3), chapter 4.

32. P.C. Smith, 'Neurasthenia, Degeneracy and Mobile Organs', *BMJ* (3 March 1906), i, 494–6.

33. For example Alfred Taylor Schofield, *The Force of Mind* (London: J.A. Churchill, 1902, 1903,1905). For an account of his career: *Behind the Brass Plate: Life's Little Stories* (London: Sampson Low, Marston & Co.).

34. T.A. Ross, *An Enquiry into Prognosis in the Neuroses* (Cambridge: Cambridge University Press, 1936).

35. See for instance T.A. Ross, *The Common Neuroses: Their Treatment by Psychotherapy* (London: Edward Arnold, 1923), 27.

36. H. Campbell Thomson & George Riddoch, *Diseases of the Nervous System* (London: Cassell & Co., 1925), 431.

37. For a very traditional reading of the subject and the view that neurasthenia was now a universally accepted term: Guthrie Rankin, 'Neurasthenia: the Wear and Tear of Life', *BMJ* (2 May 1903), i, 1017-20.

38. Trevor Turner, 'James Crichton-Browne and the Anti-Psychoanalysts', in Hugh Freeman & German Berrios (eds.), *150 Years of British Psychiatry. Volume II The Aftermath* (London: Athlone, 1996), 144–55.

39. Alfred T. Schofield, *op. cit.* (note 29), viii.

40. For instance: 'Psychological Medicine', BMJ (1933), ii, 455-7; 'Teaching of Medical Psychology', *Lancet* (1935), ii, 1185.

41. C. Lawrence, 'Still Incommunicable: Clinical Holists and Medical Knowledge in Interwar Britain', in C. Lawrence & G. Weisz (eds.), *Greater than their Parts: Holism in Biomedicine, 1920-1950* (Oxford:

Oxford University Press, 1998), 94–111.

42. Anne Digby, *The Evolution of British General Practice, 1850-1948* (Oxford: Oxford University Press, 1997), 239–40.

43 Guthrie Rankin, 'Neurasthenia: the Wear and Tear of Life', *BMJ* (2 May 1903), i, 1018; Ernest Reynolds, 'Hysteria and Neurasthenia', *BMJ* (22 Dec. 1923), ii, 1193–6.

44. Jamieson B. Hurry, *The Vicious Circles of Neurasthenia and Their Treatment* (London: J.A. Churchill, 1915).

45. E.F. Buzzard, 'The Dumping Ground of Neurasthenia', *Lancet* (1930), i, 1–4.

46. Lord (Stephen) Taylor & Sidney Chave, *Mental Health and Environment* (London: Longmans Green & Co., 1964), 117.

47. Antineurasthin is advertised for instance in *New Age*, 17 June 1909, 163.

48 Ross, *op. cit.* (note 34), 38–9.

49. D. Rapp, 'The Early Discovery of Freud by the British General Public, 1912-19', *Social History of Medicine*, 3 (1990), 217–45.

50. *The Secret Places of the Heart*, 136.

51. M. Barke, R. Fribush & P. Stearns, 'Nervous Breakdown in 20th-Century American Culture', *Social History*, 33 (2000), 565–84.

52. Shorter, *op. cit.* (note 19); Oppenheim, *op. cit.* (note 3).

53. Simon Wessely, 'Neurasthenia and Fatigue Syndromes', in German Berrios & Roy Porter (eds.), *A History of Clinical Psychiatry: The Origin and History of Psychiatric Disorders* (London: Athlone, 1995), 509-32. There is surely, however, a danger in a history which approaches this as a 're-emergence', with all that this suggests about a fixed, natural identity lying beneath shifting diagnostic language. Neurasthenia was so intimately tied to its culture that it has to be regarded as dying with that culture or at least becoming something fundamentally different as that culture evolved.

54. Peter Bartrip, *Workmen's Compensation in Twentieth Century Britain* (Aldershot: Gower, 1987), x, 121.

55. 'The Traumatic Neuroses', *BMJ* (14 Mar. 1914) i.

56. Savill, *op. cit.* (note 9), 21.

57. Guthrie Rankin, 'Neurasthenia: the Wear and Tear of Life', *BMJ* (2 May 1903), i, 1018.

58. Stephen Taylor, 'The Suburban Neurosis', *Lancet* (26 Mar. 1938), I, 759.

59. Roger Cooter, 'Malingering in Modernity: Psychological Scripts and Adversarial Encounters During the First World War', in R.Cooter, M. Harrison & S. Sturdy (eds.), *War, Medicine and Modernity* (Stroud: Sutton, 1998), 125–48.

60. Mathew Thomson, 'Status, Manpower and Mental Fitness: Mental Deficiency in the First World War', in Cooter *et al.*, *ibid.*, 149–66.

61. A significant proportion of shell-shocked British soldiers were diagnosed neurasthenic. There was disagreement, however, as to whether this was a useful label. This lack of consensus remained in the *1922 Report of the War Office Committee of Enquiry* into 'Shell-Shock'. For instance, W.H.R. Rivers, a psycho-therapeutic pioneer, reported that 'he never used the word"neurasthenia". It had become an absolutely worthless word. What was ordinarily called "neurasthenia" he called "anxiety neurosis". ' (57) This can be contrasted with Dr Arthur Hurst who believed that 'practically every man coming out of the Peninsula was neurasthenic.' (25). It was generally believed that officers were more liable to neurasthenic symptoms as a result of the strain of greater responsibility and the need to repress fear; the ranks by contrast more frequently assumed hysterical symptoms such as mutism and paralysis (68-70).

62. Eric Leed, *No Man's Land: Combat and Identity in World War I* (Cambridge: Cambridge University Press, 1977).

63. M. Stone, 'Shell Shock and the Psychologists', in W. Bynum, R. Porter & M. Shepherd (eds.), *The Anatomy of Madness* (London: Tavistock, 1985), 242–71.

64. Eric Coplans, 'Some Observations on Neurasthenia and Shell Shock', *Lancet*, 2 (1931), 960.

65. For instance: T.A. Ross, 'Some Evils of Compensation', *Mental Hygiene*, 3 (1939), 141–5.

66. James L. Halliday, 'Psychoneuroses as a Cause of Incapacity among Insured Persons', *BMJ Supplement* (9 Mar. 1935), 85–8.

67. For a report of a Ministry of Health ruling on this: 'Psychotherapy', *Lancet* (1933), ii, 262. Whether such guidelines were consistently understood or upheld is unclear. See also: Bentley Gilbert, *British Social Policy, 1914-39* (London: Batsford, 1970), 292–3; and 'Psychotherapy under the Act', *Lancet* (1933), i, 54.

68. T.A. Ross, 'Some Evils of Compensation', *Mental Hygiene*, 3 (1939), 141–5.

69. L. Beales & R.S. Lambert (eds.), *Memoirs of the Unemployed* (London: Victor Gollancz, 1934) 23–4, 43–5.

70. H.V. Dicks, 'Neurasthenia: Toxic and Traumatic', *Lancet* (1933), ii, 683.

71. 'Psychotherapy and National Health Insurance', *Mental Hygiene*, 5 (1939), 73–4.

72. Oppenheim, *op. cit.* (note 3), chapter 7.

73. M. Thomson, *The Problem of Mental Deficiency: Eugenics, Democracy*

and Social Policy in Britain, 1870-1959 (Oxford: Oxford University Press, 1998).

74. 'Neurasthenia among Europeans in India', *BMJ* (27 June 1914), i, 727–8.

75. Nikolas Rose, *Governing the Soul: the Shaping of the Private* Self (London: Routledge, 1989), 55–74.

76. H.L. Beales & R.S. Lambert (eds.), Memoirs of the Unemployed, *(op. cit.* (note 69); Max Cohen, *What Nobody Told the Foreman* (London: People's Book Cooperative Society, 1953).

77. R.D. Gillespie, 'Mental Hygiene as a National Problem', *Mental Hygiene*, 1 (1931), 1–9.

78. For a detailed analysis of the results of persuasion: T.A. Ross, *op. cit.* (note 34). For an example of the common criticism of psycho-analysis from one of the founders of the National Council for Mental Hygiene: Maurice Craig, *Nerve Exhaustion* (London: J. & A. Churchill, 1922), 125. On the First World War: Ben Shephard, 'Pitiless Psychology: the Role of Prevention in British Military Psychiatry in the Second World War', *History of Psychiatry*, 10 (1999), 491–524.

79. Shorter, *op. cit.* (note 2), 245–53.

80. For a eulogy towards psychotherapeutic treatment of neurasthenia, suggesting that the patient's main desire was to be taught how to fight the condition and to be told the truth, not simply to be placated see Doris Mary Armitage, *Challenge to Neurasthenia* (Cambridge, W. Heffer & Sons, 1935). This, moreover, clearly met a receptive audience as it was entering its fourth edition, first published in 1929. See also the postive response from former patients of psycho-therapeutic treatment in Ross, *op. cit.* (note 34).

4

'A Mob of Incoherent Symptoms'?
Neurasthenia in British Medical Discourse, 1860-1920

Chandak Sengoopta

Although much has been written on neurasthenia, the literature is rather deficient in studies of the regional transmutations of the concept.[1] This paper will summarise the history of neurasthenia in Britain and then show how the concept of neurasthenia played important and hitherto unanalysed roles in the complex professional politics of Victorian and Edwardian medicine.

Neurasthenia in Britain

The basic history of the concept of neurasthenia is well-known. From the late 1860s, Beard argued in a set of papers and ultimately, two monographs, that his country was reeling under a new plague that produced no clear physical damage but incapacitated the lives of the best and the brightest and characterised by a galaxy of symptoms ranging from headache, pervasive fatigue and sleeplessness to blushing, tooth decay and dyspepsia, all supposedly caused by the depletion of nervous energy due to the pressures of modern life.[2] Although there was no evident structural lesion in the nervous system, the pathology of the condition was considered to be entirely somatic: a depletion of nervous energy. It was a nervous disorder, but a functional one: neurological function was impaired without any discernible anatomical pathology.[3] Confined, Beard thought, almost entirely to 'brain-workers' and almost exclusively to America, neurasthenia was 'American Nervousness': savages and labourers did not suffer from nervous exhaustion. The delicate nervous balance of brain-workers was being upset by the inexorable acceleration of life, the explosive proliferation of communication networks and the oft-quoted 'mental activity of women.'[4] The idea of neurasthenia, Beard proudly declared, challenged the virtual one-way traffic in scientific ideas between America and Europe. Here was a medical concept that had originated in the New World and which the Old World would have to import.[5] He did not have to wait for long: neurasthenia rapidly became a standard medical diagnosis all over Europe. In the process, the concept became fuzzier and fuzzier, eventually incorporating at least four different identities: hysteria, the so-called 'fatigue neurosis', depression and an early stage of insanity.[6]

Britain, of course, had its own form of nervousness: the English Malady affecting the highest and the best in society described in the mid-eighteenth century by George Cheyne and Thomas Trotter's early-nineteenth-century version, to which every urban dweller was considered vulnerable. Neither Cheyne nor Trotter ever conceived of nervousness as a mental disorder: it was caused by physical and social causes and had to be combated along the same avenues. The nervous patient was not insane, nor at any particular risk of developing insanity. When neurasthenia arrived in Britain, it tapped into many of the same seams. It was seen as a disease of (caused by) modernity and initially, at least, no British physician doubted that despite some of its symptoms being mental, neurasthenia was a wholly somatic condition.[7] Perhaps the most influential supporter of the neurasthenia diagnosis in Britain was Sir Thomas Clifford Allbutt, the eminent Leeds physician, one time Commissioner in Lunacy and from 1892, the Regius Professor of Physic at Cambridge.[8] A generalist *par excellence*, Allbutt had a marked interest in nervous and mental disease: apart from his work as a lunacy commissioner, he was active in establishing the Diploma in Psychological Medicine at Cambridge in 1912 and, in the 1880s, had himself been warned by a London physician that if he continued to work as hard as he did, 'a breakdown would follow within six months'.[9]

While accepting Beard's name for the condition as well as the central tenet of his causal hypothesis, Allbutt rejected his restriction of the disease to American intellectuals. 'Neurasthenia, in its pronounced examples', he asserted,

> is common enough also in the wage-earning-classes of England; it is frequent in the West Riding, especially, I think, among colliers ... The truth is that neurasthenia is found no more in the market-place than in the rectory or in the workhouse; no more in busy citizens than in idle damsels.[10]

Many neurasthenics were 'quite dull people' and the idea that neurasthenia was the disease of the brainy and affluent was 'the prepossession of consultants occupied with the middle and upper-classes of society'.[11] Thomas Dixon Savill, physician to the West End Hospital for Diseases of the Nervous System in Welbeck Street, London, and formerly Medical Superintendent of the Paddington

Infirmary, agreed, arguing that neurasthenia and other nervous disorders were encountered as frequently among the upper-classes as among hospital outpatients and residents of workhouses.[12] If Beard had propounded an essentially Cheynean concept of neurasthenia as an affliction of the refined, then the leading British supporters of the concept revised it in the direction of Trotterian universality.

As far as gender was concerned, most agreed that men and women were affected about equally, with a slight preponderance of men – by far the majority of patients were young adults.[13] Neurasthenia, as Janet Oppenheim has pointed out, was seen to be primarily a disease of the most productive years of the most productive section of the populace.[14] Moreover, it was widely believed that although it was perfectly possible to acquire the malady, the potential for neurasthenia was often inherited in the form of a nervous constitution.[15] 'Direct inheritance', as one physician put it, 'is rare, but ... it is usually found that upon one or other side [of lineage] there is a history of some neurosis, or nervous disease, or less often of insanity'.[16] Inheritance, however, was mostly considered to be a predisposing cause and rarely sufficient to precipitate neurasthenia. Some ignored it altogether.[17]

Neurasthenia, it was acknowledged, was not always easy to diagnose, and its differentiation from hysteria was particularly difficult. Some physicians such as Clifford Allbutt even accepted that neurasthenic symptoms could be combined with clear hysterical symptoms in certain varieties of the condition.[18] The concept of male hysteria, as Mark Micale has shown, was never widely accepted by Victorian doctors, in spite of their familiarity with the work of Jean-Martin Charcot. Hysteria continued to be een as the archetypal affliction of deceitful, obstinate and unbalanced females.[19] Neurasthenia, however, was another matter. Janet Oppenheim remarks that 'the impeccably physiological origins that Beard assigned to his neurotic creation, problematic though they proved to be, made it a far more respectable affliction for British men' and many male patients were doubtless diagnosed as 'neurasthenic' simply to avoid the pejorative connotations of hysteria.[20]

Female neurasthenics, however, were not in short supply — female 'nervous' ailments that did not display standard hysterical stigmata fell quite naturally into the neurasthenic category.[21] Gynaecologist William Smoult Playfair, Professor of Obstetric Medicine at King's College London and obstetric physician to King's College Hospital from 1863 to 1898, observed:

Many of the cases occur in clever, emotional, but not fanciful
women, who would give all they possess to be well, and heartily long
for good health, if they only knew how to obtain it and in such cases
the disease is as far removed as possible from the condition known
as 'hysterical'.[22]

The number of women patients was high enough to encourage the
import of Silas Weir Mitchell's expensive rest cure, the merits of which
were proclaimed tirelessly by Playfair.[23] Other experts agreed: 'Now, as in
hysteria the key of the treatment is active impulsion', declared Clifford
Allbutt, 'in neurasthenia it is rest, rest, rest'.[24] Drugs were not considered
to be terribly efficacious but nevertheless, sedatives such as bromides and
nerve tonics such as arsenic or strychnine were fairly extensively used.
Various physicians added their own favourites to the pharmacological
armamentarium - opium, cannabis, mercury, hyoscine, injections of the
nervous tissue of rabbits, the list is endless.[25] Electrotherapy was greatly
popular and so was hydrotherapy; the two were also available in
combination as the 'sinusoidal bath'.[26] Hypnotherapy, however, was
conspicuous by its absence. Even Allbutt, who was no hypnosceptic,
asserted that 'hypnotism, effective as it often is in hysteria, is of little use
in neurasthenia. It can readjust an unbalanced nervous system, it cannot
create its energy'.[27]

Even from this highly compressed overview, it should be clear
that neurasthenia was an important issue in British medical discourse
of the turn of the century. That, however, is only part of the story.
British engagements with neurasthenia were not always neutral,
purely clinical affairs; nor were clinical opinions on the validity of the
concept always rooted only in clinical reasoning. Just as neurasthenia,
in clinical terms, was situated on the borderland of insanity, so, in
professional terms, was it located on the borderland(s) between
different sectors of the changing medical world of Victorian Britain.
Because of its multiple and diverse symptoms, different varieties of
doctors claimed to be its rightful healers. Conversely, some groups
sought to establish their own professional identities by distancing
themselves from the concept or by changing it root and branch. The
fortunes of neurasthenia in Britain were linked, in short, to the
evolution of British medicine as a whole.

The uterine connection and beyond:
neurasthenia and gynaecology

It shouldn't surprise anybody that William Playfair, a specialist in
midwifery should have been prominent in the early British debates

on a functional nervous disorder. Virtually every Victorian doctor believed that the female organism was centred on its reproductive system: the irritation of the genital tract could cause reflex irritation of the rest of the body, bringing about countless disorders, including generalised nervous disruption and full-blown insanity. This conviction justified 'local' treatment with pessaries of conditions that had no apparent link with the reproductive system. 'Nervous' disorders in women were particularly liable to be treated gynaecologically.[28] Moreover, because of the stigma associated with mental illness, upper-class women suffering from nervous or mental symptoms often consulted a gynaecologist rather than an alienist.[29] As Playfair himself reminisced, his interest in neurasthenia 'was originally almost accidentally forced upon my attention from the very frequent association of this type of disease within the gynaecological work which is my special province'.[30]

'The mobility of the nervous system, especially in the sphere of the emotions, which distinguishes the woman from the man', Playfair once wrote, 'influences the character and progress of all kinds of disease in women...'[31] Although impeccably Victorian on this issue, Playfair was no simple yea-sayer to conventional wisdom. To see Playfair as a proto-feminist would be wrong but he was not the typical Victorian gynaecologist in every respect. He had nothing but contempt for the conviction of his colleagues that functional nervous and mental disorders in women were always caused by local pelvic disorders. 'Of this alleged connection', he declared, 'I have never been able to find any reliable evidence at all'. The recent practice of removing ovaries and uterine appendages he condemned as 'unscientific, unnecessary, and often hurtful ... it is impossible to speak too emphatically in condemnation of a rash and irretrievable experiment of this kind'. In many cases of functional neuroses, Playfair emphasised, pelvic lesions existed independently or had themselves been caused by the general disorder. In such cases, local pelvic treatment 'may not only be inadmissible but, injudiciously carried out, may be intensely prejudicial and very gravely increase the general ill health'. Even if a relatively insignificant local lesion had precipitated the generalised nervous disorder, the former might, in time, 'become so over-shadowed by its own secondary consequences that the judicious practitioner will minimise any treatment of it'.[32] Sometimes, he declared, ignoring a local lesion was less injurious than its over-enthusiastic treatment.

Playfair's advocacy of the Weir-Mitchell rest cure was intertwined with his critique of thoughtless local treatment resorted to by gynaecologists. By promoting the rest cure energetically but not completely dismissing the importance of local uterine conditions in causing generalised nervous disorders, he distanced himself from his more conventional peers, positioning himself as the representative of a modern, 'scientific' gynaecology. This was a useful professional strategy in late-nineteenth-century Britain where the status of gynaecology was low in the eyes of 'generalist' consultants, who comprised the professional elite.[33]

Attitudes toward gynaecology were especially severe because women patients were seen as crucial to the success of a medical practice, whether general or special. In an 1885 address to medical students, gynaecologist James Hobson Aveling, the co-founder of the British Gynaecological Society, observed,

> The successful management of the diseases of women is the key to general practice and forms a large portion of your work. Women, as you know, enjoy, and always find time for gossip with one another... Woe to the unhappy practitioner who has failed in his treatment of their troubles; his condemnation will be widely heard. On the other hand he who has been successful will have the trumpet of fame sounded with extravagant force.[34]

Playfair's strategy retained this advantage of the gynaecological specialist over generalists, while his involvement with the generalised treatment of a generalised condition attenuated, if it did not completely neutralise, the common generalist complaint that specialists concentrated on single organs or systems and had no understanding of how every disease affected the organism as a whole.

More specifically, Playfair's engagement with neurasthenia led him into a fascinating interaction with an eminent supporter of the concept of neurasthenia and a fierce opponent of standard gynaecological treatment of women's nervous disorders. This was Sir Thomas Clifford Allbutt and his encounter with Playfair led to considerable elevation of Playfair's own status as a medical man and by implication, of gynaecology itself.

'This gynaecological tyranny':
Clifford Allbutt, neurasthenia and the reintegration of medicine

Elite British consultants were not necessarily big supporters of the neurasthenia concept. '...[T]he term "neurasthenia"', declared Sir Andrew Clark,

is unscientific, inaccurate, and misleading...the descriptions given of
it do not include a clear, concise, or distinctive account of genuine
nerve exhaustion, and do include a mob of incoherent symptoms
borrowed from the most diverse disorders...for a malady thus
constituted and containing antagonistic conditions, no rational
principles of treatment are possible....

The disavowal of neurasthenia, as Clarke made clear, was a
nosographic one: the symptoms of nervous debility were real enough
but the category of neurasthenia failed to satisfy the criteria for a
coherent disease-concept.[35] Other general physicians, such as Clifford
Allbutt, thought, as we have seen, quite otherwise. Not only did
Allbutt consider neurasthenia to be a valid clinical category, he also
found it to be virtually tailor-made for use in defending generalist,
'whole-body' medicine against the encroachments of specialists.

Unlike Beard, however, Allbutt denied that neurasthenia was
caused by 'the unrest due to living at high pressure'.[36] Nevertheless,
he acknowledged,

not only do we hear, but daily we see neurotics, neurasthenics,
hysterics, and the like: is not every large city filled with nerve-
specialists, and their chambers with patients; are not hospitals, baths,
electric-machines, and massages multiplying daily for their use;
nerve-tonics sold behind every counter, and health-resorts advertised
for their solace and restoration?

None of these Beardian signs of the times, however, impressed
Allbutt as very real or worrying. There were, he acknowledged, more
rich and idle people around than there ever had been before and 'they
run, as they always did, after the fashionable fad of the day; what was
"liver" fifty years ago has become "nerves" today'.[37] There were,
however, genuinely ill people in this group and who should take care
of them? Only the general physician possessed the wide knowledge
and 'whole-patient' perspective that was required to do justice to
such cases. Allbutt's engagement with neurasthenia was motivated by
'generalism' rather than by a simple, uncomplicated elitism. But
Allbutt was also fighting a specific battle over neurasthenia: this was
with the gynaecologists.

In his 1884 Gulstonian Lectures on visceral neuroses, Allbutt
declared that neurotic women got easily

entangled in the net of the gynaecologist, who finds that her uterus,
like her nose, is a little on one side; or again, like that organ, is
running a little ... so that the unhappy viscus is impaled upon a

stem, or perched upon a prop, or is painted with carbolic acid every week of the year, except during the long vacation, when the gynaecologist is grouse-shooting, or salmon-catching, or leading the fashion in the upper Engadine.[38]

He called upon his fellow physicians ('we of this College') to revolt against 'this gynaecological tyranny': the neuroses could only be successfully managed by doctors with 'a good all round knowledge of a kind which will enable him to take the main bearings of any case which may come to him'. That 'all round knowledge' allowed a physician to investigate every aspect of the patient, including the gynaecological, and then decide whether the patient did indeed need any specialist care. 'The speculum and the uterine sound', he proclaimed

> were invented as much for my benefit as for other people, and I feel it both my duty and goodwill to examine into every detail of a case, whether medical, surgical or pelvic. This done, I am able to judge under whose care a patient may best be placed ... If the gynaecologists pelt us with stories of long pain and sickness uncured by medical futilities, but rapidly cured under uterine medication, we can mate their stories, and check them by double the number of cases received by the physician from the sofa, the manipulations and mental abasements of narrow uterine specialism.[39]

From discord to alliance:
Allbutt, Playfair and the professional uses of neurasthenia

In response to Allbutt's attack, the British Medical Association's Section of Obstetric Medicine arranged a discussion on the 'local and constitutional treatment of uterine disease' at its next annual meeting.[40] In his opening address, Playfair acknowledged that Allbutt had privately explained to him that he was not referring in his critique to 'the practice of the instructed and scientific gynaecologist, but to that of men who do not understand thoroughly the class of disease they profess to treat'.[41] Strongly defending the scientific record of recent gynaecology – 'there is no department of medical science in which, within the last quarter of a century, more real and solid advances have been made' – Playfair stressed that local treatment could often do a lot of good. To proclaim that 'pessaries never do good' was comparable to arguing that 'castor-oil never acts as a laxative'. But even in well-selected cases, frequent pelvic examinations were not required and it was 'a gross abuse' to ask such patients to 'visit their physicians once or twice a week for a succession of months'. It was, above all, crucial to avoid dogmatism of either kind in treating nervous disorders and combine local treatment with general, constitutional approaches.[42]

In his response, Allbutt emphasised that he had nothing against well-trained gynaecologists of honour such as Playfair himself but, he added,

> provincial medical men know well what, up to the present, they have had to expect when one of their lady-patients migrated to the "London gynaecologist." It meant too often the very reverse of Dr Playfair's description; it meant lodgings in town, the doctor's brougham at the door three or four times a week, sixty or seventy guineas to pay at the end of the season, and ι deluded and neurotic patient as the end of it all.[43]

Allbutt had no wish to deny the sterling achievements of modern gynaecology as practised by the leaders of the profession but it would, he stressed, be 'absurd...to deny that modern gynaecology has led to, or has suffered, most direful abuses'.[44]

The same session of the BMA also included an address by Thomas More Madden, consulting obstetrician in Dublin and vice-president of the British Gynaecological Society. Madden did not deny the harmful effects of excessive or inappropriate local treatment but argued that the debate between physicians and gynaecologists over the appropriate treatment of nervous disorders in women was not just a clinical dispute but involved broader, professional differences over the value of specialisation. Specialisation, he declared, was inevitable for the profession and good for the patient:

> It appears an utter waste of time and energy to declaim, even as eloquently as Dr. Clifford Allbutt...against that prevailing tendency to specialism in all branches of the healing art, of which they seem to consider gynaecology the most reprehensible outcome.[45]

The 'generalist' lobby, too, had always had a clear idea of the importance of the question of local pelvic treatment in the great debate over specialisation. Sir John Russell Reynolds, a fervent opponent of medical specialisation, had considered pelvic treatments with 'all kinds of contrivances...to cure backache, vesical irritation, albuminuria, hysteria, and I know not what besides' to be among the worst examples of the evils of 'specialism'.[46]

The battle-lines, it might seem from all this, were drawn clearly over the issue. And so they were for most members of the two camps.

Nevertheless, there were negotiations across the dividing line between stalwarts of both groups. Allbutt and Playfair provide a good example of such interaction. Although the primary loyalty of each was, of course, to his respective field, the question of the local treatment of the neuroses, paradoxically, brought them together as allies. Allbutt was eager to demonstrate that he had no irrational, generalised animus against gynaecology as a whole: the 'instructed and scientific gynaecologist', he pointed out, was a worthy and valuable colleague. Playfair, on the other hand, was intent on distinguishing 'instructed and scientific' gynaecology from mere womb-doctoring: neurasthenia and the rest-cure offered him a golden opportunity to do so and his balanced but far from conventional views on the value of local pelvic treatment edged him close to Allbutt. Allbutt referred with admiration to Playfair in his works on neurasthenia and Playfair always expressed the highest respect for the man he referred to as his friend and colleague.[47]

The most solid outcome of their alliance was their co-editing of a gynaecological handbook, intended to complement the well-known *System of Medicine* edited by Allbutt himself. Its preface (signed by Playfair alone) proclaimed that

> the advances made within the last few years in Gynaecology are perhaps more remarkable than in any other branch of medicine ... a treatise on Gynaecology written twenty years ago is absolutely useless as a guide to the practice of today.

Allbutt's co-editorship of the volume was little more than decorative; it was Playfair's book in a real sense. 'I', he explained in his preface, 'am myself alone responsible for the selection of the contributors [to the volume], which my co-editor has left to my judgement'.[48]

Playfair's involvement with neurasthenia, thus, had brought him not only professional success in concrete, economic terms – he was the leading British practitioner of the rest cure, hardly an unremunerative position – but also an influential personal ally in an otherwise hostile camp, and through the good offices of the latter, the opportunity to speak to the medical world as the leading representative of a new, 'scientific' gynaecology that was far removed from ignorant womb-doctoring. As for Allbutt himself, the recruitment of Playfair as an ally on the issue of local treatment provided valuable reinforcement of his stance on neurasthenia and more broadly, for his generalist perspective on medicine, which, of course, was further reinforced by his emergence as the co-editor of a comprehensive gynaecological handbook. He could not now be regarded as a simple-minded enemy of gynaecology or even of specialism but as the enlightened preacher of an undivided medicine.

Neurology, psychiatry and neurasthenia: transformation and dissolution

British neurologists were, at best, lukewarm about the concept of neurasthenia.[49] As W. F. Bynum has shown, the language of 'nerves' and the concepts of functional nervous disorders such as hysteria had been part and parcel of British neurological discourse well into the nineteenth century. The introduction of the reflex concept, however, and the emergence of specialist neurological hospitals (and the concomitant development of localisation of neurological functions and localised surgical operations) led to a fairly rapid reorientation of neurological interests.   By the second decade of the twentieth century, British neurologists became increasingly preoccupied with organic disorders marked by structural lesions: the functional nervous disorders were now left to other medical fields.[50]

In 1904, the journal *Brain* had published an article on hysteria and neurasthenia, which was a transcript of the Presidential Address of Seymour J. Sharkey, the President of the Neurological Society.[51] By 1914, however, psychiatric elements had disappeared almost completely from the pages of *Brain*, with the content demonstrating a new alliance between neurologists and experimental physiologists.[52] Even at the height of the shell-shock epidemic, when many patients were diagnosed as neurasthenic, it was psychiatrists rather than neurologists who took charge: an out-patient psychiatric service, rather than a neurological service, developed to cater to 'over 100,000 "neurasthenic" ex-servicemen'.[53]

Sir George Henry Savage – Lecturer on Mental Diseases at Guy's Hospital Medical School, former Resident Physician-Superintendent of Bethlem Hospital and the 'nerve-doctor' of the London elite – devoted only about a page to the concept in his textbook of insanity, and that almost as an afterthought to his discussion of hysteria, with no attempt to differentiate between the two with any great rigour.[54] 'I at once say', he emphasised in his textbook, 'that I do not consider neurasthenia as a specific entity'. The symptoms of neurasthenia were common enough but the condition itself was not 'a definite and easily recognised disease with a certain pathology'. Rather, he explained, it was:

a condition of the nervous system manifesting fatigue or partial exhaustion of the nerve centres, and exhibiting different symptoms, according to the inherited or acquired peculiarities of the individual.[55]

Yet, this same George Savage diagnosed Virginia Woolf as neurasthenic and in a lecture, admitted that the term neurasthenia was useful as a euphemism for insanity, a dread word that terrorised the friends of patients.[56] For Savage, neurasthenia was no more than a convenient euphemism to soothe – and retain – the patients in his lucrative private practice.

The career of London alienist William Stoddart offers a remarkable example of the passage of neurasthenia from a neurological to a psychiatric paradigm. An assistant physician at the Bethlem Hospital for the Insane, Stoddart dedicated the first edition of his textbook of psychiatry to his 'revered teacher' John Hughlings Jackson. The book aimed 'to induce the reader to think neurologically of mental processes' and an entire chapter was devoted to neurasthenia.[57] Stoddart defined neurasthenia as a constitutional psychopathic state found most commonly among 'the poorer middle-classes' and recommended the rest cure for relief. He was pessimistic, however, about the duration of relief, remarking that the patient's 'troubles return with the absence of restraint and he is often obliged in the end to seek permanent refuge in an asylum'.[58] From the second edition began a fundamental transformation in Stoddart's orientation: acknowledging the importance of psychoanalysis, the disciple of Hughlings Jackson now incorporated two chapters on that subject in his book.[59]

In the third edition, Stoddart announced his full conversion to Freudianism (the reverent dedication to Jackson was removed silently) and adopted Freud's division of the functional nervous disorders into psychoneuroses and actual neuroses, the last being subdivided into neurasthenia and anxiety neurosis. In the first edition, neurasthenia had been attributed to bad heredity — the parents came in for censure in the third edition too but for 'abnormal behaviour ... during the infancy of the patient' which caused the neurasthenic's 'inability to engage in the battle of life in a normal way'. The section on treatment still ended with the dire observation that most neurasthenics tended to end up in the asylum but now, there was a contradictory assertion about the availability of 'one certain cure': psychoanalysis.[60] In the fourth edition, neurasthenia was not even an actual neurosis but a full-fledged psychoneurosis, classified with hysteria and compulsion neurosis.[61] Even Ernest Jones had not gone that far — he, as well as Freud himself, considered neurasthenia to be an actual neurosis found only in compulsive masturbators (caused not by the masturbation itself but by the expenditure of nervous energy in overcoming moral scruples) and that in refractory cases, 'the buried mental complexes' of the patient must be resolved through psychotherapy.[62]

Few British psychiatrists, of course, had much time for Freud. But even alienists more conventional than Stoddart did not necessarily treat neurasthenia with the respect that Allbutt or Playfair had.

Finally, let us turn to T. A. Ross, the Medical Director of the Cassel Hospital for Functional Nervous Disorders. Ross considered neurasthenia and anxiety neurosis to be identical: anxiety, he argued, could be expressed differently on different occasions by the same individual — 'one day he may react neurasthenically, on another hysterically'.[63] In the second edition, the term neurasthenia at last received its coup de grace: 'This word has ... been given so many meanings that it had better be dropped', remarked Ross, replacing it forthwith with 'anxiety reaction'.[64] Although the term itself and some vestiges of Beard's old concept survived for years in the pages of textbooks of psychiatry, its glory days were now definitely over. In 1927, the standard psychiatric textbook of the period had commented: 'Like Charcot's "grande hystérie" neurasthenia has largely died out since physicians ceased to expect it so frequently and to search for its symptoms so diligently'.[65]

The growth of psychiatric interest in neurasthenia proved, as Wessely has rightly argued, to be the agent of its dissolution. Since it was only Beard's simple, unitary pathological idea of the depletion of nervous energy that had united the 'mob of incoherent symptoms' into one nosological entity, that entity crumbled as soon as its hypothetical somatic foundation was removed. Leonard Woolf, whose wife Virginia is probably the most famous British neurasthenic, once wrote that neurasthenia was merely 'a name, a label, like neuralgia or rheumatism, which covered a multitude of sins, symptoms, and miseries'.[66] As long as doctors believed in the concept of nervous exhaustion, neurasthenia, of course, was much more than a name: it meant something accepted – at least by some – to be real. Once the cloudy notions of nervous energy and the possibility of its exhaustion went out of vogue, however, Beard's term did indeed become a name and no more than that. Over the same period, the controversies over medical specialism had also died down and the rather unfocused fears of modern industrial civilisation so characteristic of Beard's generation had come to be replaced by new anxieties and sharper fears. Every single element that had gone into the construction of neurasthenia was now gone. The name lived on but only as a pale shadow of its Beardian self.[67] Almost all the countless 'sins, symptoms and miseries' it had once incorporated had now come to be grouped differently, interpreted in new ways, and graced with novel, perhaps even more transient labels.

Acknowledgements

My thanks to Roy Porter, W. F. Bynum, Roger Cooter, Jane Henderson, Marijke Gijswijt-Hofstra, Rhodri Hayward, Chris Lawrence, Jayne Morgan and Michael Neve for their help and encouragement.

Notes

1. See, above all, Janet Oppenheim, *Shattered Nerves: Doctors, Patients and Depression in Victorian England* (Oxford: Oxford University Press, 1991); and Simon Wessely, 'Neurasthenia and Fatigue Syndromes: Clinical Section', in German Berrios and Roy Porter (eds), *A History of Clinical Psychiatry: The Origin and History of Psychiatric Disorders* (London: Athlone, 1995), 509–32.

2. For a comprehensive list of symptoms, see George M. Beard, *A Practical Treatise on Nervous Exhaustion (Neurasthenia): Its Symptoms, Nature, Sequences, Treatment* (New York: Wood, 1880), 11–85.

3. The group of functional nervous disorders (a category overlapping with that of the neuroses) was a large one in the nineteenth century: in the 1850s, it included entities such as paralysis agitans, epilepsy, tetanus, migraine, or hysteria. By the end of the century, the evolution of new diagnostic and pathological techniques had led, of course, to the redefinition of many of these conditions as organic. See Ernest S. Reynolds, 'Hysteria and Neurasthenia', *BMJ* (1923), ii, 1193–96, on 1193. It was Beard's hope that neurasthenia, too, would one day be demonstrated to be an organic disorder of the nervous system. See Charles Rosenberg, 'The Place of George M Beard in Nineteenth-Century Psychiatry', *Bulletin of the History of Medicine, 36* (1962), 245–59, on 249.

4. Beard, *American Nervousness: Its Causes and Consequences* (New York: Putnam's, 1881), vi.

5. See *ibid*, xvii–xviii.

6. See Wessely, *op. cit.* (note 1), 510–11.

7. Some believed that the condition represented 'the borderland of

insanity'; the German physician Rudolf Arndt, in his contribution to
Tuke's *Dictionary*, portrayed neurasthenia as the breeding-ground of
every serious nervous ailment. See R. Arndt, 'Neurasthenia', in D.
Hack Tuke (ed.), *A Dictionary of Psychological Medicine*, 2 vols
(London: Churchill, 1892), ii, 840–50, 843; and Thomas Stretch
Dowse, *On Brain and Nerve Exhaustion, 'Neurasthenia': Its Nature
and Curative Treatment* (London: Baillière, Tindall and Cox, 1880),
12. Beard, on the other hand, had proclaimed that 'thousands and
thousands are nervous who are not and never will be insane' (see
Beard, *op. cit.* [note 4], 16–17). See also the 1902 discussion at the
Psychological Section of the BMA, led by Clifford Allbutt, 'A
Discussion of the Relation of Neurasthenia to Insanity', *BMJ* (1902),
ii, 1208–13.

8. 'Although the dangers of insanity in neurasthenia must be indicated,
the transition is not one of ordinary anticipation. The insane person
is only too often indefatigable'. See Thomas Clifford Allbutt,
'Neurasthenia', in Allbutt and H. D. Rolleston (eds), *A System of
Medicine*, 2nd edn, 9 vols (London: Macmillan, 1905-11), 8 (1910):
727–91, 747. Allbutt was well acquainted not merely with the
American discourse on neurasthenia but also with the German,
French, and obviously, English. See the bibliography in *ibid.*,
789–91. Generally on Allbutt, see Humphry Davy Rolleston, *The
Right Honourable Sir Thomas Clifford Allbutt, KCB: A Memoir*
(London: Macmillan, 1929).

9. Rolleston, *op. cit.* (note 8), 95–6.

10. Allbutt, *op. cit.* (note 8), 738. Not every British physician agreed:
see, for instance, J. Michell Clarke, *Hysteria and Neurasthenia*
(London: John Lane, 1905), 175, for the argument that 'the more
highly civilised races suffer more from the disease ... In these islands
that part of the population which derives from the Celtic peoples is
perhaps rather more prone to it. Jews are especially often affected....'

11. Allbutt, *op. cit.* (note 8), 741.

12. Thomas Dixon Savill, *Clinical Lectures on Neurasthenia*, 2nd edn
(London: Glaisher, 1902), xi, 2–5, 85, 101–3. On Savill, see his
obituary in *Lancet*, 1910, i, 213–4.

13. Oppenheim, *op. cit.* (note 1), 141.

14. *Ibid..*, 144–45.

15. *Ibid.*, 89–92; Allbutt, *op. cit.* (note 8), 741.

16. Clarke, *op. cit.* (note 10), 176.

17. See for instance, Savill, *Clinical Lectures on Neurasthenia*, 4th edn,
x–xi, for the theory that the cause of neurasthenia was
auto–intoxication by abnormal metabolites.

18. See the discussion of traumatic neurasthenia in Allbutt, *op. cit.* (note 8), 762–7.
19. Mark Micale, 'Hysteria Male/Hysteria Female: Reflections on Comparative Gender Construction in Nineteenth-Century France and Britain', in Marina Benjamin (ed.), *Science and Sensibility: Gender and Scientific Enquiry, 1780-1945* (Oxford: Blackwell, 1991), 200–39.
20. Oppenheim, *op. cit.* (note 1), 144.
21. Nevertheless, some physicians believed that in women, neurasthenia was 'apt to be associated with hysteria ... and especially so in young women'. See Clarke, *op. cit.* (note 10), 238.
22. W. S. Playfair, 'Neurasthenia', in Richard Quain, F. T. Roberts and J. M. Bruce (eds), *A Dictionary of Medicine*, 4 vols (London: Longmans Green, 1894), iii, 205–206: 205. For reproductions and critical analyses of 'before and after' photographs of some of Playfair's rest cure patients, see Jayne Morgan, 'Eadweard Muybridge and W. S. Playfair: An Aesthetics of Neurasthenia', *Journal of Photography*, 23 (1999), 225–31. Not much biographical information is available on Playfair, but see the obituaries in *Lancet* (1903, ii, 570–75) and *BMJ* (1903, ii, 439).
23. W. S. Playfair, *The Systematic Treatment of Nerve Prostration and Hysteria* (London: Smith, Elder, 1883), 3.
24. Allbutt, *op. cit.* (note 8), 777. Allbutt's 'rest, rest, rest' was echoed in the Harley Street 'nerve specialist' Sir William Bradshaw's advice to the shell-shocked Septimus Warren Smith in Virginia Woolf's *Mrs Dalloway.* 'It was merely a question of rest, said Sir William; of rest, rest, rest....' See V. Woolf, *Mrs Dalloway,* ed. David Bradshaw (Oxford: Oxford University Press, 2000), 82.
25. See Oppenheim, *op. cit.* (note 1); and Julius Althaus, 'On Cerebrine Alpha and Myeline Alpha in the Treatment of Certain Neuroses', *Lancet* (1893), ii, 1376–8, on 1377.
26. Oppenheim, *op. cit.* (note 1), 120, 131–8; and Clarke, *op. cit.* (note 10), 274, 281–2.
27. Allbutt, *op. cit.* (note 8), 783; and Rolleston, *op. cit.* (note 8), 103.
28. Oppenheim, *op. cit.* (note 1), 187–91; and Charlotte MacKenzie, *Psychiatry for the Rich: A History of Ticehurst Private Asylum, 1792-1917* (London: Routledge, 1992), 156.
29. The restoration of menstruation was one of the major aims in the treatment of insane women with amenorrhoea. Suppressed menstruation was supposed to cause vascular congestion in the brain, interfering with thought and reason. See MacKenzie, *op. cit.* (note 27), 155–6; and Elaine Showalter, *The Female Malady: Women,*

Madness, and English Culture, 1830-1980 (London: Virago, 1987), 55-7.

30. W. S. Playfair, 'Some Observations concerning what is called Neurasthenia', *BMJ* (1886), ii, 853-5, on 853.

31. W. S. Playfair, 'The Nervous System in relation to Gynaecology', in Thomas Clifford Allbutt and William S. Playfair (eds), *A System of Gynaecology* (London: Macmillan, 1896), 220-31, on 220.

32. *Ibid.*, 229-30, 225-6.

33. Ornella Moscucci, *The Science of Woman: Gynaecology and Gender in England, 1800-1929* (Cambridge: Cambridge University Press, 1990), 57-9, 72-4; and Christopher Lawrence, *Medicine in the Making of Modern Britain, 1700-1920* (London: Routledge, 1994), 60.

34. Quoted by M. Jeanne Peterson, *The Medical Profession in Mid-Victorian London* (Berkeley: University of California Press, 1978), 129.

35. See Sir A. Clark, 'Some Observations concerning what is called Neurasthenia', *Lancet* (1886), i, 1-2, on 2.

36. T. Clifford Allbutt, 'Nervous Diseases and Modern Life', *Contemporary Review*, 47 (1895), 210-31, here 210, 211, 214-5.

37. *Ibid.*, 217.

38. T. Clifford Allbutt, 'The Gulstonian Lectures on Neuroses of the Viscera', *BMJ* (1884), i, 495-9, 543-7, 594-9, on 496.

39. *Ibid.*, 496. Allbutt was fundamentally against any division of the medical art — even that between surgery and medicine, and, indeed, admired gynaecologists for not drawing a distinction within their speciality between medical and surgical aspects. See Rolleston, *op. cit.* (note 8), 277.

40. Rolleston, *op. cit.* (note 8), 87-8.

41. W. S. Playfair, 'On the Proper Sphere of Constitutional and Topical Treatment in Certain Forms of Uterine Disease', *BMJ* (1885), ii, 587-9.

42. *Ibid.*, 588.

43. T. Clifford Allbutt, 'On Local and Constitutional Treatment in Uterine Diseases', *BMJ* (1885), ii, 589-90, here 589.

44. *Ibid.*, 589-90.

45. T. M. Madden, 'On the Correlation of Constitutional and Local Treatment in Gynaecological Practice', *BMJ* (1885), ii, 590-4, here 591, 592.

46. See J. Russell Reynolds, 'Specialism in Medicine', in Reynolds, *Essays and Addresses* (London: Macmillan, 1896), 194-207, on 202.

47. Allbutt, *op. cit.* (note 8), 776.

48. W. S. Playfair, 'Preface to First Edition', in T. C. Allbutt, W. S. Playfair and T. W. Eden (eds), *A System of Gynaecology*, 2nd edn (London: Macmillan, 1906), vii.

49. Wessely, *op. cit.* (note 1), 516.

50. W. F. Bynum, 'The Nervous Patient in Eighteenth- and Nineteenth-Century Britain: The Psychiatric Origins of British Neurology', in W. F. Bynum, Roy Porter and Michael Shepherd (eds), *The Anatomy of Madness: Essays in the History of Psychiatry*, 2 vols (London: Tavistock, 1985), 1: 89–102, 95.

51. Thomas Horder, '"Neurasthenia": A Critical Inquiry', *St Bartholomew's Hospital Journal*, February 1903, 67–73, on 68; and S. J. Sharkey, 'Hysteria and Neurasthenia', *Brain: A Journal of Neurology*, 27 (1904), 1–26.

52. For a similar shift in British cardiology, see Christopher Lawrence, '"Definite and Material": Coronary Thrombosis and Cardiologists in the 1920s', in Charles Rosenberg and Janet Golden (eds), *Framing Disease: Studies in Cultural History* (New Brunswick: Rutgers University Press, 1992), 51–82, here 74.

53. Martin Stone, 'Shellshock and the Psychologists', in Bynum, Porter and Shepherd (eds), *op. cit.* (note 49), 2: 242–71; and Showalter, *op. cit.* (note 28), 174–5.

54. George H. Savage, *Insanity and Allied Neuroses* (London: Cassell, 1884), 90–1. This brief account remained virtually unchanged in the enlarged second edition (London: Cassell, 1907), 96–7. On Virginia Woolf's illness and the opinions on it of Savage (and of others), see Leonard Woolf, *Beginning Again: An Autobiography of the Years 1911-1918* (London: Hogarth, 1964), 82 and 150–1; and Stephen Trombley, *'All that Summer She Was Mad': Virginia Woolf and Her Doctors* (London: Junction Books, 1981).

55. George H. Savage, 'A Lecture on Neurasthenia and Mental Disorders', *The Medical Magazine*, 20 (1911), 520–30, here 520.

56. *Ibid.* Since Savage's estate was valued at over £27,000 after his death (see Trombley, *op. cit.* [note 59], 107), his concerns were obviously appreciated by his patients and their friends.

57. See W H B Stoddart, *Mind and Its Disorders* (London: Lewis, 1908), v, vii.

58. *Ibid.*, 362, 366–7.

59. *Ibid.*, 2nd edn (London: Lewis, 1912), viii.

60. *Ibid.*, 3rd edn (London: Lewis, 1919), v, 212, 217, vi.

61. *Ibid.*, 4th edn (London: Lewis, 1921), 226.

62. Ernest Jones, 'The Treatment of the Neuroses, including the Psychoneuroses', in William A. White and Smith Ely Jelliffe (eds),

The Modern Treatment of Nervous and Mental Diseases by American and British Authors, 2 vols (Philadelphia: Lea & Febiger, 1913), i, 331–416, on 342–4.

63. T. A. Ross, *The Common Neuroses: Their Treatment by Psychotherapy* (London: Arnold, 1923), v, 7–8, 27, 49.

64. *Ibid.*, 2nd edn (London: Arnold, 1937), 28–29. Another eminent British physician had already declared that virtually all alleged cases of neurasthenia were actually cases of manic–depressive insanity or generalized anxiety. See Sir E. Farquhar Buzzard, 'The Dumping Ground of Neurasthenia', *Lancet*, 1930, i, 1–4.

65. D. K. Henderson and R. D. Gillispie, *A Text-Book of Psychiatry for Students and Practitioners* (London: Oxford University Press, 1927), 407.

66. L. Woolf, *op. cit.* (note 59), 76.

67. The term continued to figure in Henderson and Gillispie's textbook up to 1950. See D. K. Henderson and R. D. Gillispie, *A Text-Book of Psychiatry for Students and Practitioners*, 7th edn (London: Oxford University Press, 1950), 160–6.

5

'Uterine Mischief':
W.S. Playfair and his Neurasthenic Patients

Hilary Marland

In May 1879 Elizabeth Lovington was taken into the care of Dr W.S. Playfair suffering from exhaustion and severe pain. Three years previously, the 26-year-old woman had been playing with a little girl, and, while swinging the child about, she had been seized with weakness and violent pains in the left side of her abdomen and in her back down to her thigh.

> The next and following days the pain got worse & she was confined to her bed. At the end of a fortnight she recovered sufficiently to walk about but three days after she experienced a fall while out walking & was unable to walk home. She was confined to the house eight months...

After a period of improvement and then relapse, she was treated by one of Playfair's colleagues, Mr Wood, but worsened again, and was confined to bed for a further six months. When Lovington's case was taken over by Dr Playfair, she had been an invalid for 14 months out of the last three years, but, apart from painful menstrual periods, showed no further symptoms.[1]

In the same month Playfair treated Lydia Bennett, aged 34, who had suffered from severe palpitations of the heart and headache for over ten years. Her last pregnancy had been eight years ago. She had got out of bed eight days after her confinement and had not rested sufficiently. Three years after her confinement matters were made worse when Bennett strained herself, and went on to develop pains and weakness in her back and left side from breast to hip, which was exacerbated by any exertion. She was anaemic, had lost her appetite, had irregular and heavy menstruation, and an unpleasant yellowish discharge. She was very nervous and any excitement resulted in palpitations of the heart.[2]

These women were not neurasthenic. Nor were they Playfair's private patients. Rather they were working women who were treated

117

by Playfair in the ward for women and children at King's College Hospital, London. Lydia Bennett was a 'fairly hard working cook', who, while working in reasonable conditions, 'lacked exercise'. Elizabeth Lovington was a governess 'in an easy place' with 'easy hours'. There was a family history of ill health and weakness in both cases. Bennett's mother had died of tuberculosis and Lovington's mother was referred to as 'delicate'. In Lovington's case an abscess was suspected as causing the condition, then dismissed, but an internal examination showed a retroflexion of the uterus.[3] Bennett's case remained more of a mystery. These women, and many others like them, presented themselves at King's College Hospital with distressing, debilitating, painful, yet vague, gynaecological and 'nervous' disorders, and were admitted for treatment or brief periods of rest and care.[4]

W.S. Playfair

The focus here will be on the work of one practitioner and his neurasthenic patients. Playfair is an obvious choice. He was an early and enthusiastic British convert to Silas Weir Mitchell's rest cure.[5] Playfair began to write about how the rest cure could be applied to women with nervous exhaustion from 1881 onwards,[6] and published case notes on his neurasthenic patients in the *Lancet*, *BMJ* and in his slim volume, *The Systematic Treatment of Nerve Prostration and Hysteria* (1883).[7] The published case histories make up in detail what they lack in number, and Playfair, eager to use his case histories to solicit recognition and support for the rest cure, offers more material on his patients than most other British writers on the subject. Playfair initially linked nervous prostration to gynaecological and obstetric histories and disorders, which makes it possible to pick up on one aspect of the 'wastepaper basket diagnosis' that neurasthenia seems so often to be. Later his view on this relationship became more complex. This essay will deal only with the earliest phase of neurasthenia, the 1880s, female patients exclusively, and largely with one man's views, practice and patients. The patient's view is mediated and indirect, recorded by Playfair in his published case notes and by a succession of hospital clerks at King's College Hospital.[8] Playfair's accounts tell us little about patients' own diagnosis of their conditions, though he often pointed out that they had been poorly informed, misled, or mis-diagnosed before they came to him.

None of Playfair's hospital patients was described as 'neurasthenic'. This is not surprising. Playfair was careful to explain when writing about neurasthenia that by and large this was a condition that affected ladies of standing and great delicacy of feeling. For Playfair, the condition had powerful class and cultural dimensions. This, however, was not a view shared by all. One of Playfair's contemporaries, Thomas Stretch Dowse, described nervous disorders as being 'common amongst all classes of society'.[9] The eminent nerve doctor, Thomas Dixon Savill cited numerous cases of working-class neurasthenia in his 1899 book, his findings being largely based on observation of patients in a London Poor Law infirmary.[10] Little is known of Playfair's work and practice, aside from what he tells us in his case notes. However, by taking an approach which encompasses both his hospital practice and consulting work, it became evident that, while he did not label his poorer patients as 'neurasthenic', he saw them as presenting similar symptoms. The King's College Hospital case notes are more informative than we might expect, describing patients admitted with a wide variety of complaints, succinct but informative family, medical, obstetric and menstrual histories, and numerous women who were 'nervous', anaemic, 'losing flesh', and prey to pains and weakness, palpitations, coughs and headaches. Some of these disorders - in a similar way to those of Playfair's well-to-do neurasthenic patients - were diagnosed as having an organic origin, and they were cured or relieved of this. But for others no organic cause could be found, and, after examination and treatment, they were discharged, some a little better, but others with their condition unresolved.

William Smout Playfair (1835-1903) is credited as being responsible for introducing Silas Weir Mitchell's rest cure to Britain, but little is known of his personal life, and there appear to be no details of his private consulting practice other than his published work.[11] He was born into a medical family; his father George Playfair was Inspector-General of Hospitals in Bengal, India, and two of his brothers, Lord Lyon Playfair and Sir Robert Lambert Playfair, were eminent physicians.[12] He trained at St Andrews and then Edinburgh, graduating as MD in 1856. He worked for a brief time in the Indian Medical Service, and as Professor of Surgery in Calcutta, followed by a few months in St Petersburg, before returning to London. In 1863 he was appointed Assistant Physician for the Diseases of Women and Children at King's College Hospital, and in 1872 was promoted to head up the department and appointed Professor of Obstetric Medicine at King's College. He retired after 25 years in these posts in 1898, then becoming emeritus professor and consulting physician to the Hospital.[13]

The episode for which Playfair also became well known is unrelated to his work with neurasthenic women. In 1896 Playfair made an 'unintended contribution to medical ethics', when he became involved in a well-publicised court case, which sent 'shock waves' through polite society.[14] His sister-in-law, Linda Kitson, had been persuaded to consult him when she started suffering from gynaecological problems. Playfair found evidence that she had recently had an abortion, though she had been separated from her husband for over a year. Playfair revealed this to his wife and one of Kitson's brothers, and Linda Kitson proceeded to sue him for alleged breach of professional confidence. Not surprisingly, the case received a good deal of professional and public attention. Playfair was supported in his action by many eminent colleagues, although the medical press had a more mixed response to the case. The *Lancet* believed, despite his good intentions in protecting his family, that he had acted indiscreetly in revealing his patient's secret, and that he should have sought professional advice on the matter.[15] The jury found for Linda Kitson, who was awarded £12,000 in damages. A letter to *The Times* referred to Playfair as 'an Englishman of the very highest standing torturing a feeble and lonely woman by threats of revealing what he thought he had learned'.[16]

Overall, this episode did not have any serious implications for Playfair's professional career, and he came to be recognised for making a solid contribution to late nineteenth-century obstetrics and gynaecology. Never to become a high flyer, as his obituary concluded, he did not make any 'noteworthy advances' to obstetric medicine, but 'filled a very extremely useful place in medical literature by reason of his great clearness and ease of style'.[17] He wrote *The Science and Practice of Midwifery* (1876) which had passed through nine editions by 1898, and was joint editor with the physician, Regius Professor of Physic at Cambridge and fellow nerve specialist Sir Clifford Allbutt of *A System of Gynaecology* (1896), contributing an article on 'Treatment of Functional Neurosis in Women' to the volume.[18] He was physician-accoucheur to members of the royal family and the aristocracy, acquired a string of honorary fellowships and degrees, and during the year 1879-80 was President of the Obstetrical Society of London.

Playfair and the rest cure

It is for his introduction of the rest cure to Britain that Playfair is best known. In May and June 1881, Playfair introduced Weir Mitchell's rest cure, including his method of 'dealing with certain grave and most intractable forms of nervous disorder familiar to all who see much of the diseases of women', to the British medical profession, through the medium of the *Lancet.*

> In doing so I have no original contribution to make; I have simply followed Dr Mitchell's directions, but with results so astonishing and satisfactory to myself, in cases which were quite heart-breaking from their obstinate resistance to all ordinary management, that I am confident I shall be doing the profession a service if I can secure for Dr Mitchell's plan, which is based on sound theory and accurate clinical observation, a more extended trial than it has yet received. I am the more encouraged to do this since Dr Mitchell informs me that he is not aware that his principles of management have hitherto been tried at all in England, although well known in America.[19]

Playfair went on to outline the principles of Mitchell's treatment, based on seclusion and rest; massage and electricity; and diet and regimen. The seclusion of neurasthenic patients was absolutely essential. The woman, as the first step towards a cure, was to be removed from her usual surroundings, which were a disturbing influence, to be placed completely at rest under the care of a suitable nurse. She should not be visited by family or friends. Bed rest for a prescribed and usually lengthy portion of the day was insisted upon: 'As a rule, in bad cases this repose in bed is continued from six to eight weeks; and at first the rest is made absolute, the patient being only allowed to rise for the purpose of passing her evacuations, and is neither allowed to read, to sew, nor to feed herself'[20] (in severe cases she would not be permitted to leave bed 'to pass her evacuations, nor should she wash herself').[21] This would be combined with massage to help exercise wasted muscles 'without expending nerve force', and in some cases the application of electricity. Finally, the patient would be built up with regular and hefty amounts of nutritious food, in a regime of 'over-feeding'.[22] In his article 'The Systematic Treatment of Functional Neurosis', which appeared in *A Dictionary of Psychological Medicine* in 1892,[23] Playfair reflected on how by then he had an 'absolute preference' for a private nursing home as the best place for treatment rather than lodgings, to avoid the patient being too much at the mercy of a nurse. 'Moral management' was also emphasised, which, for Playfair, referred to the need for a doctor of great experience and 'firm kindness', one capable of 'showing that the practitioner has the superior will'. [24]

Playfair would have already come across some elements of the rest cure in connection with the treatment of cases of puerperal insanity, a severe mental disorder following childbirth, which he and many other nineteenth-century obstetricians were familiar with.[25] A key aspect of the cure was to remove the sufferer promptly from her home and the upsetting influences of husband, family and new-born infant. Moved to a private house or secluded cottage, she would be visited daily by her doctor and be tended by nurses specialising in the care of this condition.[26] Puerperal insanity shared other features with the rest cure; an emphasis on diet and building up the patient, literally 'fattening', bed rest, careful watching, patience and delicacy in handling the case, and also emphasised the absolute authority of the attending doctor which replaced that of the husband.[27] This kind of approach, and its intrinsic optimism about 'restoring' the patient, would already have been familiar to Playfair. So too was the use of electricity for gynaecological disorders, which was also resorted to sparingly in treating poor hospital patients.[28]

Playfair combined other treatments with the rest cure, seeking to put right any obvious gynaecological problems, for example, by inserting a pessary or correcting the position of the womb, and prescribing drugs, particularly in the early stages of treatment to encourage rest and sleep. A visit to a health resort or a journey to foreign parts could also be recommended in the final convalescent stage. But these therapies merely set the scene for the rest cure or, in the case of travel, were added on when it had been successfully completed. Playfair stressed that the rest cure was the only way to produce a full and permanent cure for nervous exhaustion. Other doctors also recommended Mitchell's rest cure, or components of it, modifying and adapting its use, but no other British practitioner seems to have advocated it as enthusiastically as Playfair.

The connection between nervous disorders and reproductive function which was incorporated into Playfair's analysis of neurasthenia was far from being an original one; indeed, it had 'a venerable history'.[29] Ornella Moscucci has described how women's biological, particularly reproductive, functions blurred into disease, and also unleashed 'a host of psychological disorders, from strange moods and feelings, to hysteria and insanity'.[30] Throughout the Victorian era, obstetricians, gynaecologists and specialists in women's diseases continued to be fascinated by female nerves and particularly their connection with the uterus. One of the foremost authorities on the nervous diseases of women, Thomas Laycock, believed women to be much more susceptible to hysteria and nervous disturbances than men, a result of their biology, natural susceptibility and maternal emotions.[31] According to his 'Fourth Principle' of causality, *'Hysteric Diseases appear only during that Period of Life in which the reproductive*

Organs perform their functions...'.[32] Samuel Ashwell, an authority on
women's diseases and Guy's Hospital obstetrician, described in 1844
how an irritable uterus could confine a woman to 'the sofa' without
any perceptible organic change or disease.[33] In the second half of the
nineteenth century, medical and popular literature continued to
make clear the dangers of disease and mental or nervous disturbance
to women, at risk during all stages of their reproductive lives from the
onset of menstruation to its end. In the words of the eminent
gynaecologist, Robert Barnes, 'even in the healthiest women, there is
evidence of exalted nervous action under the influence of
menstruation'.[34] He included dysmenorrhoea, painful menstruation,
as a cause of insanity, and, while hysteria and neurosis were 'words
used to conceal ignorance', both could be cured by treating the root
cause, a menstrual or uterine disorder, with retroflexion or
retroversion being more strongly implicated than uterine disease.[35]
All Victorian gynaecologists were undoubtedly interested in nerves,
but few developed such a systematic treatment as Playfair, and none
publicised their treatment as successfully.[36] What is most interesting
about Playfair, however, is not his acceptance of this link between
uterine disease and disturbance and nervous disorders, but his later
questioning of it.

Playfair and his patients: cases and cures

Even in his earliest published work, Playfair was already in a position
to present several of his success stories, giving detailed patient
histories, which became a hallmark of his advocacy of the rest cure.[37]
Many of his patients were believed to be suffering from the after
effects of pregnancies or childbirth, or from gynaecological disorders.
But the rest cure was also advocated for those, 'worn and wasted,
often bedridden woman, who had broken down, either from some
sudden shock, such as grief, or money losses, or excessive mental or
bodily strain'.[38]

Through the 1880s, Playfair sharpened his conception of 'ideal'
patients for the rest cure. In his 1892 essay he gave specific guidance
on how to select cases. He referred almost exclusively to women, and
mainly to those suffering from nerve exhaustion, but he was prepared
to try the rest cure in select cases of hysteria, eating disorders,
narcosis, and occasionally mental disease.[39] The desire to be cured on
the part of the patient was absolutely vital, and for that reason
hysterics would usually not respond to the rest cure; nor would the
nervous case 'to whom her illnesses are a source of enjoyment'.[40] The
rest cure would not be effective in most cases of mental illness (a view

shared by most nerve doctors), including chronic melancholia, where the relatives often wished to hide the true facts of the illness and disguise it as a nervous disorder. In very carefully chosen instances, it could pull the patient back from the 'edge of a precipice' with mental disease on one side, health on the other, but there was also great risk that it could push her over, especially if the symptoms included religious delusions or suicidal impulses.[41] Presented as something of a miracle cure, the rest cure was not appropriate to more than a select few cases.

There is evidence to suggest that Playfair's interest in neurasthenia was in some ways a direct response to and an extension of his obstetric and gynaecological work, rooted not just in the distressing cases he encountered in his private practice, but also in the wards of King's College Hospital. Like his neurasthenic patients, Playfair's Hospital cases were predominantly young women or women of childbearing age. However, Playfair was absolutely emphatic in insisting that neurasthenia was a disorder that befell only women of high culture and delicacy. Playfair's patients were women of 'refinement', more than delicate, they were, as Showalter puts it, 'a model of ladylike deportment and hyperfemininity, a paradigm of that wasting beauty that the late Victorians found so compelling',[42] super-sensitive women who had reached and then surpassed the ideal of Victorian womanhood. They took on the role of anorexic, too spiritual to consume food; they stopped menstruating, almost from force of will; they were sexually withdrawn. In a case reported in the *Lancet* in December 1881, Playfair detailed how one woman's nervous irritability had so increased that

> To touch her bed, the ringing of a bell, sometimes the sound of a voice, sunlight, &c., affected her so as to make her almost cry out... She cannot sit because the tip of the spine is so sensitive; any pressure on it makes her feel faint. She cannot go in a carriage because it jars every nerve in her body. She cannot lie on her back because her whole spine is so tender.[43]

The roots of her illness were varied. A severe neuralgic illness at the age of 16 was cited. Soon after marriage she had a miscarriage, then two pregnancies, ending with the delivery of dead children, and, finally, a third pregnancy resulting in the birth of a daughter now aged three. During all of her pregnancies she had suffered from nervous afflictions. Subsequently, she had several 'shocks' in the form of the deaths of near relatives. One gynaecologist diagnosed a 'uterine lesion', and her treatment included leeching, pessaries, and intracervical applications of carbolic acid, iodine, and 'fuming' nitric acid. By the time Playfair was brought in she was suffering from a whole range of symptoms: tenderness of the spine, attacks of syncope when she became deaf, blind and deadly cold, and sciatica. She was wasting away, acutely emaciated, and had developed a heart murmur. Playfair had this 'naturally fine and highly cultivated woman', removed from home, anaesthetized and brought by train some 200 miles to London, where he found no evidence of organic disease and placed her under the rest cure. In a week, Playfair reported, she could lie in a bright sunlit room, in ten days the whole spine could be rubbed rigorously from top to bottom, she gained flesh, and within five weeks she could sit up and ride out in a carriage. She recovered and remained perfectly well, setting out with her husband on a world tour.[44]

A clearer gynaecological root nervous exhaustion was specified in the case of a 32-year-old woman, who had suffered a variety of uterine troubles, since the birth of her last child: ulceration, perimetritis, and endometritis, the latter culminating in a pelvic abscess, which first opened through the bladder and then the vagina. The patient suffered from paralysis of the bladder, and a catheter had to be used to draw the urine. Her legs had become paralysed, then her left arm and back and neck, until finally the woman was only able to move her right arm. At this point, however, the pelvic abscess cleared up, and there 'were no further symptoms referable to the uterine organs'.[45] Yet her general condition remained the same.

> She was seen, from time to time, by several of our most eminent consultants, all of whom recognised the probable hysterical character of her illness, but none of the remedies employed had any beneficial effect. There was almost total anorexia, the amount of food consumed was absurdly small, and the necessary consequence of this inability to take food, combined with four years in bed with paralysis of the greater part of the body, and the habitual use of chloral to induce sleep, had reduced a naturally fine woman to a mere shadow.[46]

In October 1880 she was brought to London, seen by Playfair together with his associate the neurologist, Dr Buzzard. Together they concluded that the paralysis was 'purely functional', there was no evidence of the pelvic abscess, and the uterus was mobile and healthy. The patient was isolated in lodgings with a nurse of Playfair's choosing, and communication with her family and friends suspended. The rest cure commenced on 16 October. The patient was fed up on milk, eggs, bread, mutton chops and porridge. Within a few days 'she passed water for the first time for four years'. Chloral was discontinued, she slept through the night, she was massaged and electricity applied. By 30 October she was consuming three full meals a day, and could move in bed. By 6 November she was sitting in a chair, on 17 November she walked downstairs and went for a drive. She had by this time 'increased enormously in size, and looks an entirely different person from the wasted invalid of a few weeks ago'. On 26 November she went to Brighton to convalesce and 'since remained strong and well, and has resumed the duties of life and society'.[47]

The treatment of neurasthenia was no doubt lucrative, although we have no idea how much Playfair actually charged for his rest cure. He may have had followers and imitators, though there is little evidence of this, but in any case he cornered the market by becoming the rest cure's best advocate and one of London's leading nerve specialists, which bolstered his already lucrative gynaecological practice. He was praised for his flawless bedside manner, and his reputed courtesy towards his patients did him great financial good. Despite his costly court case in 1896, his estate amounted to £44,261 upon his death in 1903.[48]

Playfair and his patients: the relationship

Contemporary observations and reminiscences of Playfair, though few, uniformly talk of his gentle and gentile manner. He is presented as a respectful man, who had 'a kind and courteous manner in dealing with patients, doctors, and students'.[49] This is a common enough representation, but one which is confirmed by the way in which he presented his case histories, and by the King's College Hospital notes, which show his patient involvement with his poorer clientele. Unlike the hysteric who he disliked intensely, Playfair spoke admiringly of his private neurasthenic patients and their cultivated ways and ladylike demeanour, despite their wasted invalid appearance.

During the rest cure the doctor–patient relationship became intense and heightened. The doctor could not cure without the patient, the patient could not be cured without her doctor. Naming the condition and sharing a diagnosis seems to have been taken as the first step towards a cure.[50] It put a stop to the restless searching for a diagnosis, which had been experienced by many of Playfair's patients. Playfair was keen to make neurasthenia appear to be a 'species of general nervous breakdown which constitutes a very real and very important malady'.[51] Because of its precision, the cure could not be abandoned half way or deviated from, or be taken over by another practitioner. There was also a large degree of 'infantisation' and dependence involved in the treatment. The woman was fed a milk diet, was declared unable to perform her natural functions, she needed assistance to urinate and defecate, and, in some cases, was carried like a baby to the place of treatment. The authority established by Playfair was absolute. However, even if we are sceptical about Playfair's claims to cure his patients so rapidly and fully, we must assume that he had some success in order to keep acquiring them. And, given the alternative treatments on offer for nervous and gynaecological disorders, Playfair must in some cases have saved his patients from more radical interventions, including cauterisation, leeching and major surgery.

While Playfair viewed neurasthenia as a real condition with real causes, these were many and varied and sometimes difficult to explain. Many of his clients were reacting to traumatic miscarriages, pregnancies, stillbirths, and difficult deliveries, even though these events may have taken place many years previously, to painful or abnormal menstruation, or gynaecological, especially uterine, disorders. He cited other causes, for both men and women: addiction to chloral or morphine (although this seems in his case notes to be more a result of nervous exhaustion and lack of sleep than a cause), and a less surprising one between higher education, overstudy and nervous collapse, which again could occur in men and women.

Playfair seems to have felt some sympathy towards his patients and their plight, though often relating it to female weakness. His comments on the large number of doctors consulted by his patients seems to be less a criticism of them for their irresolution, than a refection of his absolute confidence that he would cure them, his contempt for 'quackery', and also a strong dislike of the regimes imposed by his colleagues which saw as being misdirected and dangerous. What Playfair did not lack was the confidence that he would cure where others had failed; he did not publish cases where he had not completely cured his patients. He illustrated his feelings and those of his patients in a transcription of a poem written by one of his patients, a lady currently under his care, who was now 'on the high road to recovery'.[52]

> PATIENT: But stay: I have prescriptions tried by scores;
> Gone out for walks, and sometimes stayed in doors;
> Was galvanised till I became much worse;

Would ride, but cannot always find a horse;
Tried German baths, and much increased my pain,
Until I fear all remedies are vain.

DOCTOR: Believe it, and from remedies abstain![53]

Oppenheim has suggested that Playfair fundamentally disliked women who suffered from nervous disorders, criticising them for being a drain on family resources, and for moving through a succession of practitioners and cures. 'Nothing', declared Playfair, 'could possibly be more hopeless than the experience of all of us of these wretched instances of broken and shattered lives, these bed-ridden, helpless creatures, who became a burden not only to themselves but to all around them, making happy homes miserable, and exhausting at once the patience, and the resources of those who are responsible for their care'.[54] Playfair also described the

> confirmed neurotic of many years standing, whose social position and means enable her to follow any advice she may have received, and consider what her probable history has been. Ever since her illness began she has been going from one health resort to another. She has tried Schwalbach, St. Moritz, and the Riviera; she has swallowed pints of drugs, iron, quinine, bromides, chloral, and anti-spasmodics; she has exhausted the virtues of hydropathic establishments; she is lucky if she has not also run the gauntlet of innumerable pessaries, and much uterine treatment; of late years almost certainly she has 'tried a little massage', and most certainly it has failed to do good; and lastly she has had hosts of sympathetic friends, many nurses, and a whole phalanx of doctors. This is no exaggerated picture. It is a simple statement of what almost all well-to-do patients of this kind have gone through, and their last state is always worse than their first.[55]

This reading of Playfair suggests more of an irritation with the range of useless cures on offer and prevailing ignorance on nervous disorders, rather than annoyance at the patient and her ultimately useless tour of them at the financial and emotional expense of her family. This approach, of supporting the patient against the opposition, was also a powerful marketing strategy and Playfair was an excellent self-publicist.

He reported a case in *The Systematic Treatment of Nerve Prostration* of a lady who was sent to him after years of illness with a note from her medical man, outlining her ill-defined symptoms of headache, nausea, spinal irritability, giddiness, etc. 'She never stirs out of the house, or moves from her bed or sofa, eats next to nothing, and is never happy unless seeing a doctor, or taking physic'. Playfair examined the patient, aged 29, who 'for nine years had been entirely on her back'. 'I need say no more about this case, than that it was as successful as the rest of the same type I have had to deal with', and indeed Playfair claimed to have restored her fully within two months.[56]

Playfair, as Showalter also emphasises, was keen to distinguish hysterics from neurasthenics. Hysterics were, he announced, putting on some kind of show: 'fat, well-feeding hysterics who thoroughly enjoy their life of inert self-indulgence', while neurasthenic invalids were desperate to be cured, and 'long for good health if they only knew how to obtain it'.[57] Neurasthenia occurred in clever, emotional and excitable women, but not the fanciful. It was a gradual and incipient disorder, often caused by a variety of obstetric occurrences, illness, and shocks and strains.[58] In his hospital case notes too, derisory references are made to women showing signs of hysterical behaviour. In 1878, one patient was admitted with heavy menstrual bleeding and pain in the right side. She was convinced that she had a tumour, 'but this is merely hysterical'. After the insertion of a pessary the woman complained of pain on her other side; again this was 'purely hysterical'.[59]

In the case of drug abuse, his stance remained sympathetic, as in a case he treated in May 1880, of a young woman, aged 31 and unmarried, who had overtaxed herself while nursing her mother five years previously, 'since which time she had been a complete invalid, suffering from backache, bearing-down, inability to walk, disordered menstruation, and the usual train of uterine symptoms'.[60] She was confined to her bed and sofa, suffering constant nausea, complete loss of appetite, and becoming addicted to chloral and morphia for relief. Playfair diagnosed retroflexion of the uterus, tried, as a colleague had previously done, to insist that she wore a pessary, but the patient pulled them out each time they were inserted. Irritated but not put off, Playfair tried another type of pessary which the patient left alone, and commenced with his rest cure, stating that he believed the retroflexion had little to do with the patient's general state. A total cure was soon achieved.

> She rapidly gained flesh and strength, and very soon I entirely
> stopped both chloral and morphia, and she never seemed to miss
> them. On Dec. 11th, when the treatment was commenced, she

weighed 5st. 9lb. On Jan. 20th she weighed 7st. On Jan. 25th she walked downstairs, and went out for a drive, and from that time she went out twice daily... On Feb. 1st she went to the seaside, looking rosy, fat, and healthy, and has since returned to her home in the country, where she remains perfectly strong and well. A few days ago she came to town, a long railway journey, on purpose to announce to me her approaching marriage.[61]

Not only cured, but about to marry, this woman was fully restored to her natural functions.

Playfair did not in any substantial way contravene the standard Victorian view of women, their role, demeanour and limitations. Yet his linking of overstudy and nervous collapse needs to be looked at more closely. He certainly was not advocating that women should not study at all. He warned of the dangerous time that the onset of menstruation represented.[62] He also stressed that girls should not be regarded or educated in the same way as boys, but many of the problems involved in teaching girls could be put down to a lack of physical and mental preparation. Care should be taken to develop 'strong-bodied and healthy-minded' young women, rather than bringing up girls like 'hothouse plants'.[63] He cited two cases of young girls, aged 14 to 16, one chlorotic whose menstruation had ceased for a year, the other suffering from menorrhagia, anaemia, and debility. They had timetables of 7-8 hours of study, 'an amount not in itself, perhaps, excessive in a healthy girl'. The problem lay in their failure to take healthy exercise, and the slackness of the school authorities in checking on 'the state of an all-important bodily function'.[64] Girls should be encouraged to play games, not football or cricket which were too violent, but tennis, which could produce 'a thoroughly healthy English girl', 'The Lawn Tennis Girl':

> Sensible people have long ago agreed to accept this new type of womanhood as being distinctly admirable... wherever we meet her we come upon an excellent example of the healthy, well-developed, and unsentimental girl - the girl who does not think it necessary to devote herself to the study of her own emotions, and who finds in active physical exercise an antidote to the morbid fancies which are too apt to creep into the mind of the idle and self-indulgent.[65]

Playfair as a modern gynaecologist

Playfair was keen to point out that functional neurosis, neurasthenia, was not well understood. The fact that he took the condition so seriously may have greatly benefited his patients; he made it real, and named it, as well as promising to treat it. Though he was keen to seek out organic disorders and deal with them - and this is best shown in his treatment of cases at King's College Hospital - he stressed that the long-term draining effects of gynaecological disorders must also be treated through the rest cure. He also argued, that even when detected, uterine problems, which he sometimes referred to as 'uterine mischief', might not be contributing that much to the condition. He took a holistic view of his patients and the cause of their disorders, and as such put himself forward as a modern gynaecologist, capable of looking beyond local pelvic conditions. He discouraged too much 'local uterine treatment'.[66] This included the insertion of pessaries, although he did resort to them, quite commonly in his hospital practice. In some cases it seemed to be the only treatment that might offer relief, and may also have satisfied Playfair's need, and perhaps that of his patients, to be seen to be doing something.[67] In 1882 he reported on 'a case under my care as I write, in which the patient may fairly be said to be suffering from pessary on the brain - so incessantly is she thinking of one or other of the seventy-nine different instruments which she has had inserted in the last few years in America and in this country'.[68]

> Nothing can be more deplorably bad for a nervous, emotional woman, whose general health is at a low ebb, than to have her attention constantly directed to her reproductive organs by vaginal examinations repeated two or three times a week, pessaries constantly introduced for 'a slight displacement', the cervix frequently cauterised, or the endometrium curetted, and the like; and yet these are things one incessantly sees in cases in which, on examination, no definite reason for such interference is found to exist. No doubt it is often done in good faith; but the results are often disastrous...[69]

He offered the rest cure as an alternative to Battey's operation: 'If the case is purely neurasthenic it cannot, under any conditions, I apprehend, be one even for the consideration of oöphorectomy', although a chronic condition of the ovaries could perhaps warrant surgical intervention as a starting point. Real mental disorder could not be treated by the rest cure,[70] but Playfair found it unreasonable to remove the ovaries or carry out other drastic operative procedures as a way of curing excessive masturbation and 'various erotic manifestations' in the mentally ill.[71]

One of the central tenets of Playfair's approach to neurasthenia was that this condition should not require operative intervention, and a survey of the King's College Hospital records has revealed Playfair to be an infrequent operator in this context too. Few surgical interventions were carried out in terms of his total workload, the bulk of which consisted of minor uterine disorders and displacements, infections and menstrual problems. He made occasional use of the speculum to carry out internal examinations and in a handful of procedures chloroform was administered. He dealt routinely with fibroids, abscesses and prolapse, removed those tumours he considered operable, and very occasionally performed an ovariotomy. In one case at least it was the patient who insisted that he 'did something' which seems to have prompted him to operate.[72] Playfair shared the interest of many of his contemporaries in retroflexion of the uterus and the condition he referred to as an 'immobile' uterus. He saw uterine displacement as being a root cause of many forms of gynaecological and nervous disorder. Yet he remained ambivalent about its full impact. Many of the conditions he described as being gynaecological in origin, had been treated or had healed spontaneously, leaving the patient in a state of debilitation and nervous exhaustion long after the initial cause had vanished. His hospital work was routine and repetitive. Rather than intervention on a grand scale, Playfair was more likely to be dealing with the insertion of pessaries, correcting the position of the uterus and clearing up vaginal discharges. There were few heroic outcomes to be had. His interest in neurasthenic patients may have presented a welcome opportunity, given the reported success of his rest cure treatment, to carry out dramatic cures in contrast to the relative drudgery and lack of results connected to his hospital work.

Conclusion

To return to my starting point and the question of the context for Playfair's work on neurasthenia, his interest in neurasthenia seems to be part of a process, which grew out of his work in gynaecology and the diseases of women. The rest cure was a way of dealing with unspecified though troubling gynaecological and nervous disorders. Playfair's awareness and response developed not just from being confronted with well-to-do ladies, suffering a range of nervous and physical symptoms in his private consulting work, but also from almost twenty years experience of working on a busy hospital ward.

Oppenheim talks of nerve doctors 'who catered to an affluent clientele' assuming 'an elitist attitude, often as much from lack of experience as from social snobbery'.[73] Playfair had much experience of working with poor women, and appears to have been sympathetic to their plight. They did not and could not fit his label 'neurasthenic', but Playfair did not deny the possibility that they too could fall prey to 'nervous exhaustion' of a kind associated with their reproductive or gynaecological problems or their lifestyles. His 'proto-neurasthenic' hospital cases were women of a very different rank and life experience, including servants, nurses, laundresses, cooks and barmaids, needlewomen, teachers and governesses. Their gynaecological and physical debility was often linked to long and hard physical work, sometimes in association with childbearing. Starvation was related more to need and poor nutrition, than to inability to eat, coughs to poor living and working conditions. They laboured excessively rather than too little, and some were forced to give up paid work because of their condition.[74] After Playfair's adoption of the rest cure in the early-1880s, it is possible (though we have no proof of this) that his approaches in treating wealthy patients may have fed back into his hospital work, bolstered his concern about over-meddlesome gynaecology, and made him reluctant to act in cases where he simply did not know what was wrong with his patients. It is hard to believe that Playfair's work went along two parallel tracks without his establishing connections between the experiences of his two sets of patients.

The symptoms reported by Playfair's well-to-do neurasthenics and his hospital patients are similar in many ways, including headaches, coughs, 'dragging' pains, anorexia, loss of flesh, exhaustion, anxiety and nervousness. Marriage was often cited as the start of the woman's problems, more explicitly for his hospital patients; they not only started producing children at this point, but often had to work much harder. As with his wealthy clientele, the poorer woman's condition could have a psychological basis, related to shock, strain or stress. Psychological and somatic causes often dovetailed, for example in the case of women becoming ill after tending for a sick or a dying relative or those beset by financial crises.[75] The language, although the hospital case notes are minimal compared with the rich detail of the published accounts of private patients, is similar. Often very vague symptoms are described in the case notes, with Playfair at a loss to explain their origins. In the case of Esther Perry, admitted to King's College Hospital in November 1880 with weakness and shooting pains, Playfair lapsed into the language of neurasthenia, 'the existence of uterine or pelvic mischief has been suspected'.[76] Playfair's work with his neurasthenic patients, it could be argued, was based in part on his accumulated experience, on what he had observed in private practice and on his busy hospital wards. His experience primed him for his warm reception of the rest cure, parts of which he was using before he came across Weir Mitchell's work. His downplaying of local pelvic conditions as a cause of nervous disorders was found in both of his areas of practice, and built into his self-presentation of himself as a promoter of a new, more subtle form of gynaecology. For his neurasthenic patients, according to Playfair, it meant certain cure, for his poor hospital patients, for whom the full rest cure was not available, a more uncertain outcome.

Notes

1. King's College Hospital (KCH), Clinical Records, Case Notes (CN), 320, March 1879 - Nov. 1881, King's College Ward: Elizabeth Lovington, admitted 29 May 1879, 24, 26.
2. KCH/CN/320: Lydia Bennett, admitted 23 May 1879, 14.
3. A backward arching of the uterus, a very common condition and not nowadays considered as an abnormality, although symptoms such as backache and menstrual disturbances can be relieved by correcting the position of the uterus. It attracted a good deal of attention in contemporary gynaecological texts: see, for example, the section on displacements of the uterus and their treatment in T.C. Allbutt and W.S. Playfair (eds), *A System of Gynaecology* (London: Macmillan, 1896), 194–210.
4. For the relationship between nerve doctors and patients in the U.S., including working-class patients in general hospitals, see Barbara Sicherman, 'The Uses of a Diagnosis: Doctors, Patients, and Neurasthenia', *Journal of the History of Medicine*, 32 (1977), 33–54, especially p. 52 which refers to very similar symptoms being presented by working-class patients.
5. For the specifications of Mitchell's rest cure, see his books, *Fat and Blood: And How to Make Them* (Philadelphia: Lippincott, 1877) and *Wear and Tear, or Hints for the Overworked* (Philadelphia: Lippincott, 1887).
6. W.S. Playfair, 'Systematic Treatment of Nerve Prostration and Hysteria Connected with Uterine Disease', *Lancet*, 28 May, 1881, 857-9, 11 June, 1881, 949-50. See also 'Some Limitations of the So-called Weir Mitchell Treatment', *Lancet*, 7 Jan. 1888, 8–9.
7. W.S. Playfair, *The Systematic Treatment of Nerve Prostration and Hysteria* (London: Smith, Elder, & Co., 1883). In addition to his case notes, with their emphasis on close description, Playfair

produced photographic representations of his rest cure patients, a
series of which were given by Playfair to the rest cure's originator
Silas Weir Mitchell with whom he had an extensive correspondence:
see Jayne Morgan, 'Eadweard Muybridge and W.S. Playfair: An
Aesthetics of Neurasthenia', *History of Photography*, 23 (1999),
225–31.

8. Cf. the patient accounts of George M. Beard, who first applied the
term neurasthenia, and Mitchell, who included lengthy transcripts of
patients' 'self'-diagnosis in their articles. See Tom Lutz, *American
Nervousness 1903: An Anecdotal History* (Ithica: Cornell University
Press, 1991).

9. Thomas Stretch Dowse, *The Brain and the Nerves: Their Ailments
and Their Exhaustion* (London: Ballière, Tindall, & Cox, 1884), 121.
See Janet Oppenheim, *Shattered Nerves: Doctors, Patients, and
Depression in Victorian England* (Oxford University Press, 1991),
104–7, 138–9 for the relationship between nervous exhaustion and
class.

10. Thomas Dixon Savill, *Clinical Lectures on Neurasthenia* (London:
Henry J. Glaisher, 1899).

11. Playfair features little in histories of gynaecology: he is not referred
to in Ornella Moscucci's *The Science of Woman: Gynaecology and
Gender in England 1800-1929* (Cambridge University Press, 1990),
and earns one brief mention in Ann Dally, *Women under the Knife: A
History of Surgery* (London: Hutchinson, 1991) (102) for his
treatment of nervous disorders.

12. Archives held at Edinburgh University Library include material on
the two brothers, but no information on W.S. Playfair. For Lyon
Playfair, see Anne Hardy, 'Lyon Playfair and the Idea of Progress:
Science and Medicine in Victorian Parliamentary Politics', in D.
Porter and R. Porter (eds), *Doctors, Politics and Society: Historical
Essays* (Amsterdam: Rodopi, 1993), 81–106.

13. Details on Playfair were taken from the *New Dictionary of National
Biography* (Ann Dally) and *Lancet*, 'Obituary: William Smout
Playfair', 22 Aug. 1903, 570–5.

14. *Lancet*, 28 March, 4 April, 9 May, 1896; *The Times*, 7 April 1896.

15. *Lancet*, 9 May 1896, 1292.

16. *The Times*, 7 April, 1896, 6.

17. *Lancet*, 22 Aug. 1903, 575.

18. See Chandak Sengoopta's contribution to this volume for the
relationship between Playfair and Clifford Allbutt and for Playfair's
advocacy of modern gynaecology.

19. *Lancet*, 28 May, 1881, 857–9, 11 June 1881, 949–50, 957.

20. *Ibid.*, 858.
21. W.S. Playfair, 'The Systematic Treatment of Functional Neurosis', in Daniel Hack Tuke, *A Dictionary of Psychological Medicine* (London: J. A. Churchill, 1892), vol. II, 854.
22. *Lancet*, 28 May, 1881, 858–9.
23. Playfair, *op. cit.* (note 21), 857.
24. *Ibid.*
25. And to which he devoted a chapter in W.S. Playfair, *A Treatise on the Science and Practice of Midwifery*, 3rd edn. (London: Smith, Elder, & Co., 1880), vol. II, 310–24.
26. Hilary Marland, 'At Home with Puerperal Mania: The Domestic Treatment of the Insanity of Childbirth in the Nineteenth Century', in Peter Bartlett and David Wright (eds), *Outside the Walls of the Asylum: The History of Care in the Community 1750-2000* (London: Athlone, 1999), 45–65.
27. Although the time required for a cure in cases of puerperal insanity was often calculated in terms of months rather than weeks for neurasthenia. For Playfair, the prognosis for both was good. See also Hilary Marland, '"Destined to a Perfect Recovery": The Confinement of Puerperal Insanity in the Nineteenth Century', in Joseph Melling and Bill Forsythe (eds), *Insanity, Institutions and Society, 1800-1914* (London and New York: Routledge, 1999), 137–56.
28. One of these rare cases, Elizabeth Locke, was admitted with 'functional paraplegia' to the King's College ward in October 1875. She was reported as suffering from sickness and retching, backache, 'dragging pains and weakness'. Her abdomen was swollen and her uterus 'antiflexed'. Belladonna and magnesium carbonate were administered, but after a couple of weeks there was no improvement and Locke complained of chilliness and shivering, 'cold and numbness in the legs, and of inability to stand on them'. She was treated with electricity to the lower extremities, a pessary introduced, and her uterus was replaced in the normal position. The variety of treatments administered and her length of stay also make Locke's case unusual. She was finally discharged 'relieved' on 13 December, two and a half months after admission. KCH/CN/315, Sept. 1873 - April 1876: Elizabeth Locke, admitted 5 Oct. 1875, 279–80.
29. Oppenheim, *op. cit.* (note 9), 187. See also Anne Digby, 'Women's Biological Straitjacket', in S. Mendus and J. Rendell (eds), *Sexuality and Subordination: Interdisciplinary Studies of Gender in the Nineteenth Century* (London and New York: Routledge, 1989), 192–220; Moscucci, *op. cit.* (note 11), esp. chs 1 and 4.

30. Moscucci, *ibid,* 102.
31. Thomas Laycock, *A Treatise on the Nervous Diseases of Women; Comprising an Inquiry into the Nature, Causes, and Treatment of Spinal and Hysterical Disorders* (London: Orme, Brown, Green, and Longmans, 1840).
32. *Ibid.* Cited in Pat Jalland and John Hooper (eds), *Women from Birth to Death: The Female Life Cycle in Britain 1830-1914* (Brighton: Harvester, 1986), 96.
33. Samuel Ashwell, *A Practical Treatise on the Diseases Peculiar to Women* (London: S. Highley, 1844), 240, 242.
34. Robert Barnes, 'Lumleian Lectures on the Convulsive Diseases of Women', *Lancet,* 26 April 1873, 585.
35. Robert Barnes, 'Uterine Disorders and Insanity', in Tuke, *op. cit.* (note 21), vol. II, 1350–1.
36. Most textbooks on the diseases of women or gynaecology would contain at least a section on nervous disorders or neurasthenia; for example, John Thorburn's, *A Practical Treatise on the Diseases of Women* (London: Charles Griffin, 1885), included a chapter on neurasthenia, including Weir Mitchell's rest cure (106–33).
37. *Lancet,* 28 May 1881, 858–9.
38. Playfair, *op. cit.* (note 7), 89. Cited in Elaine Showalter, *The Female Malady: Women, Madness and English Culture, 1830-1980* (London: Virago Press, 1987), 139.
39. Playfair, *op. cit.* (note 21), 851–3.
40. *Ibid.,* 853.
41. *Ibid.*
42. Showalter, *op. cit.* (note 38), 140.
43. *Lancet,* 17 Dec., 1881, 1029.
44. *Ibid.*
45. Playfair, *op. cit.* (note 7), 24.
46. *Ibid.,* 24–5.
47. *Ibid.,* 23–7.
48. *Lancet,* 22 Aug. 1903, 575. Not including the diamond ring presented by the Czar of Russia during his brief stay in St Petersburg: *BMJ,* 19 Sept. 1903, 677.
49. H. Willoughby Lyle, *King's and Some King's Men Being a Record of the Medical Department of King's College, London, from 1830 to 1909 and of King's College Hospital Medical School From 1909 to 1934* (Oxford University Press, 1935), 295.
50. See Nelleke Bakker's chapter in this volume for shared diagnoses. I would like to thank Nelleke Bakker for her helpful comments on this, and other, aspects of my article. See also Sicherman, *op. cit.*

(note 4).

51. Playfair, *op. cit.* (note 21), 851.

52. Playfair, *op. cit.* (note 7), 6.

53. *Ibid.*, 7.

54. Oppenheim, *op. cit.* (note 9), 230. Citing W.S. Playfair, 'Remarks on the Systematic Treatment of Aggravated Hysteria and Certain Allied Forms of Neurasthenic Disease', *BMJ*, 19 Aug. 1882, 309-10.

55. Playfair, *op. cit.* (note 21), 850.

56. Playfair, *op. cit.* (note 7), 82–3.

57. Playfair, *op. cit.* (note 21), 851; Showalter, *op. cit.* (note 38), 139–40.

58. Playfair, *op. cit.* (note 21), 850–1.

59. KCN/CN/319, April 1877 - June 1879: Mary Ann Bradshaw, admitted 5 June 1878, 92.

60. Playfair, *op. cit.* (note 6), 949.

61. *Ibid.* It is noteworthy how many times the patients' recovery is linked by Playfair to a long railway journey alone. It crops up repeatedly in case notes, whereas railway travel was often used as a symbol of the mounting stresses of the late nineteenth century (e.g. by Max Nordau), and as a cause of nerve stimulation and exhaustion.

62. Cf. the discussions of Playfair's contemporaries, including Michael Ryan and E.J. Tilt, in Jalland and Hooper (eds), *op. cit.* (note 32), 60–76.

63. Playfair, 'The Nervous System in Relation to Gynaecology', in Allbutt and Playfair (eds), *A System of Gynaecology*, 220–31, quote on 220.

64. *Ibid.*, 221–2.

65. Cited by Playfair from 'The New Woman and the Old', *The Speaker*, 12 Jan. 1895. In *ibid.*, 222.

66. *Lancet*, 22 June 1903, 575.

67. Many of his case notes record the use of pessaries particularly in cases of retroflexion, though his patients often reported difficulty or pain in connection with them, and he had to reinsert them frequently.

68. *BMJ*, 19 Aug. 1882, 309.

69. Playfair, *op. cit.* (note 63), 226.

70. *Lancet*, 10 Dec. 1881, 991.

71. Playfair, *op. cit.* (note 63), 230. He was far from being alone in his views, his colleague T.C. Allbutt warning how women could become 'entangled in the net of the gynaecologist'. See Dally, *op. cit.* (note 11), 190.

72. The case of Florence Baker, aged 34, admitted in November 1880,

138

suffering from dysmenorrhoea. By 7 December the pain was worse, and she 'is very anxious to have something done'. Playfair undertook an internal examination, found nothing abnormal in the uterus, but incised the posterior lip of the os uteri. Since the operation the pain was declared much better, though the os uteri was irritable, and Florence Baker was discharged on 22 December. KCH/CN/322, Nov. 1880 - Oct. 1882: Florence Baker, admitted 24 Nov. 1880, 78.

73. Oppenheim, *op. cit.* (note 9), 104.

74. As in the case of Francis Farrim, aged 21, who, within three years, had given birth to one child and had three miscarriages. Pale, anaemic and weak, with a severe cough, she had to give up her occupation at a seed factory. Farrim, who Playfair referred to as being 'delicate' and sickly as a child, came to him with severe pain in the ovarian region, for which he could find no cause or cure. KCH/CN/326, Sept. 1883 - May 1890: Francis Farrim, admitted 10 Dec. 1883, 36.

75. Cf. Sicherman, *op. cit.* (note 4), who points to purely somatic interpretations for poor neurasthenic patients, 52.

76. KHC/CN/322, Nov. 1880 - Oct. 1882: Esther Perry, admitted 23 Nov. 1880, 64.

6

Public Views of Neurasthenia:
Britain, 1880–1930

Michael Neve

The British setting

This is a difficult historical story to speak of with certainty, hidden as
it still is in a mass of lost doctor/patient encounters, hundreds of
pages of magazine advertising, a blizzard of advice literature on
tonics, fats, electricity and – for the wealthy – recommendations of
luxury cruises and very specific kinds of mineral water. For the less
affluent patients there was the rest cure, perhaps a sea bath or – a
modest but an important innovation at the end of the nineteenth
century – regular rides on a bicycle. Preliminary research on public
perceptions of neurasthenia in Britain vindicates earlier work by W.F.
Bynum and Simon Wessely: that the history of the neurasthenia
diagnosis is that of somaticism becoming increasingly supplemented
by the language of psychological explanation and therapies from
about the 1870s onwards. This psychological addition is occurring
whatever the details of the agreements and disagreements between
elite neurologists, gynaecologists and others. By the 1920s at the
latest, the 'nervous patient' was fully in the charge of psychiatrists and
general practitioners, with British neurologists concentrating on
other things. From the late 1870s the established place of the general
physician in the 'moral therapeutic' aspects of neurasthenia was set.
Trust in the physician had of course been at the core of the rest cure
itself but it remained so in therapeutic encounters not based on Weir
Mitchell's methods.[1]

Did these changes of emphasis, these psychological
developments, owe anything to the patient's own involvement in the
discussion and treatment of neurasthenia? And did it make a
difference if the patient or sufferer in the last years of the century was
female? This is important to ask in the light of Lutz's timely reminder
that Charlotte Perkins Gilman was both an active feminist and 'a
believer in the validity of neurasthenia until her death in the 1930s'.

Likewise, Mathew Thomson's discussion of the involvement of the state is equally important. But so is the place of the patient in the market-place, whether it be as a purchaser of coca wines or indigestion pills or seeking active collaboration with certain esteemed, covertly advertised doctors and their methods. Here if anywhere the question of public perception might be settled, although it would indeed be an indefatigable historian who could manage to write a social history of nineteenth-century fatigue! The possibility that for the 'public' there was just some general sense of a long experience of being tired, anxious but genuinely not insane and that a multitude of remedies helped a little but not much more than that: this historical possibility may be all too real.

Equally historically visible are the emergence of general practitioner and psychiatrist-based therapies at the end of the nineteenth century, allied first to a moderate feminism and then, especially in Britain, to diluted forms of psychotherapy and psychological medicine. Diluted because in Britain there was no J.M.Charcot, no George Beard and certainly no Sigmund Freud. Even more to the point there was no Marcel Proust, no doctor's son acutely aware of his father Adrien's writings on neurasthenia who then made his asthma and his fatigue the vantage point from which to expose an entire social class in a novel, written in a race against time and fading health. In Britain there was instead a cluster of practices around mental and moral hygiene and advice literature; there were Boy Scouts and Girl Guides; there was school milk and physical education.[2] There was the novelist E.M. Forster (in lieu of Proust) and there was that small but interesting conversation between Allbutt and Playfair described elsewhere in this collection, notably by Chandak Sengoopta.

The British story may well be a very limited and confined one. A good history might be written as to how various Continental practices and discourses - from sexology, criminology, hypnotism and psychoanalysis – developed in Britain in diluted, limited and watered down forms: the history of neurasthenia might share in this restriction and re-working, this suspicion of fashionable American and Continental extremes and extreme remedies.[3]

Elsewhere in the growing suburban world from the 1920s onwards that was one of the subjects of that poet who was also a doctor's son, W.H. Auden, it is possible to detect the way in which neurasthenia was the continuing name for mysterious fatigue and daily anxiety, almost the modern version of 'this long disease, my life'. Far away from Queen Square and its neurologists and from the

Harley Street addresses of doctors like Thomas Stretch Dowse (Fellow of the Royal College of Physicians of Edinburgh and based at 14 Welbeck Street, off Cavendish Square) and his book of 1880 and its various editions, the rhetoric and the metaphors for both disease and cure were traditional. The British call was still to the old stalwarts of 'manliness and no nonsense', 'women and children first' and 'play up and play the game'. The rest cure combined, as Thomson shows in his article, with standard moral therapy ideals and these were extended rather than altered with the growth of psychological persuasion and suggestion. Summoning the collaborative will of the patient, central to moral managerial alienists like John Conolly, was deployed in precisely the same way in later therapies, with no concession to indulging the patient's passivity or to making alterations in the doctor–patient relationship.

With regard both to class matters and gender concerns, the application of the neurasthenia diagnosis in Britain had both similarities and differences with other European countries.[4] Unlike Holland there was little sense of avoiding applying the category to proletarians, including male proletarians. Unlike Germany, the category itself was mostly shunned by elite doctors and instead utilised by alienists and general practitioners.[5] There was considerable British concern about degeneration – in the work of Henry Maudsley the psychiatrist, in fears about military weakness after the South African Wars, about growing alcoholism and the end of the large bourgeois family but the continuation of the large proletarian one. Equally if not more powerful were public health environmentalists, medical officers of health and disciplinarian, mental hygienist, paediatrically-focused psychiatrists such as the Scotsman Sir James Crichton-Browne. Crichton-Browne could not follow Maudsley down a pessimistic and secular road, where Maudsley pondered what point there was in attempting regeneration at all. Public health officials had every reason to argue for anti-hereditarian solutions to degenerationist concerns: cleaner water, better housing and purity of food, infant feeding, improved mother's health. Furthermore, psychological therapies that were introspective would lead to will-lessness and exhaustion. Crichton-Browne famously remarked that Freud resembled Socrates 'as much as a toadstool does a British oak'.[6] He denounced the motor car, the writings of Zola and Tolstoy, the growth of feminism. He defended Thomas Carlyle as the great Scotsman of the age against allcomers and contributed forcefully to the debate on brain exhaustion and exam pressures in early schooling. This last issue – mental and physical exhaustion in the young – has been described by other historians and was especially important, jeopardising the brain at a crucial time in its development and leading to disorder and perhaps insanity in later life. Crichton-Browne was an important figure in a whole range of educational, psychiatric and mental hygienist campaigns in the course of a long life. His deliberate Scottish reactionary (or as he would see it heroic) stand would be revised and contested, especially by feminists. But the commitment to practical solutions as against degenerationist pessimism was part of a wider movement in which the neurasthenia debates and remedies also figured.[7]

The absence in this article of full evidence from asylum records or the personal correspondence of doctors requires a brief, compensatory glance at the printed British medical sources. What did books like Dr Hugh Campbell's *The Anatomy of Nervousness and Nervous Exhaustion*, (four editions – 1886, 1887, 1889 and 1890) or T.S. Dowse's *On Brain and Nervous Exhaustion* of 1880 or Edwin Ash's *Mind and Health: the Mental Factor and Suggestion in Treatment* of 1910 or Andrew Scott Myrtle's 1888 lecture, reprinted in 1889 as *Neurasthenia: True and False* actually say?

Textual evidence

Dowse first. In fairly familiar ways, the neurasthenic patient here is on the borderline of insanity, thus requiring a careful family history. This would be non-trivial, since (as with Virginia Woolf) the neurasthenic was not insane and could with time be rescued. For Dowse, the patient was probably a businessman or clergyman. Iron was useless, electricity pretty useless, opium useful.[8] As were arsenic, phosphorous, strychnine and the salts of bromine and iodine. Patients must be assured that the drugs would work because otherwise they would resort to mesmerists and quacks. Or myriad other doctors. As to travel and its benefits, Dowse agreed with Beard – this often made things worse, especially in spinal and brain neurasthenia. Seaside residence was not useful but a 'lengthened sea voyage is *par excellence* the best chance of a cure in a confirmed and protracted case of neurasthenia'.[9] Cannes and Nice and other southern European resorts were not suitable but the upper Engadine was fine because of its pure, dry and bracing air. As to daily regime: rise after 8am. Tepid bath then recline in a damp sheet; dry with a coarse towel. Breakfast on fish or rump steak and above all eat slowly. Toast not bread. Read the paper but not about politics or finance. Stroll for an hour or perhaps have a gentle ride. Luncheon at 1.30 with oysters four times a week a requirement: tankard of stout or Bass pale ale allowed, or whisky with Apollinaris water. Afternoon exercise, followed by dining at 7pm but with a Turkish bath first. No more than four courses at dinner and no pastry or drinking of drams. An hour before bed take a bottle of seltzer or Apollinaris water with fresh lemon juice. Sleep on a hard bed with the head toward the north and the feet toward the south with the window closed before 3pm. in the winter and 7pm. in the summer. Never despair: trust your practitioner entirely.[10]

It is worth noting the proximity of this language to that of Crichton-Browne and to note the specific Scottish place in his neurasthenia story. Scottish accounts of avoiding neurasthenia put great weight on the need for vigorous exercise throughout life, careful diet and varieties of muscular Christianity, that old Victorian ideal of combining religious devotion with robust physical exercise and natural history hobbies. It is also worth pointing out how the title of Dowse's book altered in the later editions of 1887, 1892 and 1894. Here was added '...and the exhaustions [sequelae] of influenza'. For those searching for the past connections to present taxonomies, this early version of post-viral fatigue syndrome may be of interest. One cannot but be struck by the level of affluence assumed in the patient and to ponder once again whether the development from the 1870s/1880s onwards of more psychological remedies, seen by orthodox - or at least more senior doctors - as quackeries, might not mark the beginnings of affordable remedies for a bourgeois or petit-bourgeois clientele, for whom the Upper Engadine was a world away.

Myrtle in 1888/90, speaking in Leicester, saw the neurasthenic as in the grip of a slow process, frail and free of their 'lower natures'. The strings of the instrument have snapped, although the true neurasthenic will regret the trouble they cause and be grateful for all assistance. 'False neurasthenics' want attention and care not about the nuisance they make.[11] If 'false neurasthenics' were to be treated it should be away from friends and family. Myrtle does seem to have class focus : for him it is not the machine workers, the factory workers, who suffer but 'the inventors of the machines'. Again, no real news comes from this four page printed lecture except that the doctor/patient relationship is at the heart, combined with a clichéd view of the angelic innocence of the female patient. Myrtle again recommends sedatives, bromides and a long sea voyage in a high-class steamer.

Dr Hugh Campbell of 23 Wimpole Street, near Harley Street, spelt out a familiar story in the various editions of *The Anatomy of Nervousness* mentioned above. Here we have the disease as one of refinement and civilisation, with a strong hereditarian component. Remedy: diet, regimen, improving the blood. Less brain-work and as many fats as possible. As a vegetable, sea kale was especially good. But above all, patients needed peace: 'Sexual excitement has a most pernicious influence upon persons suffering from nervous exhaustion and should be studiously avoided.'[12] It brings on a 'nervous perturbation and malaise quite out of proportion to the momentary exaltation'. Arsenic was especially useful because of enriching the blood, and bathing in sea water was also useful. A douche for spinal exhaustion might be used in the home. Campbell also spelt out conventional objections to rail travel while stressing his concerns about muscular and blood quality by endorsing faradism and galvanism at considerable length.

T.S. Dowse, as indicated earlier was a Fellow of the Royal College of Physicians of Edinburgh and from a position of professional prominence insisting on building a firm foundation for medical treatment, based on complete authority and trust in the doctor in the late 1870s. Suggestion remedies ran alongside the moral/managerial throughout our period and formed a continuous story in the tradition of Pinel, Esquirol and Conolly.[13] The authority of the medical practitioner could only be enhanced by the growing emphasis on psychological matters. This would come to include the difficult matter of sexual problems, difficult, that is, if sex might be a possible cure rather than part of the problem. Sex might have to be avoided as part of the remedy in a sexual neurasthenia diagnosis, i.e. one where sexual feelings contributed to fatigue – this is clear from European as well as from American sources such as Margaret Cleaves's autobiography of 1910. Cleaves was of course a doctor herself. Radkau in his essay in this volume has found a large and hidden world where the sexual story is central to the male patient's experience and here a novel will be cited – by an American woman who spent long periods in Europe – which explicitly addresses the sexual question regarding neurasthenia. Was there a time when one aspect of moral therapy, that sexual problems could be dealt with by diverting the mind away from such matters, was reversed? Not just a matter of women getting physically stronger before returning to marriage and children, but of the cure for sexual neurasthenia being sex itself - outside marriage if needs were urgent and obvious? If it is true throughout the main neurasthenia literature and practice that the road back to sexual health was in the first instance a road that led away from sex, on established grounds and because rest or exercise were preliminary requirements; and if it is also true that when the road returned to the departure point the aim then was marriage and reproduction, what might be another history, where the deliberate sexual deprivations of (mainly female) patients required a more straightforward solution, a solution that contradicted earlier practice? A writer like Campbell (as mentioned earlier a Wimpole Street, private practitioner) clearly makes the case for the debilitating dangers of sexual excitement and a variety of British and Continental authors stress that no one should assume that marriage was always the answer. Was there a counter-argument, where sexual excitement was seen as the cure where other doctors construed it to be a contributor to neurasthenic disease?

The moral agency of the doctor who admitted a sexual component in neurasthenia (let alone its possible cure by him) would obviously be different to that of Dowse or Myrtle or Campbell. But this difference would not be in terms of his power. In a very conventional way, he might be seen as a mountebank but the quack doctor would as always be seen by orthodoxy as more authoritarian and unreliable than they. The citing of the sexual as part of a cure rather than a source of stress does not require an accompanying historical revision of the power of the doctor. It simply requires a historical sense of the changes in the neurasthenia diagnosis at the turn of the century and the remedies for it. A doctor involved in the practice of sexual healing had not in any sense evacuated or altered or lessened the position of authority that moral therapy had always insisted on.

The novel taken later in this article as an example, *A Dark Lantern* (1905) by Elizabeth Robins, explores the question of the place of physical love in the recovery of a rest cure patient. This example from fiction is best supplemented by examining the world of the market-place and the growth of self-help and self-education; it is also important to remember the origins of the electrical apparatus which took all the discussion of electricity in works like Campbell's to a logical if initially sanitised conclusion: the commercial manufacture of the vibrator for women.[14] Various steam powered massage and vibratory devices were developed in America in the 1870s, but by the early-1880s the British model designed by the physician Joseph Mortimer Granville was patented by Weiss and battery run. As Maines tells the story, Granville insisted that the device be only used for male skeletal muscles. But in the United States such doubts were not so strong, culminating in the 'Cadillac of the vibrators', the Chattanooga, which cost $200 in 1904. Designed for both sexes the vibrator became a 'home appliance', although women's magazines hinted at the power to bring pink cheeks and bright eyes. This 'social camouflage' to use Maines's words continued until the 1920s when the true vibrator, but not the massager or electro-convulsive devices, disappeared from doctor's surgeries. Re-emerging forty years later, the vibrator was no longer a medical instrument, but a sex aid.

The fact that this is partly a history of the way devices for all the body, whether male or female later become exclusively designed for female vaginal and clitoral stimulation may seem obvious. But that would be to leave aside the history as to why the mechanical devices were de-medicalised; what kinds of needs they met in the period both up to 1920 and after then; and also to fail to ponder whether doctors simply saw them as labour-saving devices in pelvic massage before suddenly rumbling the hedonistic calculus and distancing themselves from the sexual use of artificial massage, respectable though that was in all other regards. If the use of electrical devices suddenly took off its physiological, health as 'efficiency and balance' facade and were also overtly reviving the body through pleasure, why did the doctors abandon them? Or were men in danger of now becoming technologically obsolete? The story of how drives towards vibratory 'health' for both sexes became specifically 'sexual' health for women is a conundrum in the medical sciences of the early-twentieth-century and adds a Foucauldian dimension to some of the elements in the neurasthenia debates. Research is still needed on the missing British dimension, looking at the commercial marketing of 'home electrical devices' in ways that Maines has done for the United States, with particular reference to self-help remedies in neurasthenia.

The market in medicines

Even when it forms part of the familiar account of medical men coming close to advertising medicines, remedies and practices when formally not supposed to, the growth of the commercial domain in other neurasthenia aids is huge. Going through the pages of advertisements in the medical press indicates the advertised products that had a public profile in Britain, some of the most interesting being Tidman's Sea Salt; ' VISEM' (seed of strength) a phospho-protein combined with three per cent pure lecithin and some glycerophosphate of soda; and Allen and Hanbury's well known 'BYNO' hypophosphites, a popular nerve tonic. Similar was Clay and Paget's 'Glycolactophos' – ninety-five per cent pure Casein and recommended for neurasthenia, tabes dorsalis and neuralgia. Armbrecht's Coca Wine was advertised as one that avoided the distressing symptoms associated with opiates, chloral hydrate and bromides. It cost four shillings and sixpence. Pages of the *BMJ* routinely carried adverts for Marienbad and various sanatoria. A survey of the sources also brought forward 'The Odo-Magnetic Treatment of nervous debility and all diseases resulting from poorness of blood and enfeebled constitution'. Here, 'Odo-Magnetic apparel' for both men and women was worn on various parts of the body – the abdomen, the knee, the legs, the knee caps. Belts cost £4 and knee caps £1,10 shillings. The idea was that – invisible from the outside – the sufferer went into the world dressed in wool bound magnets, in a private magnetised world of their own, with the magnetism working on the body and thus the blood and the glands. Magnetism was superior to galvanism and far less expensive, as well as avoiding the dangers of drugs. A rash of testimonial letters comes at the end of this small Odo-Magnetic volume, from Bethnal Green, Stoke Newington, South and North London, Manchester, Canterbury and Middlesborough. Such is the material of public responses and gratitude for cures for insomnia, asthma, neurasthenia, liver trouble, and general weakness.[15] Bernarr [sic] MacFadden's diet books – all thirty-three chapters, as well as his magazines for showing how to make men virile – were accompanied by advertisements for his pneumatic facial massage roller for women.[16] And although one might argue how far this was genuinely self-help, let us take a glance at the work of Eugen Sandow, (1867-1925), author of a series of books on physical strength and how to obtain it (1897), neurasthenia (1921), a designer of dumb-bells and the founder of an institute that bore his name. One of his books is called *Life is Movement: the Physical Reconstruction and Regeneration of the People (a Diseaseless World)* of the early-1920s. The institute was in London and the books published there. The neurasthenia text emphasised that this was a disease of malnutrition. His system allowed the sufferer to 'put by an abundant Reserve of Life Capital'.[17] Sufferers were businessmen, shell-shocked soldiers, the student, the victims of nerve-strain, the victims of life's severities from all classes. 'My methods' he writes, 'strengthen the digestive machinery'. The point to stress is that while obviously luring people into his system and his Institute, Sandow's book contained consultation forms at the back for home correspondence and that on the back cover there is a message 'You will be doing a public service by passing this book on to a friend when you have finished with it'. One need not doubt the claim to medical omnipotence here, but that old claim was clearly situated within a commercial growth industry which solicited the collaboration of patients as advertisers.

Alongside this literature was the British version of suggestion therapies. In 1903 Richard Ebbard published a title in a 'new self-help series' from the London Modern Medical Publishing Company.[18] It is uncertain whether he was a qualified doctor although he is named as a 'professor' but in his preface Ebbard says he will not be talking of physical ailments because these are matters for the physician and surgeon. He continually warned against quackery and kept quoting from reputable authorities. Ebbard talked about will power and suggestion. Suggestion was not connected to mysticism or occultism and he did not discuss hypnotism. Suggestion was liberating; it allowed the will to be exercised and the agent free: it was like trusting a friend and the beginnings of a 'thought-cure'. Women were screened from the world and more vulnerable and needed to be persuaded to socialise: here Ebbard quoted approvingly of a case from Bernheim. Further on he says that sexual neurasthenia was not a special case except that its consequences were especially far reaching.[19] And patients often believed (because predisposed to do so) that the effects of masturbation were fatal: Ebbard here quotes a professor from Lund in Sweden, writing on sexual hygiene, that people were terrified of trashy literature expounding wrong views. A proper diet, exercise coupled with consistent psycho-therapeutic suggestion would work, because neurasthenia 'is hardly attended with any real danger' and 'neurasthenics are the prey of undue timorousness, afraid that they are going to die without cause'.[20] Importantly, the cure was based on diverting the mind from sexual matters, ending day-dreaming and masturbation and endorsing work, walking, riding, swimming, entomology, bee-culture and conchology. Here – aside from the Nabokovian charms of entomology, butterflies and conchology – the diversionary tasks set out are very conventional moral management and moral therapies. Marriage may be the answer but as with other authors was not always so and anyway it had its purpose and hence its burdens: 'the procreation of strong and healthy offspring'. Again, a fairly conventional eugenics can be detected. For impotence, Ebbard suggested the injection of morphia and cocaine into the seminal ducts and the wearing of a suspensory bandage.

The wonderfully-named Edwin Lancelot Hopewell-Ash MD continued this mixed refrain, this mix of old and new in his *Mind and Health* of 1910.[21] Again, hypnotism was not necessary: the less extreme, the more acceptably British method of suggestion was quite sufficient. An idea could be repeated until it became fixed by either simple or indirect suggestion. In cases of muscular pain there should be direct suggestion and massage, perhaps with mild faradic current. But 'to isolate a patient with disordered nerves...in deadly dull and unsympathetic surroundings with the idea of supplying him with milk and slops is but a poor parody of a cure'.[22] And again, the manner and methods of the physician play a central and vital part in awakening hope in his patients.

This illustrates how the period around 1870 to about 1920 sees an additional psychological approach to neurasthenia and that suggestion is one key therapy. In Britain, this might be construed as a diluted form of more radical and Continental practices, including hypnotism and eventually Freudism. At the same time and in the mass market, a whole barrage of cures and advertised medicines was present. One may still see the patient as heavily controlled within this commercial market but there was nonetheless an appeal to an idea of self help and in some examples displays of neurasthenic cures that were not the work of medical men. As discussed earlier, this seems best described as an extension on conventional ideas of moral therapy but with small but visible additions, many of them showing the impact of changes in the human sciences and the object of their enquiries. Suggestion was an acceptable innovation but did not alter the moral therapeutic template.

Women as commentators and activists

One key context for aspects of the psychological developments at the end of the century was the position of women, the 'women's movement' and the complicated matter of a possible sexual aetiology for neurasthenia. Did it matter if the patient was a 'new woman', with different expectations of the doctor–patient relationship? And even if that involved a new kind of intimacy with the doctor or the physical trainer or whomever, was there any real change in the power relations even when sex was allowed to be part of the answer and not part of the problem?

Here, it is appropriate to consider Elizabeth Robins (1862-1952).[23] Born in America she began her acting career in 1880 and married in 1885. Her husband committed suicide after two years and from 1888 Robins began travelling, including coming to England where she settled in 1889. When in London she started acting the major parts in the plays of Ibsen, having visited Scandinavia in the meantime. She always attributed her interest in the 'woman question' to Ibsen: in the summer of 1893 she played Hedda Gabler (having first played it in 1891), Rebecca West in *Rosmersholm* and Hilda

Wangel in *The Master Builder*. Robins was well connected, knowing Henry James and the Bloomsbury circle, especially Julia Stephen, and the Hogarth Press also published her in later life. Her feminist address 'Woman's Secret' was first published by the Pankhurst's Women's Social and Political Union in 1907. Max Beerbohm saw her at dinner in London: 'Altogether a rather pleasing meal – save for the Robins...conceive! Straight pencilled eyebrows, a mouth that has seen the stress of life...She is fearfully Ibsenian and talks of souls that are in nerve-turmoil and are seeking a common platform. That is literally what she said! Her very words! I kept peering under the table to see if she really wore a skirt'.[24] Henry James was more intrigued and more dubious (as he was famously dubious about Ibsen). Aware of Robins's skill as an actress and as a theatrical force at a time when he was concerned about his own plays being staged in London and whether she might act them, he responded to her suffragist pamphlet in 1907. The 'secret' that Robins spoke of in her pamphlet was this : women were really equal with men, in thought and feeling, but since the origins of human society, woman had voluntarily kept this secret from man in order to protect her children and to flatter men as food-gatherers and defenders of the family. This arrangement was out of date and it was time to speak out the truth 'so long and religiously upheld'. James wrote a complicated reply, suggesting that the history was more involved than that. Women may have had a card up their sleeve, but 'indirectly they were in the game, through an effect upon men and through a limit to their separateness from them...to which I suggest you don't do justice'. James goes on to say that the Robins 'card' is the way things are going, that it's bound to happen, 'part and parcel of the whole current drift of things' and that when it comes '...the thing will be enormously interesting. Only all the novels will become bad thereby – all yours and mine, or at least all the novelists; and the new ones, poor things, will have to learn a new trade altogether'.[25] Robins nonetheless consulted James about her play *Votes for Women* that same year before she published it as a novel entitled *The Convert*.

The neurasthenia novel *A Dark Lantern* has the heroine Katharine Dereham, a poet who has worked too hard, take to her bed, especially after she has refused suggestions of an extra-marital affair with a Prince Anton Waldenstein. She burns the midnight oil by reading a lot and sees a variety of doctors 'and learned by that sure means to believe herself very ill'.[26] Distressed at the same time by her father's illnesses, her knowledge of some of his deviant ways, and the possibility that they shared some kind of identity and fate, all further consultations make her steadily weaker. At last she decides to give the rest cure a chance and encounters Dr Garth Vincent. Vincent is rude to his patients, cuts off Katharine's mail, only allows unproblematic, light reading, makes his hired nurses curt and sour: at one point he finds a patient's dinner hidden up a chimney, rescues it and makes the (female) patient eat it. The nurse tells Katharine that this worked well and that after leaving the nursing home this particular patient married and had a baby.

Now all this might make one concur with Henry James's anxieties about the 'novel of the future', except that Robins makes Vincent liberal with regard to writing; has him express the view that the reason 'neurasthenia had the foremost nations in its grip' was that 'people spend more and more every year on mere movement', that even the poor imitate the journeys of the rich and the 'essential unrest' was the same. When Vincent asked Katharine where she lived, she replied 'London'. At which point Vincent reeled off all the other places she had lived and told her she had never stopped anywhere for more than twelve months. Hence the rest cure. Robins shows Vincent to be high-handed, eugenist, insistent on countering the patients wishes – on massage for example – and a fully paid up creator of dependence. But Robins then turns the Ibsenite screw: in an argument, Katharine reveals that she had no wish to have been Prince Anton's lover and had not been. Vincent says it were better for her had she given in, since she had not had the sense to marry. When the doctor and the patient visit the countryside in spring, as the cure begins to work, Katharine has a question to ask the doctor based on a question she asked herself 'What is it I have lacked? A man'.[27] After sex, after spring and after marriage to the doctor in the summer, there is a powerful scene of the doctor-husband breaking down the door to Katharine's room after a quarrel. But as Elaine Showalter rightly notes, he is 'clearly meant to represent life-giving passion...and not rape or violation of her spirit. Although Robins's novel is lurid and sentimental, it shows that even for feminists the rest cure might have had creative and sexual advantages'.[28] Something of the urgency and radicalism of Robins's neurasthenic scenes can be sensed when recalling Virginia Woolf's reaction to the novel after reading it at one sitting. Woolf speaks of the novel's 'morbidity' and says: 'It explains how you fall in love with your doctor if you have a rest cure. She [Robins] is a clever woman, if she weren't so brutal.'[29]

It would be wrong to make too much of a novel published by Heinemann and written by an American as part of an account of public perceptions of neurasthenia in Britain. But the connections that Robins makes with the rest cure and with the abuse that it allowed are of interest, because the return of the will and the power of the will allows the heroine to make the doctor part of the cure. Outside marriage, at least in the first place and - despite its sentimental ending – very unsentimental about the rest cure itself. The rest cure was an opportunity and a safe harbour from the Ibsenite storms of heredity and sexual exploitation. But only because Robins's heroine fights back, seducing the doctor who then breaks down her out of date door.

Later developments

The commercial scale of neurasthenia cures was enormous. To return to the publicity blizzard mentioned at the beginning: pluck some pages from *The Medical Annual: a year book of treatment and practitioners index* (Bristol and London) for 1909 (its twenty-seventh year) and we see sanitoria advertisements for places for inebriety, narcomania, minor mental ailments and then hotels from Bournemouth to Ullapool in Scotland for general neurasthenia. The Peebles Hotel Hydropathic was a 'German Kuranstalt in Scotland' with Nauheim baths and Schott exercises, Weir Mitchell treatment, Turkish baths, Russian baths, brine baths, sulphur baths, douches, electricity vibration, massage, special dieting etc. etc. Such treatments were available in Matlock, Derbyshire, Great Malvern and Harrogate. The class focus here (as with the private mental homes whose advertisements follow) is middle and upper-middle-class, perhaps less affluent than the ones making the journey to Switzerland and Germany. What is not advertised are the psychological methods that developed from the early part of the century. One place where that approach receives a semi-commercial airing is Doris Mary Armitage's *A challenge to neurasthenia* of 1929, 4th edition 1935. Here, Armitage establishes her authorial status on account of having been one of the patients of the Hertfordshire general practitioner Leonard Stewart Barnes. Barnes died in 1927 having practised in the town of Whitwell and Armitage takes up his cause. Always remembering the social distance from here to the Harley Street addresses of Dowse and company mentioned at the beginning and remembering too that even those sympathetic to Freud, such as W.H.B. Stoddart and Bernard Hart were at Bethlem and St Thomas's hospital and in private psychiatric work (Hart worked at Northumberland House, north London where the first Mrs T.S. Eliot was admitted), what does Doris Armitage bring to the story from semi-rural Hertfordshire?

First she speaks from experience. Barnes was trained in medicine and psychotherapy although his actual status was as a surgeon (MRCS) and an LRCP from 1891 at St. Barts. He was a public vaccination and medical officer for the 3rd division of the Hitchin Union; a surgeon to the Odd fellows and Foresters. In 1900 he acted as a police surgeon and from 1905 he was surgeon and physician at the Queen Victoria Memorial Hospital in Welwyn. Barnes received an OBE in 1925 and was also editor of Martin's book on first aid and home nursing. He had an address in Witwell near Welwyn as well as one at 16 South Audley Street, London W1 – part of affluent Mayfair. On neurasthenia his position was simple. Fear was at the root of all neurasthenic troubles. Public perceptions that what was needed was expensive stays in homes and hence the seeing off of a 'nervous illness' missed the point. Fear was the key, to be reached and subdued not by Freudism (one patient, whose gender was not specified came to Barnes precisely because they had received no benefit from psychoanalysis) but by a simple admission that the 'subconscious' was an active agent and that there was 'no idea causing fear or distress to his patient too absurd or trivial for consideration and close analysis'.[29] Armitage had spent two years in a home for neurasthenics and her own observation of patients had helped her see the acumen of Dr Barnes's method. The 'real self' could be summoned and healing begin, especially as Barnes stressed two things. One was the truth of Sir Frederick Treves's maxim, that 'The physician who is able to conceive of a disease not only as his art should show it to him but as it appears to the view of his patient has grasped the foundation of therapeutics'. The other was that general practitioners needed to study neurasthenia because specialists in large towns could not be reached by more than one in a hundred patients.[30] There are the usual statements about diet and exercise and relaxation and once again the political economy metaphor is invoked: quiet times may seem nothing but they are in fact times when 'you are banking credit, which is no small thing'. At the back of the book we see once again an advertisement suggesting the use of the Barnes methods for self-help. There is no mention of sexual neurasthenia and no mention of any psychological core ideas other than fear and the subconscious. As a doctor–patient relationship, Armitage cannot convey the same drama as Robins in her novel. But both sources have something to tell us about the move towards combining the psychological with the somatic as well as contextualising neurasthenia within feminism and non-specialist medicine and more concretely, the accessibility of a general practitioner based psychotherapy as against the costly hydro-hotels, rest cures and visits to metropolitan consultants.

This growing new context for the treatment of neurasthenia is further illustrated by the history of the Lady Chichester Hospital in Hove, Sussex. Founded in 1905 and specialising in the treatment of nervous disorders in poor women and children, the force behind it was Dr Helen Boyle (1869-1957) who pioneered a non-asylum approach to mental disorders in 'borderline' patients. Boyle believed that the asylum could be avoided if cases were treated early enough. Her feminist commitments were illustrated by the election of Elisabeth Garrett Anderson to the vice-presidency of the Hospital – Anderson of course being one of the first women doctors in Britain and the founder of her own hospital. Speaking in 1906 to the Hospital annual general meeting, Anderson singled out the need to deal with the non-affluent neurasthenic patient; they were peculiarly difficult to reach as general hospitals did not admit them and it was not easy to help them properly as outpatients.[31] Further research on such new kinds of small but innovative hospital and the female medical professionals who worked in them may well reveal hitherto unknown and pioneering feminist involvement with neurasthenia as suffered by mostly female and often poorer patients. Lady Chichester Hospital catered exclusively for women and children but it seems likely that a small archipelago of less specifically focused and less professional contexts for neurasthenia treatments have yet to be uncovered. It is intriguing for example that a close friend of the novelist and actress Elizabeth Robins, mentioned earlier was Octavia Wilberforce, a general practitioner also based in Brighton, Sussex. Wilberforce superintended a rest-home for women based at Elizabeth Robins's Sussex farmhouse in the late 1930s. While there is every likelihood this catered for more affluent patients than the Lady Chichester Hospital, it adds another detail to the slowly growing map of feminist and non-hospital based neurasthenic practices. Combined with public perceptions of advertised remedies, future research will open up this 'borderland' between elite neurological clinics, the asylum (both public and private) and the general hospital.

The jury still seems to be out on the sociology of the disease: businessman or housewife? W.S. Playfair at King's may have thought of neurasthenia as strictly confined to women of refinement but also drew lessons from busy hospital wards about the exhaustion of poorer women, the kind of women targeted by Helen Boyle. Rest cures rescued the affluent but not the poor. Meanwhile we see the slow utilisation of psychological approaches within general practice, sometimes – as with Doris Mary Armitage – precisely to enable an approach to the troubles of neither the affluent patient nor the patient admitted to hospital. Add to this the sense that even if Playfair and Allbutt were on a limb within elite practice, the general population might actually know of, experience and seek help for something called 'neurasthenia' and the possibility arises that located between mental illness on one side and serious physical injury or disease on the other, neurasthenia was the people's illness, however precise the medical attempts to isolate, define or discard it. A genuine example of Freud's 'ordinary unhappiness' but experienced by a far larger community than could afford to seek his particular, lengthy and expensive solutions.[32] The everyday nature of this strange exhaustion, this truly social illness was both omnipresent in the advertising press, part of everyday speech and embodied in characters from the popular novel: Sherlock Holmes – thin, cocaine-dependent, sexless, vigilant but anti-social; and Svengali in George du Maurier's massively successful novel *Trilby* of 1894 – the hypnotist, the alien, the Jew, the bringer of a new power to frail Trilby, who was transformed from a mere artist's model to a sublime international concert singer, but only when performing unconscious and hypnotised – a zombie. Trilby must escape Svengali but when she does, she is a nothing, a husk. Both Conan Doyle and du Maurier set their stories in Britain and the Continent and part of the fate of their characters was determined by the new and strange powers that lurked in the one rather than the relative safety, the moderate, cheerful, healthy 'Britishness' of the other.[33] Both Holmes and Svengali entered British public perceptions and public senses of new forms of power and illness, strength and weakness in long-lasting ways.

Notes

1. W.F. Bynum, 'The nervous patient in eighteenth- and early-nineteenth-century Britain: the psychiatric origins of British neurology', in W.F. Bynum, R. Porter and M.Shepherd (eds), *The Anatomy of Madness, 1: People and Ideas* (London: Tavistock, 1985) 89-102; Simon Wessely 'Neurasthenia and fatigue syndromes: clinical section' in G.E. Berrios and R.Porter (eds) *A History of Clinical Psychiatry* (London : Athlone Press,1995), 509–532.

2. D. Dwork, *War is Good for Babies and other Young Children* (London: Tavistock, 1987); Greta Jones, *Social Hygiene in Twentieth Century Britain* (London: Croom Helm, 1986).

3. Michael Neve, 'Degenerationist categories in nineteenth-century psychiatry with special reference to Great Britain', in Y. Kawakita

Michael Neve

(ed.) *History of Psychiatric Diagnoses* (Tokyo: Ishiyaku EuroAmerica Inc., 1997), 141–163.

4. There was no popular perception in Great Britain of working-class patients being beneath the dignity of the condition, although during the First World War some commentators did see neurasthenia as being experienced by officers rather than ordinary soldiers.

5. Chandak Sengoopta's article in this volume makes this point clearly.

6. On Crichton-Browne and his Scottish resistance to the over-pessimistic views of Maudsley and others see Michael Neve and Trevor Turner, 'What the Doctor Thought and Did: Sir James Crichton-Browne (1840-1938)', *Medical History*, 39 (1995), 399–432.

7. General guides to the British situation and to differing pessimisms and optimisms can be found in Janet Oppenheim, *'Shattered Nerves': Doctors, Patients and Depression in Victorian England* (New York and London: Oxford University Press, 1991); Richard A. Soloway, *Demography and Degeneration: Eugenics and the Declining Birth-rate in twentieth-century Britain* (Chapel Hill, London: University of North Carolina Press, 1995); Jose Harris, *Private Lives, Public Spirit: Britain 1870-1914* (Oxford: Oxford University Press, 1994); Dorothy Porter, *Health, Civilization and the State* (London: Routledge, 1999).

8. T.S. Dowse, *On Brain and Nerve exhaustion: Neurasthenia, its Nature and Curative Treatment* (London: Ballière, Tindall and Cox, 1880), 50–51.

9. *Ibid.*, 57.

10. *Ibid.*, 65–69.

11. Andrew Scott Myrtle, 'Neurasthenia – true and false', *Provincial Medical Journal*, 8 (1889), 85.

12. Hugh Campbell, *The Anatomy of Nervousness and Nervous Exhaustion*, fourth edition (London: Henry Renshaw, 1890), 90.

13. Sonu Shamdasani's excellent work suggests the need to jettison the 'psychological' component that I am historically arguing for; my view is that a sexual liberalising physician with a more emphatic sense of the sexual and the psychological is a real historical figure but not one whose authority differed from the moral managerial strictures of the earliest years of the nineteenth century.

14. Robins's novel is discussed by Elaine Showalter in *The Female Malady* (London: Virago, 1987) and further contextualised in some of the letters of Henry James collected in Philip Horne's *Henry James: a life in letters* (London: Allen Lane, 1999). I wish to thank Abigail Bishop for her help with Robins and with related

neurasthenia literature. Despite containing what can only be called 'howlers' – such as believing that Wilhelm Griesinger was a 'well known American physician of the second half of the nineteenth century' (37) the monograph on the vibrator and its pre-history by Rachel P. Maines *The Technology of Orgasm* (Baltimore: Johns Hopkins University Press, 1999) indicates the outlines of future and deeper research.

15. Anon., *The Odo-Magnetic Treatment* (London: Magnetic Health and Appliance Company, 1906).

16. Bernarr MacFadden, *Strength from Eating* (London: MacFadden's Physical Development, 1901).

17. Eugen Sandow, *Neurasthenia and Nervous Diseases* (London: Sandow's Curative Institute, 1921), 5.

18. Richard J. Ebbard, *How to Restore Life-giving Energy to Sufferers from Sexual Neurasthenia* (London: Medical Publishing Co., 1903).

19. *Ibid.*, 59–60.

20. *Ibid.*, 88–9.

21. E. Hopewell-Ash, *Mind and Health* (London: Henry J. Glaisher, 1910).

22. *Ibid.*, 67.

23. On Robins see Angela V. John, *Elizabeth Robins: staging a life* (London: Routledge, 1995).

24. Rupert Hart-Davis (ed.), *Letters of Max Beerbohm 1892-1956* (London: John Murray, 1988), 56.

25. Horne, *op. cit.* (note 14), 451.

26. E. Robins, *A Dark Lantern* (London: Heinemann, 1905), 118.

27. *Ibid.*, 215.

28. Showalter, *op. cit.* (note 14), 143.

29. N. Nicolson and J. Trautmann (eds) *Letters of Virginia Woolf: Volume 1* (London: Hogarth Press, 1996), 43.

30. D.M. Armitage, *A Challenge to Neurasthenia* (London: Williams and Northgate,1929), 34.

31. *Ibid.*, 52.

32. East Sussex Record Office, Lewes, England: boxfile HB63/1A, annual report, November 1906. I am grateful to Dr Trevor Turner for information and data from the medical records of the LCH.

33. Dean Rapp, 'The Early Discovery of Freud by the General Educated British public,1912-1919', *Social History of Medicine*, 3 (1990), 217–43. On Octavia Wilberforce see Hermione Lee, *Virginia Woolf* (London: Chatto and Windus,1996), 733–34. On Trilby see Daniel Pick, *Svengali's Web: the Alien Enchanter in Modern Culture* (New Haven and London: Yale University Press, 2000).

7

Neurasthenia in Wilhelmine Germany: Culture, Sexuality, and the Demands of Nature

Doris Kaufmann

This chapter approaches neurasthenia in Wilhelmine Germany from two different angles. The first part outlines the general context in which neurasthenia gained and lost its special importance in German society.[1] Neurasthenia played a significant role in the psychiatric discourse, it became a tool for expressing discontent and suffering and it served as a fashionable code for the Zeitgeist during the last two decades of the nineteenth and the first decade of the twentieth centuries, only to disappear then from medical and public attention.

The second part of this article asks for the meaning of what was thought to be an important neurasthenic symptom: sexual problems that male patients in particular confessed to their doctors. It investigates the close link between the German discourse on neurasthenia before the First World War and the emergence of a 'sexual question'. This 'sexual question' was produced and followed by the establishment of the new psychiatric field of scientific sexual knowledge. This was one important starting point for psychiatry to claim authority for the order of everyday life. The rise of a sexual reform movement and the occupation of politicians, writers, artists, feminists and 'the public' with the so-called sexual question reflected society's response to this development and demonstrated the struggle over the definition of sexuality and of sexual behaviour.

The coming into being and passing away of neurasthenia in German psychiatry

Neurasthenia's coming into being was a story of an immediate success. George Beard's concept was fully adopted in German psychiatry after 1880. Already contemporary medical contributors to the rising tide of literature on neurasthenia[2] tried to explain this phenomenon. One of the repeatedly mentioned reasons was Beard's bold deed of having finally presented a disease entity that covered a broad range of symptoms, already existing various descriptions, names and set of ideas and assumptions on nervous illness.[3] Furthermore, contemporary doctors appreciated the distinct 'clinical picture' of neurasthenia that enabled them to draw a clear line at mental disease. This especially helped them to quieten their neurasthenic patients who were usually very frightened to become mentally ill or get mixed up with insane persons.[4] According to the medical debate on neurasthenia another consequence of Beard's concept was that persons suffering from hypochondria and hysteria now joined the camp of neurasthenics and were partly responsible for their increasing number. Although even the small guide books on how to recognise and to treat neurasthenia written by and for medical practitioners always reserved some space for discussing the differences between neurasthenia and hysteria, the similarities between these so-called functional neuroses clearly prevailed.[5] The discourse of mainstream psychiatry – in spite of Charcot's 'discovery' of male hysteria and later of Freud's studies – did not markedly differ from the common non-medical assumption that neurasthenia and hysteria were mixed-gender twins. Hysteria was mainly reserved for women and the lower-classes – linked from the beginning with a 'hereditary psychopathic personality' – and neurasthenia for the male members of the middle-classes plus some nice and well-behaved women from this very strata who should be spared the diagnosis of hysteria, although several psychiatric writers expected an increase of female neurasthenics should women be dragged into the '*Kampf ums Dasein*' (struggle for survival).[6]

Most medical authors agreed that neurasthenia was a condition close to health. In fact it became quite common to point to the 'floating border' between health and nervous illness.[7] But this image only underlined what seemed to have been the most important outcome of the adoption of Beard's concept of neurasthenia: its establishment as a 'real' serious disease within the whole psychiatric scientific community.

In 1883, Dr Holst, a physician from Riga, complained that there had been no place for neurasthenia in neuropathology before Beard. He hoped that functional neuroses would no longer be treated as step-children in science and that the gap between medical research and the practical needs of doctors and patients would be closed or at least diminished.[8] This gap existed, he explained, because of the different access of psychiatrists to patients who suffered from functional neuroses. Bowing to the academic establishment Dr Holst wrote that the university clinics and hospitals certainly represented the place where scientific progress was achieved, but neurasthenic patients did not go there because of their middle-class background and visited physicians with a private practice like him instead.

Apart from that there remained another problem: academic 'exact' research used to dismiss 'subjective complaints of patients' instead of making them an object of scientific inquiry. So, according to Holst, it was left for practitioners to find a way to analyse these 'subjective expressions' of their patients in an objective, i.e. scientific manner. Holst's self-confidence as well as his critical stance were no exception. Obviously Beard's concept of neurasthenia gave some assurance to practitioners about their importance as the decisive group of doctors who were confronted with the vast number of patients they could now at least provide with a consistent and accepted psychiatric diagnosis. Additionally, the somatic explanation of neurasthenia as exhaustion and over-stimulation of the central nervous system that could be traced in damaged nerve tissue was sufficient to build a theoretical bridge to the brain-oriented academic neurological and psychiatric community in Germany and to pave the way for more attention to functional neuroses. As a further consequence clinical psychiatric research came under criticism for failing to adequately examine the whole patient with all his of her expressions of suffering.

In 1896, Otto Binswanger, professor of psychiatry and director of the psychiatric university clinic in Jena, admitted in his textbook *Die Pathologie und Therapie der Neurasthenie* (On the Pathology and Therapy of Neurasthenia) that psychiatric clinical research might have been focused too much on the study of 'objectively detectable' symptoms, only paying attention to physical and chemical reactions and microscopic methods.[9] Other approaches to the examination of patients had been underestimated. Therefore Binswanger wanted to draw his students' attention to the importance of 'subjective' symptoms. As long as the physio-pathological basis of neurasthenia remained indeterminate, psychiatrists should try to gain as much experience as possible through observation of the intellectual and affective disorders which were characteristic of functional neuroses.[10] At the end of his book Binswanger felt obliged to give his students some advice about how to handle their future neurasthenic patients, namely with firmness, persuasive power and with caution. In any case, they should avoid spending unnecessary effort on 'the not small number of neurasthenic slowcoaches who use their ailments as a welcome excuse to get rid of all duties and who cannot be shaken out of their poor way of life'.[11] Professor Binswanger's remarks are significant in two aspects: first, the psychiatric elite had opened a door to the investigation of 'non-objective' symptoms and second, the chances of the new and expanding neurasthenia-market for psychiatry had been realised.

While neurasthenic patients remained a minority in the developing system of state-run public psychiatric hospitals and university clinics, that were mainly filled with poor patients suffering from severe mental disorders,[12] a growing number of middle and upper-class neurasthenics visited the practices of doctors who specialised in nervous diseases replacing the internists who had been previously consulted. This development clearly supported and promoted the discipline formation of psychiatry.[13] Also very important was the emergence of a profitable neurasthenia business around the new establishment of private clinics, including water-cure clinics, spa-clinics, and sanatoria from the 1880s till the First World War.[14] In a medical publication 500 private clinics for nervous diseases were listed for the year 1900.[15]

At the end of the nineteenth century an initiative led by the famous neurologist Paul Möbius fought for the setting up of clinics for working-class patients (*Volksnervenheilstätten*) who suffered from neurasthenia as a result of the worsening working conditions due to the rapid changes of industrialisation.[16] These clinics were meant to be financed by patrons and health insurance companies; some were indeed established. Connected to the hygiene-movement the activists for *Nervenheilstätten*, mostly social reformers and social-democratic physicians, 'democratised' neurasthenia by extending this diagnosis to the lower-classes. Thus they tried to include them in the official medical institutions and treatment.[17] Behind this 'democratisation' stood the demand to broaden the psychiatric investigation to the worker's way of living and everyday life. From the end of the nineteenth century onwards psychiatry as an institutional system and field of knowledge gained a decisive role in interpreting the social crisis phenomena that accompanied German industrialisation in terms of medical illness. Psychiatry became the key science for criminal anthropology and criminal justice and it influenced the eugenics movement as well as the German state's social welfare activities.

This impact of psychiatry and its establishment as a cultural authority before 1914 can only be explained against the background of two developments: first, the growing importance of natural sciences and of the process of handing over to scientific experts the job of identifying and solving problems caused by social crisis in general[18] and second, the development and early separation of psychoanalysis and related approaches as a distinct field of knowledge that covered the so-called psychogenetic, functional neuroses. This 'division of labour' within psychiatry meant also a broader acceptance of psychoanalysis in scientifically-oriented psychiatry than is usually assumed.[19] This does not mean acceptance here in the sense of professional acknowledgement, but refer to the implicit and sometimes also explicit handing over of a particular field of nervous disorders to the psychoanalytic approach. This development became very obvious during the First World War in the German-speaking countries when the interpretation and responsibility for the so-called war neurotics or war hysterics shifted to psychoanalysis.[20] This process already started under the umbrella of the discourse on neurasthenia in Wilhelmine Germany.

Beard's concept presumed an organic cause of neurasthenia. Not only did the afflicted patients cling to this assumption, but most of the medical literature dwelt more-or-less at length on this topic. It unfolded the idea of a relationship between a damaged central nervous system and the demands of modern life on a very general level, only then to continue with what really interested most writers and their readers, namely the medical experience with different methods of treatment. Ultimately, positive results could all be ascribed to the required strong personality of the psychiatric doctor who had to act as adviser and leader towards a better, healthy, emotionally-balanced economic and rational life. The practical therapeutic proposals physicians provided their readers with, corresponded to the ideas of the life-reform movement, such as fresh air, sports, no tight clothing, light food, a regular daily working schedule.[21] Though displaying great sympathy for the neurasthenic overstrained 'brain-worker' and less for his female counterpart, the well-off, idle woman suffering from lack of work, medical authors usually spent little effort on exploring the brain–nerve culture connection more concretely. Psychological phenomena – especially the great suggestibility of the patients – played an increasingly dominant part in the debate. It fitted into this picture that prominent psychiatrists pointed to the great adaptability of the brain – in the double sense as material and as organ of the mind - to cultural and historical change.[22] Consequently they underlined the cultural, technological and scientific progress of mankind in general and of the German Empire in particular.[23] The pessimistic thesis of the growing number of mentally ill in present society as an indication of general decline was rejected. Oswald Bumke, professor of psychiatry, wrote in 1912 that their actual increase in numbers

Doris Kaufmann

should rather be connected to the growing professional impact of psychiatry, to its broader capacity of observing, diagnosing and interpreting mental disorders and to its improved institutional presence.[24]

After the turn of the century a psychological explanation of the causes of neurasthenia and hysteria in the psychiatric discourse came to prevail. Hidden damage to the central nervous system was thought to play a role only in traumatic neuroses. This manifested itself after combined physical and mental shock and was observed particularly after railway accidents.[25] The underlying causes for an outbreak of neurasthenia and hysteria in contrast were thought to be due to an hereditary or acquired 'psychopathic constitution'; social factors were dismissed.[26] Certain behaviour, labelled before as neuropathic or hysterical symptoms, became a personal reaction not clearly distinguishable from health, but judged to be characteristic mainly of psychopathic *'Minderwertige'* (persons of inferior value) whose willpower was not properly formed, as Emil Kraepelin wrote in 1913.[27] Professor Kraepelin, who in 1917 became first director of the *Deutsche Forschungsanstalt*, the prestigious research institute for psychiatry in Munich and whose revision of psychiatric diagnosis is still in use, incorporated the symptoms of neurasthenia and hysteria into the description of psychosis.[28] That meant that neurasthenia and hysteria lost their status as independent disease entities in scientific research, which focused on the elucidation of the connection between physiological and psychic functions and functions of the brain. Medical occupation with neurasthenia shifted to the investigation of the border area between 'normal' and 'pathological' emotional behaviour and affective processes.[29] So the area for psychiatric investigation and intervention was extended to basically all expressions of personal life and everyday problems. In the following part, the connection between the discourse on neurasthenia and the emergence of a 'sexual question' in Wilhelmine Germany as an important example of this process will be investigated.

Neurasthenia and the 'sexual question'

In 1908, Sigmund Freud published an article whose title *Die 'kulturelle' Sexualmoral und die moderne Nervosität* ('Civilised' Sexual Morality and Modern Nervous Illness) offered a special explanatory context for modern nervousness.[30] Referring to the actual psychiatric discourse on neurasthenia, Freud criticised some of the prominent protagonists – Wilhelm Erb, Otto Binswanger, Richard von Krafft-

166

Ebing – for their rather general and unspecific description of the connection between modern times and neurasthenia. Freud accused them to neglect neurasthenia's most important aetiological cause: the damaging repression of sexual life through culture and its sexual morals. Though the psychiatrists Freud quoted in his article did certainly not fully share his opinion of the sexual aetiology of neurasthenia and certainly rejected his earlier broader *Drei Abhandlungen zur Sexualtheorie* (Three Essays on the Theory of Sexuality)[31] published in 1905, Freud's picture of the psychiatric disregard of the harmful impact of social conditions and cultural ideas on sexual life in the discourse on neurasthenia is rather misleading. Not only the authors mentioned in his *Sexualmoral* integrated the theme of sexual ailments as symptoms as well as cause into their concept of neurasthenia and offered ideas about the 'nature' of sexuality and its relation to culture. This topic was from the beginning extremely visible and stayed in the centre of psychiatric and public attention. Starting with Beard, psychiatrists and neurologists also wrote special books on *Sexualleben und Nervenleiden* (Sexual Life and Nervous Ailments), to quote the title of a successful publication by Dr L. Löwenfeld.[32]

Michel Foucault has argued that sex as a field of knowledge was constructed in the second half of the nineteenth century especially by psychiatrists who interpreted and defined the normality and the pathology of sexual behaviour by medicalising the sexual confessions people were driven to give.[33] Indeed, according to Professor Binswanger for example, the psychiatric consulting rooms were overcrowded with:

> patients of both sexes who complained about symptoms in the genital sphere, lamenting in epic length or in a secret, shy manner, and displaying the great importance of these phenomena for them.

Binswanger noticed further that mainly male neurasthenics loved 'to observe their sexual emotions and sexual life meticulously, to brood about it, and then to ask their doctors whether or not their sexual functions conformed to the norm'. He advised his students,

> to calm down such fearful persons and to strengthen their self-confidence, for clinical investigation often shows that the complaints about their exaggerated or reduced sexual activity are unfounded.[34]

How was the bodily and mental awareness or perception of the individual - of his or her pain and suffering - linked to the medical discourse? The discourse on neurasthenia provided a set of cultural tools, that means a cultural reservoir of images and of patterns of language and behaviour that could be used by persons who suffered and were discontented with their life. Especially the growing importance of medical experts and of psychiatric explanation of social phenomena in the German Empire suggests its increasing adoption and significance for patients to frame their suffering. There existed a twofold process. On the one hand psychiatry constructed and in a way produced neurasthenia, for instance through the new genre of the neurasthenic case study with sexual ailments at the centre. On the other hand our historical subjects, the many persons who expressed their distress in the language of neurasthenia, lived in a specific historical context which they formed but which also caused them distress – both are apparent in the discourse on neurasthenia.

Now to briefly return to Binswanger's remark that male patients were anxious whether or not their sexual life conformed to the norm and turned to psychiatric doctors for assurance. It was there where middle-class men who believed that something was wrong with their sexual life could go, talk and request help. The big umbrella of neurasthenia provided a medical framework for their 'subjective' difficulties as doctors liked to call them. Their problems appeared in the medical literature as nervous impotence, *ejaculatio praecox, spermatorrhoea* and sensitive disorders of the sexual organs. These ailments were explained along the already-introduced line of over-stimulation and exhaustion or weakness of the nervous system and were thought to cause immense depression and to make fearful, insecure individuals.[35] The many case histories of neurasthenic patients Joachim Radkau presents in his book on German nervousness,[36] also confirm that patients very often emphasised their anxieties of being unable to fulfil professional and sexual expectations, both closely linked in their narratives.

The idea of sexuality – or, in Richard von Krafft-Ebing's words of 'the psychology of love' – as a measurable process of anatomical and physiological substrata[37] obviously gained ground in late-nineteenth-century Germany and found its way into individual awareness, at least of the educated social strata, and into public debate. The emergent field of sexology,[38] whose representatives were mainly psychiatrists who treated neurasthenic patients in their practices or clinics, laid down fundamental tenets: that sexual life was the most powerful cause of individual happiness or of pathology, that sexual functions and behaviour had to follow the demands of health and nature, and that social circumstances that blocked such a scheme had to be reformed, also in the wider interest of racial hygiene.

But what was characteristic of a 'normal' sexual life? And consequently, how could sexual neurasthenia, as it was sometimes labelled, be prevented? These questions needed an answer, and they became an important topic in the medical literature on neurasthenia that contained a central statement about the different cases of wrong sexual behaviour. The violation of the 'economy' of sexuality, i.e. the failure to establish a balance between production and consumption of the energy of the nerves, would always result in nervous illness. This was true for sexual excesses as well as for sexual abstinence. Though there were some doctors who believed in a hereditary 'immoderate' *libido sexualis* like the psychiatrist and sexologist Freiherr von Schrenck-Notzing, who saw neurasthenia as the first step on the way to 'abnormal' psychopathic sexual behaviour,[39] others judged the substance and manifestations of the sexual drive as dependent on external social circumstances which 'fed or suppressed it'.[40] Under the subtitle 'Sexual life and nervous illness' in his book on *Nervousness and Culture* psychologist Willy Hellpach, for example, characterised his era as one of change in sexual matters.[41] The capitalist culture offered a whole host of sensory stimuli, especially in big cities, without providing satisfaction, he wrote. This situation put the nervous system that as a further consequence of the Zeitgeist had also become increasingly refined permanently at risk. For Hellpach the age of abstinence and prudishness had finally gone; as indicator he mentioned the increase of extramarital sexual intercourse. Hellpach and his colleague psychiatrists, occupied with sexual neurasthenia, all more or less agreed that this was essentially a positive development, because the (male) sexual desire was a powerful force and should be fulfilled in the interest of a sound nervous system. But here they confronted a problem.

The change in sexual behaviour, Hellpach mentioned, was indicated by an increase of prostitution and of illegitimate children. The danger for men to pay with syphilis for their nerves' health was very present in the literature on neurasthenia and sexuality. Additionally, the campaigns of the abolitionist groups of the German women's movement after the turn of the century led to a certain public attention to the social problems that forced women into prostitution, to their abuse and to common sexual hypocrisy (*Doppelmoral*).[42] As a training ground for sexual practice Hellpach therefore openly proposed the less dangerous '*Verhältnis*',[43] an already existing institution that meant a relationship of·an unmarried young upper-class and upper middle-class man with a lower-middle-class woman before his marriage. Hellpach's suggestion, certainly an expression of what the leader of the German Abolitionists called '*Herrenmoral*' (master's morality),[44] reflected a demographic development. An early marriage had become rather impossible for middle-class men – still the main subject of the discourse on neurasthenia – for a career and a promotion demanded many years of education and service with a limited income.

Though especially the single male was the first candidate for suffering from the symptoms of sexual neurasthenia[45] – a single woman was supposed to be able to cope much better with abstinence – after marriage the sexual life of a couple did not always become a satisfying one, according to the contemporary discourse on neurasthenia. The psychiatric literature declared that especially the most often used measure to take precautions, *coitus interruptus*, caused nervous disorders and led to neurasthenia.[46] Doctors who wrote about this topic generally supported birth control - more and more common in the educated middle-classes after the turn of the century, when the two-children-family started to gain acceptance.[47] Dr Löwenfeld approved of 'the wish to maintain an orderly and appropriate living for the family in the face of more-or-less limited means'.[48] But the same author criticised that mostly women often suffered from the particular preventive measure of *coitus interruptus* because it denied them sexual satisfaction, only producing constant sexual tension without release; the fear of getting pregnant also added to the danger of getting neurasthenia.[49] The medical discussion of *coitus interruptus* brought women's sexuality for the first time prominently into the discourse on neurasthenia. Cautiously, doctors conceded them a *libido sexualis* and some criticised men for egoistic sexual behaviour.[50] These 'feminist' tendencies – psychiatrists had obviously gained from treating neurasthenic patients – became very apparent when Dr Dornblüth even counted the development of middle-class women's employment among the advances of the German Empire:

> The disorders especially of nervous origin that had been serious and widespread among those women of the educated middle-classes, whom need had forced into the teaching professions some decades ago, are now gone. Women do have the same right to education and achievement like men.[51]

Other psychiatrists on the contrary saw in this very development and in other issues connected with the women's movement the opening up of a dangerous field: the eroding of gender boundaries, that had to be prevented at all costs.[52] Dr Freiherr von Schrenck-

Notzing[53] for example made clear that the question of neurasthenia and sexuality was by no means only a 'technical' one of properly working reproductive organs, but a question of the constant establishment and reestablishment of the gender order. The 'traditional' division of labour and the two distinct female and male '*Geschlechtscharaktere*', i.e. the allegedly innate character traits including (hetero)sexual behaviour should be maintained. Starting in childhood, education had to prevent that the individual developed a so-called inverted sexual instinct, for it could already have a pathological meaning if boys liked 'female' activities and girls 'male' activities like horseback riding, hunting and studying academic books.

If the realm of the sexual question therefore contained the much broader space of the gender order including the teaching of the 'appropriate' gender roles, then the task for psychiatrists in their own opinion was obvious. They had to be scientific advisors in sexual matters and related fields that ultimately covered almost the whole area of everyday life problems. Neurasthenic symptoms were a good starting point for this psychiatric claim because they were a widespread culturally accepted language or phenomenon and belonged into the border area between 'normal' and 'pathological' emotional behaviour.

Such psychiatric reasoning initiated and influenced the different branches of the sexual reform movement from its beginning. Prominent members and supporters came from the psychiatric profession like the sexologists Max Marcuse, Iwan Bloch, Leo Löwenfeld, Sigmund Freud and August Forel. In the name of science, the sexual reform movement fought for the reform of social conditions and juridical laws that repressed individual sexual self-determination and prevented a healthy sexual life.[54] This was expressed for example by Helene Stöcker, leader of the radical feminist League for the Protection of Motherhood and Sexual Reform (*Bund für Mutterschutz und Sexualreform*), which propagated a new morality (*Neue Ethik*) centred around the demand for women's equality in their freedom to determine and enjoy their sexual life and which postulated sexual education in schools, availability of contraceptives, legalisation of abortion, recognition of 'free marriages', and state support of unmarried mothers and illegitimate children. In 1905, she wrote in a programmatic article *On the Reform of Sexual Morality*:

> Nowadays, when the higher goal of mankind is no longer oriented to the next world, to distant eternity, but towards our own life and

the way to make it worth to be lived forever, we do need to find a morality that could lead us now to this highest goal. To it all *Wissenschaften* (the sciences and humanities) have to help us, for it had been the *Wissenschaften* which had proved the old morality and *Weltanschauung* untenable and damaging.[55]

This opinion was not shared by all participants in the debate on the sexual question. The major part of the German women's movement regarded the idea of free love based and justified by sexual science as failing to consider the social circumstances women had to cope with. Women (and men) should not be forced to follow natural instincts and scientific laws in order to prevent serious nervous damage, but should live according to a 'morality of responsibility' (*Verantwortungsethik*) and follow an own individual set up of values (*Wertsetzung*).[56]

Conclusion

The attempt of these critics of the sexual reform movement - the latter in our case represented by the radical part of the German women's movement led by Helene Stöcker - to change the frame of reference from science back to (feminist) politics had little chance to succeed in the long run. The further historical development shows that social movements and political parties would continue to use the growing authority of *Wissenschaft*, especially of science, to support and justify their demands for change. The discourse on neurasthenia in Wilhelmine Germany shows that scientific concepts became an important cultural tool and language to express individual discontent and suffering. Moreover, the discourse on neurasthenia promoted different developments for psychiatry as an institutional system and a field of knowledge like the general discipline formation, the division of labour between brain-oriented psychiatry and psychoanalytic approaches, the emergence of a new psychiatric field of sexual knowledge and the widening of the psychiatric sphere into everyday life.

Notes

1. For an overview, see J. Radkau, *Das Zeitalter der Nervosität. Deutschland zwischen Bismarck und Hitler* (München: Hanser, 1998); V. Roelcke, *Krankheit und Kulturkritik. Psychiatrische Gesellschaftsdeutungen im bürgerlichen Zeitalter 1790-1914* (Frankfurt/Main: Campus, 1999), 101–179; Andreas Steiner, *Das nervöse Zeitalter. Der Begriff der Nervosität bei Laien und Ärzten in*

Deutschland und Österreich um 1900 (Zürich: Juris, 1964).

2. See, for instance, the extensive bibliography of literature on neurasthenia in F.C. Müller (ed.), *Handbuch der Neurasthenie* (Leipzig: Vogel, 1893), 1–18.

3. Müller mentions 11 different names in Germany alone before Beard's term neurasthenia took over, *ibid.*, 37.

4. See E. Shorter, *A History of Psychiatry. From the Era of the Asylum to the Age of Prozac* (New York: John Wiley & Sons, 1997), on the renaming of psychiatric institutions (*Irrenanstalten*) which became clinics for nervous diseases (*Nervenkliniken*), quoted from the German translation *Geschichte der Psychiatrie* (Berlin: Fest, 1999), 181–3.

5. For example T. Dunin, *Grundsätze der Behandlung der Neurasthenie und Hysterie* (Berlin: Hirschwald, 1902).

6. F.C. Müller, 'Die Uebergangsformen der Neurasthenie in psychische Erkrankungen und die strafrechtliche Verantwortlichkeit der Neurastheniker', in *Handbuch der Neurasthenie, op. cit.* (note 2), 212–60, here 238f.

7. See, for example, O. Binswanger, *Die Pathologie und Therapie der Neurasthenie. Vorlesungen für Studierende und Ärzte* (Jena: Gustav Fischer, 1896), 32.

8. V. Holst, *Die Behandlung der Hysterie, der Neurasthenie und ähnlicher allgemeiner functioneller Neurosen* (Stuttgart: Enke, 1883), 3–8, also for the following.

9. O. Binswanger, *op. cit.* (note 7), 1f. Cf. F. Schiller, *A Möbius Strip: Fin-de-siècle neuropsychiatry and Paul Möbius* (Berkeley: University of California Press, 1982), 69ff.

10. O. Binswanger, *op. cit.* (note 7), 3.

11. *Ibid.*, 371.

12. D. Blasius, *'Einfache Seelenstörung'. Geschichte der deutschen Psychiatrie 1800-1945* (Frankfurt/Main: Fischer, 1994), 64–79.

13. E. Shorter, *op. cit.* (note 4), 129, refers to the outstanding number of 1400 German physicians specialised in psychiatry in 1911.

14. J. Radkau, *op. cit.* (note 1), 107–21; E. Shorter, 'Private Clinics in Central Europe 1850-1933', *Social History of Medicine*, 3 (1990), 159–95.

15. Quoted by J. Radkau, *op. cit.* (note 1), 107.

16. P. Möbius, *Ueber die Behandlung von Nervenkranken und die Errichtung von Nervenheilstätten* (Karger: Berlin, 1896); J. Radkau, *op. cit.* (note 1), 107–21.

17. For this context, see A. Labisch, *Homo Hygienicus. Gesundheit und Medizin in der Neuzeit* (Frankfurt/Main: Campus, 1992), 164–87;

Doris Kaufmann

E. Shorter, *Moderne Leiden. Zur Geschichte der psychosomatischen Krankheiten* (Reinbek: Rowohlt, 1994), 377–9 (German translation of *From Paralysis to Fatigue. A History of Psychosomatic Illness in the Modern Era*, New York: The Free Press, 1992).

18. L. Raphael, 'Die Verwissenschaftlichung des Sozialen als methodische und konzeptionelle Herausforderung für eine Sozialgeschichte des 20. Jahrhunderts', *Geschichte und Gesellschaft*, 22 (1996), 165–93.

19. See also H. Decker, 'The Medical Reception of Psychoanalysis in Germany, 1894-1907: Three brief studies', *Bulletin for the History of Medicine*, 45 (1971), 461–81.

20. See D. Kaufmann, 'Science as Cultural Practice: Psychiatry in the First World War and Weimar Germany', *Journal of Contemporary History*, 34 (1999), 125–44; for a broad analysis P. Lerner, *Hysterical Men: War, Neurosis and German Mental Medicine, 1914-21* (Columbia University, Ph.D. thesis, 1996).

21. For example W. Wilke, *Nervosität und Neurasthenie und deren Heilung. Vom naturwissenschaftlichen Standpunkt aus bearbeitet* (Hildesheim: Borgmeyer, 1903); T. Dunin, *op. cit.* (note 5); *Handbuch der Neurasthenie*, chapter 9, containing nine articles on therapy, 260–584.

22. F.C. Müller, 'Geschichte', in *Handbuch der Neurasthenie*, 19-50, here 22.

23. See O. Bumke, *Über nervöse Entartung* (Berlin: Springer, 1912), 83ff.; O. Dornblüth, *Die Psychoneurosen. Neurasthenie, Hysterie und Psychasthenie. Ein Lehrbuch für Studierende und Ärzte* (Leipzig: Veit, 1911), 386.

24. O. Bumke, *op. cit.* (note 23), 97ff.

25. See, for example, E. Fischer-Homberger, *Die traumatische Neurose. Vom somatischen zum sozialen Leiden* (Bern: Huber, 1975); H.-P. Schmiedebach, 'Post-traumatic neurosis in nineteenth-century Germany. A disease in political, juridical and professional context', *History of Psychiatry*, 10 (1999), 27–57.

26. On this shift, see V. Roelcke's article in this volume.

27. E. Kraepelin, 'Über Hysterie', *Zeitschrift für die gesamte Neurologie und Psychiatrie*, 18 (1913), 261–79; already containing his later judgement, idem, 'Die Diagnose der Neurasthenie', *Münchener Medicinische Wochenschrift*, 49 (1902), 1641–4.

28. See the relevant chapters in the nine editions of Kraepelin's textbook *Psychiatrie*, which appeared between 1883 and 1927; cf. M. Micale, 'On the "Disappearance" of Hysteria. A Study in the Clinical Deconstruction of a Diagnosis', *Isis*, 84 (1993), 496–526.

174

29. For example O. Dornblüth, *op. cit.* (note 23).
30. S. Freud, *Das Unbehagen in der Kultur - und andere kulturtheoretische Schriften* (Frankfurt/Main: Fischer, 2000), 109–32.
31. *Idem, Drei Abhandlungen zur Sexualtheorie* (Frankfurt/Main: Fischer, 1999).
32. G. Beard, *Die sexuelle Neurasthenie, ihre Hygiene, Aetiologie, Symptome und Behandlung* (Vienna: Toeplitz und Deuticke, 1885); L. Löwenfeld, *Sexualleben und Nervenleiden. Die nervösen Störungen sexuellen Ursprungs* (Wiesbaden: Bergmann, second edition 1899). On Löwenfeld's reception of Freud's work, see H. Decker, *op. cit.* (note 19).
33. M. Foucault, *Sexualität und Wahrheit. Vol. I: Der Wille zum Wissen* (Frankfurt/Main: Suhrkamp, 1977).
34. O. Binswanger, *op. cit.* (note 7), 266 (for all quotations).
35. R. von Hösslin, 'Symptomatologie', in *Handbuch der Neurasthenie*, 87–190: **180**.
36. J. Radkau, *op. cit.* (note 1).
37. R. von Krafft-Ebing, *Psychopathia sexualis* (München: Matthes & Seitz, 1993), Introduction to the first edition 1886, III-IV.
38. For a comparative perspective, see R. A. Nye, 'The History of Sexuality in Context: National Sexological Traditions', *Science in Context*, 4 (1991), 387-406; R. Porter and L. Hall, *The Facts of Life. The Creation of Sexual Knowledge in Britain, 1650-1950* (New Haven: Yale University Press, 1995).
39. F. von Schrenck-Notzing, 'Die psychische und suggestive Behandlung der Neurasthenie', in *Handbuch der Neurasthenie*, 518-84, here 522f.
40. O. Dornblüth, *op. cit.* (note 23), 172.
41. W. Hellpach, *Nervosität und Kultur* (Berlin: Räde, 1902), 159-83.
42. A. Pappritz, *Einführung in das Studium der Prostitutionsfrage* (Leipzig: Barth, 1919).
43. Hellpach, *op. cit.* (note 41), 167f.
44. A. Pappritz, *Herrenmoral* (Leipzig: Frauen-Rundschau, 1903).
45. R. v. Hösslin, 'Aetiologie', in *Handbuch der Neurasthenie*, 62–86: 67.
46. *Idem*, 85; F.C. Müller, 'Geschichte', in *Handbuch der Neurasthenie*, 19–50: 46; O. Dornblüth, *op. cit.* (note 23), 400ff.; L. Löwenfeld, *op. cit.* (note 32), 116ff.
47. See P. Marschalk, *Bevölkerungsgeschichte Deutschlands im 19. und 20. Jahrhundert* (Frankfurt/Main: Suhrkamp, 1984), 53ff.
48. L. Löwenfeld, *op. cit.* (note 32), 119.
49. *Ibid.*, 125ff.; O. Dornblüth, *op. cit.* (note 23), 397ff.
50. *Ibid.*, 404ff.

51. *Ibid.*, 386. Cf. Elizabeth Lunbeck, *The Psychiatric Persuasion: Knowledge, Gender, and Power in Modern America* (Princeton: Princeton University Press, 1994) for a similar process in the United States of the 1920s.

52. For the general context, see Ute Planert, 'Antifeminismus im Kaiserreich: Indikator einer Gesellschaft in Bewegung', *Archiv für Sozialgeschichte*, 38 (1998), 93–118; J. C. Fout, 'Sexual Politics in Wilhelmine Germany: The Male Gender Crisis, Moral Purity, and Homophobia', *Journal of the History of Sexuality*, 2 (1992), 388–421. A good example for antifeminism from the literature on neurasthenia is W. Wilke, *op. cit.* (note 21), 102ff.

53. F. v. Schrenck-Notzing, *op. cit.* (note 39), 529ff.

54. Cf. R. A. Nye, *op. cit.* (note 38); J. C. Fout, *op. cit.* (note 52); M. Jansen-Jurreit, 'Sexualreform und Geburtenrückgang. Über die Zusammenhänge von Bevölkerungspolitik und Frauenbewegung um die Jahrhundertwende', in A. Kuhn/G. Schneider (ed.), *Frauen in der Geschichte* (Düsseldorf: Schwann, 1979), 56–81.

55. H. Stöcker, 'Zur Reform der sexuellen Ethik', in M. Jansen-Jurreit (ed.), *Frauen und Sexualmoral* (Frankfurt/Main: Fischer, 1986), 110–18. On Stöcker and the Mutterschutz League, see R. J. Evans, *The Feminist Movement in Germany 1894-1933* (London: Sage, 1976), 115–143; Ann Taylor Allen, 'German Radical Feminism and Eugenics, 1900-1908', *German Studies Review*, 11 (1988), 31–56.

56. See the publications by Marianne Weber, leader of the major 'moderate' branch of the feminist movement and Helene Stöcker's main opponent within the women's movement, e.g. M. Weber, *Frauenfragen und Frauengedanken. Gesammelte Aufsätze* (Tübingen: Mohr, 1919); *idem, Die Ideale der Geschlechtergemeinschaft* (Berlin: Herbig, 1929).

8

Electrified Nerves, Degenerated Bodies: Medical Discourses on Neurasthenia in Germany, circa 1880-1914

Volker Roelcke

The decades between 1880 and 1914 were decisive in the formation of psychiatry as an academic discipline in Germany: around 1880, the field represented an important factor of public order in the service of state authorities, and at the same time a sphere of institutionalised reflection on the dangers to the bourgeois self. However, only very few university departments of psychiatry existed, and within the curriculum of medical schools the subject became obligatory only in 1906. Compared to most disciplines of somatic medicine, psychiatry could not draw on the 'cultural capital' ascribed and the financial resources allocated to the new laboratory sciences, such as physiology and bacteriology. Most of the representatives of psychiatry lamented about the missing consensus on terminologies, classification, and therapeutic procedures for the postulated mental disorders. In contrast, for the period around 1910, a theoretical and institutional consolidation may be diagnosed. This consolidation was associated with a strong orientation towards the natural sciences and somatic medicine, and also with plausible answers to concerns of the public on the strains and health hazards of life in 'modern', industrialised society. The subspecialty of neurology, which during this time also emerged in particular from internal medicine, was for the time being integrated into psychiatry.[1]

Within these three decades, the concept of neurasthenia as formulated by Beard (1869 and 1880) experienced a rapid career which is closely related to the developments in psychiatry. Furthermore, it is indicative of the public demand for professional interpretation of individual discomforts and social concerns. In this perspective, the discussions on the concept of neurasthenia are inseparable from the broader debates on the relationship between life in 'modern' civilisation, and health.

The following chapter will reconstruct this story, subdividing it into three stages. First, the intellectual and institutional resources for this career as present in the last decades of the 19th century will be sketched. The second part describes the early use of the neurasthenia-concept up to the early-1890s when the debate focused on frequent individual pathology strongly associated with the electrophysiology of the nervous system. During the third stage, the concept of neurasthenia converged with notions of heredity and degeneration, suggesting the collective pathology of the nation.

Intellectual and institutional resources

An ensemble of intellectual and institutional factors constituted the disposition that contributed to the rapid reception of the concept of neurasthenia in Germany.

Amongst the intellectual resources, three elements appear to be of particular relevance: the 'electrification' of the nervous system during the preceding decades of the 19th century; the combination of this perspective with the idea of limited energy reservoirs of an individual's body; and the availability of the category of 'neuropathic disposition' applicable to states of discomfort situated between health and disease.

Between circa 1830 and 1880, the work of physiologists and clinicians such as Hermann Helmholtz, Emil Du Bois-Reymond, Guillaume Duchenne, and finally the brain stimulation experiments by Eduard Hitzig and Gustav Fritsch, established a consensus about the importance of electricity for the functioning of the nervous system. Alongside with this, for the public, the manifold uses of electricity in the newly industrialised and urbanised world suggested the importance of this medium of energy for all kinds of processes associated with 'modern' life. Thus, during the last decades of the 19th century, it seemed very plausible and in accordance with the results of the most advanced sciences to understand the nervous system as a set of interrelated pipes and fibres activated by electrical impulses and energetic streams floating from the centre (brain) to the periphery (nerves and organs), and back.[2]

Similarly, the concept of the conservation of energy in a closed system had been legitimised by results of physics and physiology, and had a considerable plausibility through experiences in everyday life. The formulations of the two laws of thermodynamics around 1850 by Helmholtz, Julius Robert Mayer, and Rudolf Clausius found a prominent public reception in particular from the 1880s onwards when the initial hopes in the unlimited potentials of industrialisation began to be succeeded by reflections on the prize of this process for the 'human motor', and its physical economy.[3] Applied by Beard to the nervous system, the idea was that expenditure of the limited amounts of energy in one area of the body would result in the inability to meet needs in others. Increased mental activity by the demands of hectic commercial life, or by biologically weak and untrained women would thus lead to an excessive consumption of 'nerve force' in the brain, and consecutive loss in the periphery, resulting in fatigue, or various somatic symptoms.[4] Withdrawal from the settings of overriding demands, a balanced diet, baths, and electrical stimulation of the nerves would help to restore the reservoir of energy.

A third resource, perhaps most specific for the German speaking context, was the medical category of 'neuropathy', or 'neuropathic disposition' as introduced by Wilhelm Griesinger. This category referred to all those disorders with transient mental and physical discomforts which were the result of an interplay between hereditary and environmental factors. The core pathogenic feature was - according to Griesinger - an 'irritable weakness' (*reizbare Schwaeche*) of the nervous system. This condition led to manifest symptoms only in those individuals who were exposed to the demands of 'modern' bourgeois society, i.e. those who, 'well-educated and with thorough culture of their mind (*mit sorgfältiger Geistesbildung*), but without much financial resources have to rely upon a regular return of their only capital, their mental faculties and capacities'.[5] The category of 'neuropathic disposition', already introduced in the first edition of Griesinger's classical textbook in 1845,[6] received an aetiological underpinning after the publication of Morel's *Traité des Dégénérescences* in 1857: the notion of degeneration was immediately picked up in the second edition, albeit in a very specific version. It was stripped of its sociopolitical, moral, and collectivist aspects that from the outset had dominated the trajectory of the concept in France and other European societies.[7] Instead, it was used in a narrow sense to indicate the hereditary aetiology of individual pathology.[8] In this individual-centred meaning, the notion of degeneration was applied first to states of 'neuropathic dispositions', to become an increasingly more generalised aetiological substitute for most neuro-psychiatric categories in the generation of psychiatrists following Griesinger.[9]

Amongst the institutional factors contributing to the career of 'neurasthenia', the introduction of outpatient departments at university hospitals, and the establishment of private clinics for

'nervous' patients was probably the most important aspect. The case
of the Charité in Berlin may illustrate this point. In his negotiations
with the university of Berlin in 1864, Griesinger had made the
establishment of an outpatient clinic for psychiatric and 'nervous'
patients a necessary condition for his acceptance of the
professorship.[10] This allowed him to get access to those individuals
who suffered from minor, transitional complaints which were not
covered by the conventional categories of insanity, or madness, and
who were usually not amongst the clientele seen by those
psychiatrists working in the asylums. This group of sufferers
overlapped with those labelled 'neuropathic'. Griesinger was
interested to have this new 'material' at hand both for teaching and
research purposes.[11] This decision directed the focus of attention of
psychiatrists, in particular within university settings, to the group of
well-educated, socially integrated middle-class individuals who later
were to become the prime target, interested audience, and reservoir
of active participants in the discourse on neurasthenia. Parallel to this
shift of attention, private institutions for the in-patient treatment of
this clientele were established throughout central Europe, with
particular concentration in the surroundings of urban centres, such
as Berlin, the Rhineland, or Vienna.[12] Thus, there existed a social
space and a cultural plausibility for both patients and physicians to
present and negotiate the ill effects of modern urban life on mind
and body, and to find relief in specialised institutions.

A sociological model of individual pathology

At this point, it may be useful to recall that Beard's notion of
neurasthenia represented a predominantly sociological conceptualisation of disease causation. His electrophysiological model of
the nervous system, equalling the requirements of life in modern
civilisation with applications drawing energy from a battery,
suggested as the core mechanism of pathogenesis an interaction
between a strenuous environment, and the individual concerned. For
patients as well as physicians, this model offered the opportunity to
focus their explanations on the multitude of phenomena supposedly
characteristic for the way of life in the most advanced stages of
modern civilisation. Whereas in previous psychiatric theories,
'civilisation' regularly turned up as one causative factor amongst
many, and valid not for a specific, but in general for all mental
disorders, it was now upgraded as the most important single cause of
the specific condition of neurasthenia.[13] In contrast to Beard's lengthy
considerations on the individual's social environment, the ideas of

heredity, and of degeneration were only of marginal importance to his conceptualisation. Interestingly, the term degeneration is used quite inconsistently in both *Nervous Exhaustion*, and *American Nervousness*. In the latter, Beard talks about the 'cerebral degeneration' of old age, without any context of hereditary disposition, or a progressive pathology across generations.[14] In the introduction to the chapter on causes, Beard even uses the term in exactly the opposite way as set out in Morel's theory. Elaborating on the 'nature' of American society, he evaluates 'the activity and the force of the very few [civilised Americans]' as a desirable, but endangered phenomenon: 'if, through degeneracy, the descendants of these few revert to the condition of their not very remote ancestors, all our haughty civilisation would be wiped away'.[15] Thus, in this context, civilisation is depicted as artificial, but also as a positive achievement. The representatives of modern civilisation, the college educated inhabitants of big cities, are particularly active and sensitive, but not degenerated. Degeneration is identified with the loss of the mark of civilisation, sensitivity, and with an undesirable return to historically earlier states where individuals were physically stronger, but characterised by intellectual and emotional coarseness. Thus, in contrast to Morel and his followers like Magnan, for Beard the process of degeneration does not result in mental and physical impairment, but is associated with pre-modern life and physical rigour.

It is exactly the 'original' conceptualisation of Beard focused on the electrophysiology of the nerves and on the sociology of the disorder which was apparently most attractive in the initial phase of reception in Germany after 1880, whereas from the mid-1890s onwards, the aspect of degeneration (in Morel's reading), and the hereditary component in the causation of neurasthenia gained increasing importance. This is not to say that there was a clear-cut first stage of the reception in which the historical actors exclusively drew on the electrophysiological paradigm, followed by another clearly demarcated stage only focusing on the concept of degeneration. Rather, the development might be understood as a continuously ongoing shift of plausibilities, and expectations towards the medical category of neurasthenia, a shift correlated with developments within the professional field, but also in the wider public sphere.

Beard himself repeatedly stated, that his ideas had fallen on particularly fertile ground in Germany.[16] His own explanation for this had to do with the state of medical sciences, and especially electrotherapy, which he – together with many of his contemporaries – perceived as particularly advanced in Germany.[17] Proclaiming a positive resonance of his theories amongst the German scientific community may thus be interpreted as a strategy to advance his credibility and scientific standing in the American context.

But in addition to Beard's own remarks, there is complementary evidence from German sources about the great attractiveness of his concept of neurasthenia. His monograph from 1880 was translated in 1881 and went through three editions until 1889. The posthumous edition of Beard's Sexual Neurasthenia (1884) was also translated in the following year, and received similar attention in the professional journals. As early as 1893, a *Handbuch der Neurasthenie* appeared in print. It was introduced by an eighteen-page, small print bibliography on the subject.[18]

One of the key figures in the early reception was Wilhelm Erb, professor of internal medicine in Leipzig, later in Heidelberg, and one of the protagonists in the emerging fields of neurology and electrotherapy. Beard had visited Erb on his tour to Europe in 1879, and appreciated Erb's remarks on 'neurasthenia spinalis' in his chapter on the spinal chord in Ziemssen's *Handbuch der speciellen Pathologie und Therapie* (1878).[19] In return, Erb never failed to credit Beard with the 'discovery' and theoretical conceptualisation of neurasthenia.[20] In his 1882 *Handbuch der Elektrotherapie*, Erb devoted one chapter to the new disorder. According to him, neither the multitude of complaints presented by the eloquent patients, nor the clinical examination allowed a clear diagnosis of the disease, and in particular the differentiation from 'true' structural neuropathological states with an observable morphological substratum. It was only the 'objective' language of the electrode which allowed to distinguish between the structural lesions of neuropathology, and the functional disturbances attributed to neurasthenia. In coherence with the 'electrical' nature of the disorder, Erb was convinced of the value of electrotherapy in treating neurasthenia. Further, electricity was the feature which allowed a differentiation from another related, and ambiguous condition, hysteria, since this was not amenable to electrotherapy.[21]

Paul Julius Möbius, another neurologist in Leipzig and editor of the influential review journal *Schmidt's Jahrbücher der gesammten in- und ausländischen Medizin*, also identified the human 'nerve force' with the current of an electric machine, and nervousness with the flickering of an electric bulb in an overloaded electrical circuit.[22] The frequency of neurasthenia he saw as 'directly proportional to the height of civilisation' which might therefore be counted as 'the main cause of nervousness'.[23]

In the early-1890s, Erb outlined not only the medical, but also the political dimensions of the condition when he delivered a public lecture for the opening of the academic year. It was titled 'On the growing nervousness of our times' (*Ueber die wachsende Nervosität unserer Zeit*), and addressed the relationship between social conditions and the occurrence of nervousness, and neurasthenia. Similar to Beard, Erb stressed the nervous system as the central organising constituent and functional structure of the human body.[24] Its understanding would also reveal the pathogenesis of neurasthenia (which he perceived as the more severe form of nervousness). Erb considered degeneration not as a relevant mechanism, and even did not mention it as an explicit term. The admittedly massive dangers of modern 'culture'[25] put those individuals at risk (in each generation anew), who were exposed to the hectic life in urban centres. Similar to Beard, he listed urbanisation, railway traffic and steam power, telegraph and telephone amongst the most important characteristics of this life, and the foremost causes of the condition. Another prominent factor was the highly competitive world of industry and commerce with its crises,[26] an echo of the various drawbacks in Germany's struggle for gaining a leading position in the international economy.

According to Erb, the nervous system's ability to adapt to new challenges, and the progress of the sciences justified hopes that the challenges posed by nervous exhaustion would be kept under control in the future.[27] The idea of interventions in the realm of procreation, e.g. in form of marriage restrictions, is explicitly rejected.[28] This implies, however, that Erb accepted a hereditary component in the causation of the disorder. Indeed, following a Lamarckian conception, he assumed that the acquired hypersensitivity of the nervous system might create a 'nervous disposition' that in turn could be inherited by the next generation.[29] However, Morel's idea of a progressive deterioration of the germ plasma is completely absent in Erb's texts, as is the focus on alcohol or other material substances harmful for the genetic outfit. The hint to the possibility of an unspecific hereditary disposition for neurasthenia made it possible to link the concept to the discourse of degeneration which went into a new stage during these years. But before addressing this development, another difference between Beard and Erb is worth mentioning: it concerns the way in which 'modern life' is politically evaluated.

As one of the factors contributing to the condition, Erb points to 'the coming up of completely new socialist ideas of the state which threaten to upset all existing order, and confuse the dull minds of the masses'.[30] Neuropsychiatric arguments are now used to classify the liberal idea of participation in political life as potentially hazardous. Instead, military service is evaluated as 'a beneficial remedy for the nervous system'.[31] It is the authority of the nation state, and the Kaiser, that will have to guarantee the protection of the endangered youth, and carry through a paternalistic social policy to combat the increasing health risks.[32]

The gradual shift from the paradigm of external causation to heredity and degeneration, and from a sceptical to a rather pessimistic evaluation of the future, is well illustrated in the case of Richard von Krafft-Ebing, professor of psychiatry in Graz, later in Vienna. In his first text on the topic in 1883, he presented a number of cases of 'transient alienation' that he attributed to neurasthenic states. The causation of these states was 'obvious' to him: the patients had no history of alcohol abuse, trauma, or syphilis, and no constitutional 'burden' (*Belastung*). They rather suffered from previous 'mental or physical overburdening'.[33] In a more comprehensive treatise *On healthy and diseased nerves* (*Ueber gesunde und kranke Nerven*, 1885), he argued that nervous weakness was the hallmark of a whole generation, and that this weakness found its expression in a widely prevailing timidity. Such a generalised condition was associated with a 'deteriorating constitution of the masses'.[34] However, Krafft-Ebing pursued this collectivising approach to the phenomenon not in a systematical matter at this stage.

Ten years later, in a further treatise, Krafft-Ebing focused his aetiological considerations on the 'pathological disposition of the nervous system', resulting in a 'neuropathic constitution'. The hereditary aspect of the condition was now summarised by using the notion of degeneration. According to the author, 'it is legitimate to estimate the hereditary factor [in the causation of the disorder] to about eighty per cent.'[35] His argument included the inheritance of acquired states of nervousness, and the toxic effects of alcohol for the following generations. In contrast to this, the paradigm of electrophysiology remained completely marginal.

Interestingly, during this first stage of the discussions on neurasthenia, the concept was put forward mainly by representatives of the new field of neurology emerging particularly from internal medicine, like Erb, Möbius, and Ziemssen. They were successful in using the new category to make an inroad into the potential patient population that since Griesinger's time had been claimed to be within the sphere of competence of psychiatrists. However, psychiatrists also used the opportunity to access a wider clientele and to stabilise or increase their public and academic standing. New outpatient clinics for 'disorders of the nerves' were set up at universities, and private clinics created ample facilities for the diagnosis and treatment of the new disorder.[36] Amongst the methods of therapy, the rest cure propagated in particular by Weir Mitchell and introduced to Europe by Playfair found little resonance. Electrotherapy in the form of faradisation was among the foremost means advocated. Here again, physicians with a background in physiology could rely on extensive experiences both in university and private practice settings.[37] Other treatments recommended were bromides for symptomatic relief, and in particular the withdrawal from the strenuous environment, if possible to mountain or seaside spas.[38] The many private and (from the 1890s onwards) also public institutions for nervous individuals offered a broad range of therapies. However, foremost among them was the therapeutic application of water in the form of cold showers and baths. It was no coincidence that Franz C. Müller, the editor of the *Handbuch der Neurasthenie*, was also editor of the journal *Archiv der Hydrotherapie und Balneotherapie*, and director of a private institution for disorders of the nerves.

Degenerated bodies

From the beginning of the 1890s, the public discussions about the consequences of urbanisation, industrialisation, and the issues related to the political impact of the rapidly increasing labour forces began to develop a new quality. Whereas before, a discourse of pragmatic social reform, and paternalistic humanitarian activities dominated the public arena, now the immediate challenges were not any more seen as problems of social policy, but as indicators of a fundamental crisis of bourgeois culture.[39] This development was related to an increasing disillusion amongst the *Bildungsbürgertum* about the possibilities of political participation, in a situation when the Prussian government had successfully launched an informal coalition between the small group of wealthy industrialists, and the aristocratic big landowners, and when on the other hand, the labour movement gained rapidly in momentum.[40] Now, traditional norms and paradigms of interpretation, like the notions of Bildung and Kultur, came increasingly under attack from two sides: the propagators of the public importance of the natural sciences, and the representatives of a pessimistic critique of bourgeois values, and civilization. The enthusiastic reception of the philosophy of Nietzsche and Schopenhauer, and the immediate success of the physician and journalist Max Nordau's pessimistic two volume essay Degeneration are indicators of these developments.[41]

During this time, the key figure in psychiatry was Emil Kraepelin, whose career between 1880 and 1914 took him from the post of an assistant at a provincial mental asylum to the chair of psychiatry and directorship of a newly designed hospital at the University of Munich. Kraepelin reformulated psychiatric theory and disease categories with an apparent coherence and immediate plausibility for his contemporaries. At the same time, he also contributed to the restructuring of psychiatric institutions following the needs of quantitative empirical research, and to the reshaping of the discipline's public image fitting the expectations of Wilhelmine society and state authorities.[42]

In his *Compendium of Psychiatry* (1883; the first edition of his later Textbook) Kraepelin reformulated the structure of nosology by attempting to organise all disease entities according to their supposed causation. In addition, he reorganised the intrinsic structure of aetiology: external causes, and amongst them somatic causes, were now placed first in the chapter on general aetiology.[43]

From the outset, Kraepelin had declared that his central aim was to create a nosology that would provide a basis for successful prognosis, therapy, and prevention. Using the experimental design of contemporary laboratory psychology, and the principle idea of bacteriology (monocausality) as a model, Kraepelin concluded that psychiatry could only develop an equally powerful approach if clinical features were sorted out and grouped together in such a way that a common underlying cause could be assumed. In addition, this cause - which was to be focused on as the organising principle of nosology - had to be accessible to manipulation in a way similar to the germs identified by Louis Pasteur and Robert Koch.[44]

The new nosology as outlined in the *Compendium* was as yet only programmatic in character. The actual disease categories described here were still the conventional ones, constituted generally by their symptomatology. It was only in the later editions of the textbook that the postulated diseases which had emerged from empirical research conformed to the pre-empirically outlined categorical boundaries. They were the result of a research strategy selectively directed towards assumed disease entities which were constituted by specific causes and a distinct pathological anatomy. As a matter of fact, Kraepelin's theoretical reorientation towards the laboratory sciences shaped not only his further conceptualisations, but also the structure of institutionalised discourse and practice in his department. For example, when Kraepelin had taken over the chair of psychiatry in Munich in 1903, he organised regular internal discussions and public seminars on a number of topics which he enumerates in his autobiographical notes: histopathology, questions of heredity and degeneration, metabolism and serology.[45] As a result of this theoretical reorientation and the ensuing research strategy, the psychiatric tradition inaugurated by Kraepelin was dominated by a somatic-biological perspective, whereas the biographical-psychological and the socio-cultural dimensions were marginalised. Psychopathological phenomena were conceived to be the expression of discrete nosological entities, with specific somatic causes, clinical features, and pathological anatomy.

What were the consequences of this nosology for Kraepelin's conceptualisation of neurasthenia? In the *Compendium* of 1883, Kraepelin described neurasthenia as one of the 'functional neuroses' all of which had in common 'functional' alterations of the nervous tissue. This was in agreement with the prevailing theory which assumed that these alterations were material in character, but that it was not yet possible to identify them with the available methods.[46] In 1881, the German translation of Beard's monograph had been published, and - as mentioned before - in the following two decades, publications on neurasthenia as the result of modern life became almost a literary genre, elaborating on the influence of various social factors on mind and body. But in contrast to these considerations of the social factors contributing to the aetiology of the condition, Kraepelin kept firmly to his programme which implied to look for disease entities constituted by a specific somatic cause. The result was that in the 5th edition of his *Textbook* (1896), neurasthenia as a distinct entity had disappeared. Clinical phenomena which previously had been attributed to neurasthenia were now scattered abroad: they only showed up as asides or subheadings in two newly constructed and completely different disease categories: 'insanity of degeneration' (*Entartungsirresein*), and 'disorders of exhaustion' (*Erschöpfungszustände*). Whereas the first condition was - according to Kraepelin – due to degeneration, a particular form of heredity (see below), the second disorder was conceived as being caused by physical exhaustion or mental excitation, which in turn would have its effects by way of an intoxication through the accumulation of the products of catabolism. The pace and irritations of modern life, and their psychological implications, were mentioned in passing; but 'since we shall not be able to remove these general causes, it is our task to make the coming generations strong and resistant and to prepare them for the struggle for existence [*Kampf ums Dasein*]'.[47] Thus, the social causes of the condition were explicitly set aside, and intervention in the form of prevention was to concentrate on the (physical) strength of the potentially affected individuals. This was to be achieved by physical exercise in youth, abstinence, and political measures to guide or restrict marriages according to assumed hereditary disposition.[48]

The dismantling of the category of neurasthenia was continued by Kraepelin in an article published in 1902. Here, he conceded retaining the label, if at all, for conditions of physical exhaustion with neurological and psychopathological manifestations - the 'disorders of exhaustion' outlined in the textbook.[49] Although other authors, arguing from different points of view, also criticised the vague boundaries and the inflationary use of the nosological category,[50] none of them had explicitly shrugged away the social dimensions in the causation and symptom formation of the condition.

But Kraepelin even went one step further: Being himself concerned with the ambivalences of life in a rapidly changing world, he began interpreting behaviour and institutions which did not correspond to his traditional outlook on societal life as consequences of degeneration, i.e., of quasi-biological laws. The first instances of this sort of interpretation can be identified in the publications about his journey to south-east Asia in 1903, in which he set out his ideas for a 'comparative psychiatry'.[51] Kraepelin made considerable efforts to fit all phenomena with which he was confronted into his own nosological categories which implied a priority of biological over social variables. Thus, deviations from the clinical pictures with which he was familiar Kraepelin interpreted as consequences of the different nutrition, climate, and racial attributes in the region. For example, the scantiness of delusions (in patients identified by Kraepelin as suffering from dementia praecox) he attributed to a racially determined deficiency of psychological differentiation of both the affected individuals and their culture.[52] Kraepelin also assumed that the peculiarities of indigenous religion and culture might in the future better be understood as expression of racial characteristics.[53]

In this view of Kraepelin, social variables had no place in the aetiology and nosology of psychiatry, but – on the contrary – were themselves more and more seen as determined by biological processes. The interpretation of social life in terms of Darwinian biology was, of course, not novel at this time. In Germany, by the turn of the century, the ideas of Social Darwinism had mainly been propagated by biologists, representatives of hygiene, economists, and politicians.[54] Within the psychiatric profession, Kraepelin was among the first to take up these arguments and in particular to apply biologically based psychiatric categories not only to individuals, but also to social groups and institutions.

The specific assumptions of Kraepelin's approach to social phenomena had also their impact for his contribution to the debate on the relation between life in modern society and the occurrence of 'functional neuroses'. This contribution is formulated in a paper 'On Degeneration' (1908) and in the publications about his experiences abroad. Here, Kraepelin identified a bundle of medically relevant features of modern civilisation: the increased frequency of insanity including the 'functional neuroses', an increase in the suicide rate, the decline in the birth rate, and a rapid spread of sexual 'aberrations'.[55] The main thrust of Kraepelin's argument was to explain these characteristics as results of the process of degeneration. He emphasised in particular the role played by alcohol and syphilis as toxic agents to the 'germ'. These two factors he conceived as the main threat to the individual's, and, more important, to the nation's genetic pool. In contrast to Morel, Kraepelin (together with most of those of his contemporaries who adopted the theory of degeneration for their conceptualisations) did not assume a necessary link between increasing degeneration and decreasing fertility of the affected families. Whereas according to Morel, degeneration would thus be a self-limiting process, Kraepelin believed that the degenerated individuals were more likely to contribute to the spread of the hereditary evil, with their alleged tendency to uncontrolled and promiscuous sexual behavior, and their inability to live within the rules of convention. The new serological method for the diagnosis of syphilitic infection apparently confirmed Kraepelin's already earlier existing assumption and worries about the high prevalence of the infection.[56]

Thus, as perceived by Kraepelin, degeneration was a condition not limited to a small segment of the population, but one that threatened an ever-increasing proportion of the whole nation.[57] This logic allowed him to diagnose not only individuals but social groups or even the whole nation as suffering from degenerative conditions. He arrived at the conclusion that to counteract the 'undoubtedly threatening dangers', urgent 'measures' had to be taken. Since no efficient therapy was available, Kraepelin advocated a preventive strategy: the fight against alcohol and syphilis, and 'sensible racial hygiene'.[58] To assess the current state of affairs first, large-scale investigations into questions of the epidemiology and heredity of the degenerative disorders should be undertaken.[59] Welfare programmes were seen by Kraepelin as highly dubious since they secured the survival and longevity of individuals and populations of 'low value' and thus were likely to result in the deterioration of the genetic pool, an idea he had already formulated in the *Compendium* of 1883.[60]

Kraepelin's contribution marked a turning point in the whole debate: it implied a major shift in the focus of concern, namely from the social origins of a disease that affected individuals (neurasthenia), to the biological processes that threatened the collective 'culture' or 'folk body' (degeneration). Neurasthenia was now a category still in use in medical teaching, everyday medical practice, and in the context of health policy and administration. But it had vanished from the agenda of contested issues in theoretical debates of the discipline. Heredity and degeneration substituted it as the central questions of the field.

Kraepelin's propositions triggered off a debate which focused the presuppositions of his theory of disease entities, as well as his arguments about the impact of heredity, and the 'nature' of degeneration.[61] His ideas developed in this context were also the starting point of a long-term research programme in psychiatric genetics carried through by Kraepelin's pupil Ernst Rüdin which found widespread acclaim in the international scientific community, but also resonated with the aims of the racial hygiene movement, and the later health policy of Nazi Germany.[62]

In regard to the specific concept of neurasthenia, Kraepelin had as a matter of fact just given a sharp and authoritative formulation of the most recent state of the professional debates. Even authors sympathetic with sociological interpretations of the disorder, like Max Laehr, agreed with Kraepelin that the term indicated not any specific disease, but rather a group of syndromes; that the hereditary component was the one most discussed in recent literature on its aetiology; and that analyses on the disorder's impact for the national economy were deserving more interest than conceptual or clinical considerations.[63] Indeed, the medical aspects of neurasthenia were not any more discussed in psychiatric or neurological journals around 1910 (in contrast to the two decades between 1880 and 1900). Instead, the heredity of psychiatric disorders, and the more specific question about the continuity or transformation of inherited ills gained rapidly in importance: was it only the general disposition for disorders of the brain that was inherited? Was it possible that the offspring of nervous degenerates were predisposed to develop other forms of insanity? A further question discussed in relation to neurasthenia was its apparently increasing use in cases of simulation, thus causing a massive financial burden to health insurance and the general economy.[64] With these issues, psychiatrists had managed to link their debates to the ongoing discourses in somatic medicine and the laboratory sciences, and to the concerns of the public and the state authorities. This does not imply that the concept of neurasthenia was not used any more in psychiatric practice: on the contrary, it was still a widely used category in doctor–patient interactions, both in private practices and various sorts of clinics and sanatoria,[65] and finally in the official statistics of the Reich (cf. the contributions by Radkau and Schmiedebach in this volume).

Conclusion

The professional debates about neurasthenia in the decades following 1880 are an integral part of the broader discourse on the relationship between life in 'modern' civilisation and health hazards. Whereas during the first years after the 'discovery' of neurasthenia, the concept was interpreted predominantly in the context of an electrophysiological paradigm, and not necessarily linked to the discussions about heredity, and degeneration, this changed during the last decade of the century. Professional discourse and public debates converged to build up a dynamic that led to a marked change in the conceptualisation of the relationship between 'modern' life and health: the focus of the discussion shifted from the social causes of a disease that affected many individuals, to the biological processes that threatened the collective 'culture', or nation. Now, neurasthenia became one of a number of disorders perceived as the result of degeneration, which in turn was understood as a biological phenomenon. Parallel to this, the aspect of prevention gained in importance, complementing and eventually superseding the former recommendations for rest, and the application of hydro- and electrotherapy. The preventive measures proposed were rigid public health strategies against alcohol and syphilis (two main factors which supposedly triggered off the degenerative process), and marriage restrictions to preclude the procreation of those already affected by hereditary conditions.

The interpretations and suggested interventions by contemporary physicians did not only reflect scientific discussions and public concerns of the time, but in turn reinforced pessimistic 'diagnoses' about the threat to the German 'culture' and nation, and later served to legitimate far reaching decisions both in the realm of politics, and scientific institutions which had considerable impact for the next decades of German history. However, the reconstruction of these developments is beyond the scope of the present paper.

Notes

1. *Cf.* Hans-Heinz Eulner, *Die Entwicklung der medizinischen Spezialfächer an den Universitäten des deutschen Sprachgebietes* (Stuttgart: Ferdinand Enke, 1970), 257–282; Eric J. Engstrom, *The Birth of Clinical Psychiatry: Power, Knowledge, and Professionalization in Germany, 1867-1914* (unpublished Ph.D. thesis: University of Chapel Hill, North Carolina, 1997); *Volker Roelcke, Krankheit und Kulturkritik. Psychiatrische Gesellschaftsdeutungen im bürgerlichen Zeitalter, 1790-1914* (Frankfurt/M.: Campus, 1999), esp. 101–79.

2. *Cf.* Christoph Asendorf, *Ströme und Strahlen. Das langsame Verschwinden der Materie um 1900* (Berlin: Anabas, 1989); and Roelcke, *op. cit.* (note 1), 101–11.

3. *Cf.* Anson Rabinbach, *The Human Motor. Energy, Fatigue, and the Origins of Modernity* (New York: Basic Books 1990); Maria Osietzki, 'Körpermaschinen und Dampfmaschinen. Vom Wandel der Physiologie und des Körpers unter dem Einfluß von Industrialisierung und Thermodynamik', in Philipp Sarasin and Jakob Tanner (eds), *Physiologie und industrielle Gesellschaft. Studien zur Verwissenschaftlichung des Körpers im 19. und 20. Jahrhundert* (Frankfurt/M.: Suhrkamp, 1998), 313–46.

4. George M. Beard, *A practical treatise on nervous exhaustion (neurasthenia), its symptoms, nature, sequences, treatment* (New York: W. Wood, 1880), 10-11.

5. Wilhelm Griesinger, 'Ueber Irrenanstalten und deren Weiter-Entwickelung in Deutschland', *Archiv für Psychiatrie und Nervenkrankheiten*, 1 (1868), 8–43: 13.

6. Wilhelm Griesinger, *Die Pathologie und Therapie der psychischen Krankheiten* (Stuttgart: Adolph Krabbe, 1845), 117–8.

7. *Cf.* Daniel Pick, *Faces of Degeneration. A European Disorder, c. 1848-1918* (Cambridge: Cambridge University Press, 1989).

8. Wilhelm Griesinger, *Pathologie und Therapie*, 2nd, rev. ed. (Stuttgart: Adolph Krabbe 1861), 162–3, 211–3.

9. *Cf.* Roelcke, *op. cit.* (note 1), 96–100.

10. Wilhelm Griesinger, 'Vortrag zur Eröffnung der Klinik für Nerven- und Geisteskrankheiten in der Königl. Charité in Berlin' (1866), in *Gesammelte Abhandlungen*, vol. 1, ed. by Carl August Wunderlich

(Berlin: Hirschwald, 1872), 107–26; *cf.* also Engstrom, *Psychiatry,* ch. III.

11. Engstrom, *op. cit.* (note 1), ch. III.
12. Edward Shorter, 'Private Clinics in Central Europe, 1850-1933', *Social History of Medicine,* 3 (1990), 159–95.
13. George M. Beard, *American Nervousness. Its Causes and Consequences* (New York: G. Putnam's Sons, 1881), vi. In this context, the notion of 'disease of civilization' was coined: cf. Roelcke, *op. cit.* (note 1), ch. 5.
14. Beard, *op. cit.* (note 13), 27.
15. *Ibid.,* 97.
16. *Ibid.,* Preface, xiv, 8, 11; George M. Beard, *Die sexuelle Neurasthenie, ihre Hygiene, Aetiologie, Symptomatologie und Behandlung* (Wien: Töplitz und Deuticke, 1885), 8.
17. For this widely shared image, *cf.* e.g. Thomas N. Bonner, *American Doctors and German Universities. A Chapter in International Intellectual Relations* (Lincoln: University of Nebraska Press, 1963).
18. George M. Beard, *Die Nervenschwäche (Neurasthenie),* ihre *Symptome, Natur, Folgezustände und Behandlung,* (Leipzig: F.C.W. Vogel, 1881); Beard, *op. cit.* (note 16); Franz Carl Müller (ed.), *Handbuch der Neurasthenie* (Leipzig: F.C.W. Vogel, 1893).
19. Beard, *op. cit.* (note 13), 11; *cf.* Wilhelm Erb, 'Krankheiten des Rückenmarks und seiner Hüllen', in Hugo Ziemssen (ed.), *Handbuch der speciellen Pathologie und Therapie,* Bd. 11, 2. Hälfte (Leipzig: F.C.W. Vogel, 1878), 389–403.
20. *Cf.* e.g. Wilhelm Erb, *Ueber die wachsende Nervosität unserer Zeit* (Heidelberg: J. Hörning, 1893), 10, 22.
21. Wilhelm Erb, *Handbuch der Elektrotherapie* (Leipzig: F.C.W. Vogel, 1882), 201-3, 572; cf. also Andreas Killen, 'Influencing Machines. Electrotherapy and Neurosis in Nineteenth Century Germany', in Eric Engstrom, Matthias M. Weber, Paul Hoff (eds), *Knowledge and Power. Perspectives in the History of Psychiatry* (Berlin: VWB, 1999), 131–41.
22. Paul J. Möbius, *Die Nervosität* (Leipzig: Weber, 1882), 86.
23. *Ibid.,* 23, 86; similar Hugo von Ziemssen, *Die Neurasthenie und ihre Behandlung* (Klinische Vorträge, 7. Vortrag) (Leipzig: F.C.W. Vogel, 1887), 3.
24. Erb, *op. cit.* (note 20), 4.
25. Erb preferred the term 'culture' to 'civilisation'; on the contemporary use of the two terms, cf. Jörg Fisch, 'Zivilisation, Kultur', in Otto Brunner, Werner Conze, Reinhart Koselleck (eds), *Geschichtliche Grundbegriffe,* vol. 7 (Stuttgart: Klett-Cotta, 1992), 679–774.

26. Erb, *op. cit.* (note 20), 6–7.

27. *Ibid.*, 38

28. *Ibid.*, 32–3.

29. *Ibid.*, 21.

30. *Ibid.*, 5, 7.

31. *Ibid.*, 36.

32. *Ibid.*, 34–7.

33. Richard von Krafft-Ebing, 'Ueber transitorisches Irresein auf neurasthenischer Grundlage' (1883), in *idem, Arbeiten aus dem Gesamtgebiet der Psychiatrie und Neuropathologie*, vol. I (Leipzig: Johann Ambrosius Barth, 1897), 13.

34. Richard von Krafft-Ebing, *Ueber gesunde und kranke Nerven* (Tübingen: Laupp 1885), 7.

35. Richard von Krafft-Ebing, 'Nervosität und neurasthenische Zustände', in Hermann Nothnagel (ed.), *Handbuch der speciellen Pathologie und Therapie*, vol. XII, part 2 (Wien: Alfred Hölder, 1895), 16.

36. One indicator for the emergence of the new field was the launch of the journal *Neurologisches Centralblatt* in 1882, founded by the Berlin Privatdocent Emmanuel Mendel (director of a private nervous hospital), with various representatives from internal medicine (Erb, Strümpell), psychiatry (Emminghaus), physiology (Remak), and anatomy/pathology on the editorial board. On the new institutions, cf. Shorter, *op. cit.* (note 12); Joachim Radkau, *Das Zeitalter der Nervosität* (München: Hanser, 1998), 107–21.

37. *Cf.* e.g. Erb, *Handbuch* (note 21), and as an example for the private setting Sigmund Th. Stein, *Die allgemeine Elektrisation des menschlichen Körpers. Elektrotechnische Beiträge zur ärztlichen Behandlung der Nervenschwäche* (Nervosität und Neurasthenie) (Halle: Wilhelm Knapp, 1883) who considered the core pathophysiological mechanism of neurasthenia to be a 'disorder of the electrical balance in the body', 43.

38. Rudolph Burkart, *Zur Behandlung schwerer Formen von Hysterie und Neurasthenie* (Leipzig: Breitkopf 1884); cf. also the review in *Neurologisches Centralblatt* iii (1884), 559; Ziemssen, *op. cit.* (note 23), 22–7.

39. *Cf.* Rüdiger vom Bruch, Friedrich W. Graf, Gangolf Hübinger (eds), *Kultur und Kulturwissenschaften um 1900. Krise der Moderne und Glaube an die Wissenschaft* (Stuttgart: F. Steiner, 1989), introduction; Georg Bollenbeck, *Bildung und Kultur. Glanz und Elend eines deutschen Deutungsmusters* (Frankfurt/M.: Insel, 1994), 225–89.

40. Cf. Hans-Ulrich Wehler, *Deutsche Gesellschaftsgeschichte*, vol. 3

(München: C.H. Beck, 1995), 902–61.

41. Max Nordau, *Entartung* (Berlin: Duncker & Humblot, 1892/93); *cf.* Wehler, *op. cit.* (note 37), 745–50; Hans-Peter Söder, 'Disease and Health as Contexts of Modernity. Max Nordau as a Critic of *Fin-de-siècle* Modernism', *German Studies Review*, 14 (1991), 473–87.

42. *Cf.* Eric Engstrom, 'Psychiatry and Public Affairs in Wilhelmine Germany', *History of Psychiatry*, 2 (1991), 111–32; Eric Engstrom, 'Die Heidelberger psychiatrische Universitätsklinik am Ende des 19. Jahrhunderts. Institutionelle Grundlagen der klinischen Psychiatrie', *Jahrbuch für Universitätsgeschichte*, 1 (1998), 49–68; Volker Roelcke, 'Biologizing Social Facts. An Early 20th Century Debate on Kraepelin's Concepts of Culture, Neurasthenia, and Degeneration', *Culture, Medicine, and Psychiatry*, 21 (1997), 383–403; Volker Roelcke, 'Laborwissenschaft und Psychiatrie. Prämissen und Implikationen bei Emil Kraepelins Neuformulierung der psychiatrischen Krankheitslehre', in Christoph Gradmann and Thomas Schlich (eds), *Strategien der Kausalität. Konzepte der Krankheitsverursachung im 19. und 20. Jahrhundert* (Pfaffenweiler: Centaurus 1999), 93–116.

43. In contrast, one of the most widely read textbooks of the era, by Krafft-Ebing, published in its first edition four years before Kraepelin's *Compendium*, represented the hitherto traditional structure of the section on general aetiology. This section is divided into: I. Predisposing causes: 1. General predisposing causes (such as civilisation, climate, gender); 2. Individual predisposing causes (such as heredity, education); and II. Accessory, or precipitating causes: 1. Psychological causes; 2. Somatic causes (such as infections, trauma, internal diseases): Richard von Krafft-Ebing, *Lehrbuch der Psychiatrie auf klinischer Grundlage* (Stuttgart: Ferdinand Enke, 1879).

44. *Cf.* Roelcke, *op. cit.* (note 42).

45. Emil Kraepelin, *Lebenserinnerungen* (Heidelberg/ New York: Springer, 1983), 149; *cf.* Roelcke, *op. cit.* (note 1), 152–65.

46. Emil Kraepelin, *Compendium der Psychiatrie* (Leipzig: Ambrosius Abel, 1883), 356–64.

47. Emil Kraepelin, *Psychiatrie. Ein Lehrbuch für Studirende und Ärzte* (Leipzig: Ambrosius Abel, 1896), 349.

48. *Ibid.*, 256-262; Emil Kraepelin, *Die psychiatrischen Aufgaben des Staates* (Jena: Fischer, 1900), 2–6, 16.

49. Emil Kraepelin, 'Die Diagnose der Neurasthenie', *Münchner Medizinische Wochenschrift*, 49 (1902), 1641–44.

50. Cf. Simon Wessely, 'Old Wine in New Bottles: Neurasthenia and ME', *Psychological Medicine*, 20 (1990), 35–53.

51. Emil Kraepelin, 'Vergleichende Psychiatrie', *Centralblatt für Psychiatrie und Nervenheilkunde*, 27 (N.F. 15) (1904), 433–7; and Emil Kraepelin, 'Psychiatrisches aus Java', *ibid.*, 468–9.

52. Kraepelin, *op. cit.* (note 51), 436.

53. *Ibid.*, 437.

54. Paul Weindling, *Health, Race, and German Politics between National Unification and Nazism, 1870-1945* (Cambridge: Cambridge University Press, 1989).

55. Emil Kraepelin, 'Zur Entartungsfrage', *Zentralblatt für Nervenheilkunde und Psychiatrie*, 31 (= N.F. 19)(1908), 745–51.

56. *Ibid.*, 747.

57. *Ibid.*, 750–1.

58. Kraepelin, 'Java', 469; *cf.* also Kraepelin, *op. cit.* (note 48), where marriage restrictions are discussed.

59. Kraepelin, *op. cit.* (note 55), - a programme later to be carried out at the German Institute for Psychiatric Research; *cf.* Volker Roelcke, 'Quantifizierung, Klassifikation, Epidemiologie: Normierungsversuche des Psychischen bei Emil Kraepelin', in Werner Sohn and Herbert Mehrtens (eds), *Normalität und Abweichung. Studien zur Theorie und Geschichte der Normalisierungsgesellschaft* (Opladen: Westdeutscher Verlag, 1999), 183-200; Volker Roelcke, '"Rasse" zwischen Wissenschaft und Politik. Programm und Praxis der psychiatrischen Epidemiologie und Genetik an der Deutschen Forschungsanstalt für Psychiatrie', in Doris Kaufmann and Hans-Walter Schmuhl (eds), *Rassenforschung im Nationalsozialismus. Konzepte und wissenschaftliche Praxis unter dem Dach der Kaiser-Wilhelm-Gesellschaft* (Göttingen: Wallstein 2001)(in press).

60. Kraepelin, *op. cit.* (note 55), 747.

61. These debates are analysed in Roelcke, *op. cit.* (note 42); and Volker Roelcke, 'Naturgegebene Realität oder Konstrukt? Die Debatte über die "Natur" der Schizophrenie, 1906-1932', *Fundamenta Psychiatrica*, 14 (2000), 44–53.

62. *Cf.* Volker Roelcke, 'Psychiatrische Wissenschaft im Kontext nationalsozialistischer Politik und "Euthanasie": Zur Rolle von Ernst Rüdin und der Deutschen Forschungsanstalt für Psychiatrie', in Doris Kaufmann (ed.), *Geschichte der Kaiser-Wilhelm-Gesellschaft im Nationalsozialismus. Bestandsaufnahme und Perspektiven der Forschung* (Göttingen: Wallstein, 2000), 112–50.

63. Laehr was the director of the Berlin sanatorium Schönow which was especially designed for nervous patients and funded by private charity; *cf.* Max Laehr, 'Die Nervosität der heutigen Arbeiterschaft',

Allgemeine Zeitschrift für Psychiatrie, 64 (1909), 1–18.

64. *Cf.* Wilhelm Tigges, 'Untersuchungen über die erblich belasteten Geisteskranken', Allgemeine Zeitschrift für Psychiatrie, 64 (1907), 1–47; *idem*, 'Die Gefährdung der Nachkommen durch Psychosen, Neurosen und verwandte Zustände der Aszendenz', *Allgemeine Zeitschrift für Psychiatrie*, 63 (1906), 448–81; Robert Sommer, 'Psychiatrie und Familienforschung', *Allgemeine Zeitschrift für Psychiatrie*, 64 (1907), 463; Ernst Rüdin, 'Einige Wege und Ziele der Familienforschung, mit Rücksicht auf die Psychiatrie', *Zeitschrift für die gesamte Neurologie und Psychiatrie*, 7 (1911), 487–585.

65. Ernst Beyer, 'Die Heilstättenbehandlung der Nervenkranken', *Allgemeine Zeitschrift für Psychiatrie*, 65 (1908), 535–9.

9

The Neurasthenic Experience in Imperial Germany: Expeditions into Patient Records and Side-looks upon General History

Joachim Radkau

'Patient records? Throw them away, for God's sake!' (*Patientenakten? Um Gottes willen, wegschmeißen!*) That is the usual attitude of many archivists, I was told when I started in the late 1980s to investigate authentic documents of neurasthenics from the decades around 1900. Indeed, research on the history of neurasthenia frequently has the charm and likewise the trouble of path-finding work. A lot of most useful records are not to be found in public archives, but in more hidden places, if these records are preserved at all. And besides, there is the problem of data protection, which has become increasingly critical in Germany during the last two decades! For reasons of this kind, there is a widespread tendency to advocate the annihilation of patient records that are no longer needed for medical use. Experience with historical research on neurasthenia is sometimes useful in the context of the discussion of whether to conserve or to destroy these documents.[1] The conservation of patient records can only be justified if a scholarly historical interest in these records is demonstrated in a convincing way. Until recently, this task does not seem to have been clearly achieved. Patient records have been used by historians in an extremely sporadic way, if they have been used at all. It is not difficult to explain this omission. As Guenter B. Risse and John Harley Warner have remarked with a sigh, 'a careful reading of every file is a herculean task.'[2] I can confirm their deep sigh. To say nothing of the physicians' handwriting! And the problems of evaluating these documents are very likely to drive to despair graduate students who want to finish their dissertation within a limited time.

But the task is worthwhile. That was my experience over several years. In the following chapter, I will first survey the provenance of my sources. Later on, I will present a decade of observations, starting usually from case stories, but arriving at conclusions with regard to general history.

In the course of my pathfinding years I had occasion to study patient records from the following eight asylums:

First was the Karl Bonhoeffer Nervenklinik in (West) Berlin – formerly 'Dalldorf', the proverbial lunatic asylum of Imperial Germany – by which I got the idea to look into these records. The *'Städtische Irrenverpflegungsanstalt'* Dalldorf had been established in 1862 and was expanding steadily during the following decades to a capacity of much more than a thousand inmates.[3] In the cellar of the present Bonhoeffer Nervenklinik, all patient records are well preserved. They had previously been mainly used for publications on Nazi extermination policy. But in that context they served merely as documents of victimisation. Unfortunately for me, at the former Dalldorf, neurasthenic patients – who were not only victims, but actors – were like a needle in a haystack: one had to look long to find some of them.

After 1989, I was saved by the fall of the Berlin wall. Now the way was open to the famous Charité Hospital in former East Berlin where the neurasthenics were much more frequent since they, unlike the Dalldorf out-patients, were treated as well. The Psychiatric Department of the Charité had been founded in 1806 and had become famous after 1865 by Wilhelm Griesinger who combined psychiatry with neurology and enlarged the department into the Psychiatrisch-Neurologische Klinik.[4] I found the records in the heating cellar where they were waiting to be burnt. They were covered by the dust of many decades, and looking into them, though not very healthy, was rewarding, sometimes even exciting. I wondered whether the Charité records contained evidence that Berlin, that roaring metropolis, was the stronghold of modern nervousness as so many contemporary publications had asserted. The result was not wholly negative. Until the 1890s, however, the diagnosis 'neurasthenia' was not very frequent at the Charité; but it increased after 1900, especially after 1904, when Theodor Ziehen, an authority in neurasthenia, became the director of the Psychiatrisch-Neurologische Klinik.

The records of the Hessian lunatic asylum Eichberg are preserved at the Hauptstaatsarchiv Wiesbaden. The Irrenanstalt Eichberg had been established in 1849 and had been rapidly expanding during the late nineteenth century, like most German public asylums.[5] Here, the neurasthenic patients are easy to find because since the 1970s, the old records have been registered according to diagnosis. The attempt has even been undertaken to classify many patients who did not get a diagnosis in their time! It was a unique endeavor, not without delicate problems, of course, but surely helpful for the historian of today.

The Stadtarchiv of Frankfurt am Main preserves the records of the former lunatic asylum, called Affenstein, once famous for its director Heinrich Hoffmann, the author of *Struwwelpeter*, the most popular German children's book of the nineteenth century. Under Hoffmann's leadership, Affenstein had become after 1851 a modern institution. At Frankfurt, the diagnosis neurasthenia was used rather cautiously. Here as elsewhere, neurasthenia seems to have been no mere *Verlegenheitsdiagnose*, no mere hotchpotch or blanket diagnosis, as later on has been frequently claimed and had been asserted already at that time by T. C. Allbutt and others.[6]

Carl Alexander von Ehrenwall's former '*Kuranstalt für Gemüts- und Nervenkranke*' at Ahrweiler, situated in a romantic tributary valley of the Rhine, is presumably the only major private Nervenheilstätte of Imperial Germany which has survived until today within the original buildings, with the same intentions, and under the management of the same family. It was founded about 1880 at first as asylum for psychotic patients; but in the course of an enlargement of the buildings in 1886/88, the Kuranstalt discovered nervous people as a new source of clients. Before 1898, the number of neurasthenic patients increased to 65 persons (50 men and 15 women). From 1898 to 1909, 210 neurasthenics (119 men and 91 women) were treated at Ahrweiler.[7] At the top of an old tower, all patient records have been preserved. For the history of neurasthenia, this is a real bonanza. The founder had close connections with the commercial bourgeoisie of Rhineland-Westphalia and with the Catholic Alexianer Brethren. He seems to have had only a short psychiatric training, and apparently he relied more on common sense than upon medical theories.

A somewhat different regional and intellectual profile was that of the Kuranstalt of the Binswanger dynasty situated at Lake Constance, today mainly known because of Bertha Pappenheim who became under the pseudonym 'Anna O' the most famous patient of Sigmund Freud's though she was not treated by him with real success. Also the Binswanger sanatorium called Bellevue is a wonderfully rich source for the history of neurasthenia. Founded in 1857, at first for psychotic patients, it was directed from 1880 to 1910 by Robert Binswanger, whose brother Otto Binswanger, professor at Jena, included among his patients the philosopher Friedrich Nietzsche as well as Emperor William II. Otto Binswanger published perhaps the most renowned manual on neurasthenia.[8] In 1910 the new director

Ludwig Binswanger introduced psychoanalysis and prohibition to Bellevue, while Ahrweiler was rather renowned for its electrotherapy and its excellent Ahr wines. At Bellevue, the diagnosis neurasthenia began as early as 1880, immediately after the publication of Beard's manual. It is interesting to note the ratio between 'neurasthenia' as an initial in-coming diagnosis and as a dismissal diagnosis: at Bellevue, during the 1880s the relation was 10:50; during the 90s, 49:119; and between 1900 and 1909, 24:164.[9] One might state that in the time of Robert Binswanger, neurasthenia was produced at the lake Constance on a major scale. However, even at Bellevue, the neurasthenics made up only a small minority of the total patient population, many of whom were given no diagnosis at all. Also at the Binswanger sanatorium neurasthenia was more than a pure blanket diagnosis!

The Volksnervenheilstätte Roderbirken near Solingen, opened in 1906 and financed mostly by the Landesversicherungsanstalt Rheinland, was by far the biggest German public nervous sanatorium for female patients of the lower-classes. In its first year, it received no less than 286 neurasthenic women and 193 women with other nervous inconveniences, mostly unmarried, in work and not older than forty years. Unfortunately only admission records, but no detailed patient records have been preserved. However, many documents on Roderbirken are to be found in public archives. After long and intensive discussions the Landesversicherungsanstalt decided to limit the asylum for the time being to women. It was a remarkable decision. Initially neurasthenia was conceived in Germany as an illness of overworked men by the notorious antifeminist Paul Julius Möbius, ill-famed till today for his pamphlet *Über den physiologischen Schwachsinn des Weibes* (On the physiological feeble-mindedness of the female, first published in 1900). But the discourse on neurasthenia developed its own dynamics that removed it far from its one time anti-feminist beginnings. If Tom Lutz has stated for the United States that 'neurasthenia was a highly gendered discourse',[10] I can – at least on the whole – perceive no sharp gender discrimination in Germany. On the contrary, the literature upon nervousness repeatedly emphasises the similarity in suffering between the two sexes.[11] The female patients at Roderbirken were mostly workers from the textile industry of that region, but also in many cases needleworkers, housemaids, and saleswomen.

The von Bodelschwinghsche Anstalten at Bethel close to Bielefeld – a truly holy city founded initially for epileptics – built the House

Bethesda in 1886/87 for nervous women and at the same time the Eichhof for nervous men. At least the foundation of the Eichhof had in part financial motives; old Bodelschwingh called it ironically a *'Schlingelheim'* ('lazybones' home'). The records of Bethesda are preserved at the Bethel Archives. The diagnosis of neurasthenia spread quickly from the big cities into the depth of the province! In 1889, a protestant priest justified the establishment of Bethesda by 'our nervous age'.[12] Sometimes nervousness appears as an illness appropriate for the *'Pastoralmedizin'* (pastoral medical care).[13] To be sure, Bodelschwingh entertained the hope to cure ill people by the force of faith; but at the same time, he was a realistic man. On the whole, there is no marked difference between the records of the pietist Bethel asylum and the usual secular records. The role of religion within the therapy of nervous illness was less significant than I had expected from the literature. Contrary to the suspicion of some psychiatrists, even the deeply pious Friedrich von Bodelschwingh does not seem to have replaced the usual medical therapies with religious exorcism!

Neurasthenia and religion

Did neurasthenia have something to do with religion? Or did religious faith prove to be a good remedy against nervous disease at that time? Möbius, though a descendant of Martin Luther, regarded the Catholic monastery as the best model for the *Volksnervenheilstätten* he propagated with some success in the public.[14] But Wörishofen, the therapeutic center of Sebastian Kneipp, was visited by many neurasthenic priests; and Alfred Baumgarten, Kneipp's medical co-worker, wrote in his book on neurasthenia that the celibate life was one of the causes of that illness.[15] Neither was the protestant rectory a safe prophylaxis against nervous weakness. A well-known nervous clergywoman of Bodelschwingh's surroundings was Marie Schmalenbach (1835-1924) who documented her pains in her diaries. As early as 1871 she complained of her 'destroyed nerves'.[16] But at that time, she had still 53 years to live until she died at an age of 89 years. According to her diaries, faith does not appear to be a remedy against nervous weakness. But she composed a hymn which deeply moved pious people of her region: *'Brich herein, süßer Schein selger Ewigkeit!'* (Break in, sweet glimpse of blessed eternity!) It was a vision of redemption from the pains of time! Here on earth, she sang, *'Angst, davon die Augen sprechen'* (Everywhere angst is seen in the eyes).

The neurasthenics of that time were not silent. After some digging around one can find patient records in hundreds and even more. But are they of real historical interest? Or are they mere documents of the asylum apparatus: of the system of manipulation and constraint that we know sufficiently from other sources? Ironically, it is precisely the followers of Foucault postulating most provocatively that we listen to the authentic voice of the so-called mentally ill, who usually have the least confidence that they can discover this voice through historical research because they believe in the omnipotence of the medical system.[17] But, undoubtedly, there does exist a huge mass of authentic material within patient records. And it seems that it is precisely the decades before and after the turn of the century, the great age of neurasthenia, that is a fortunate period for studying the patients' view of illness using authentic sources. For by that time, the bureaucratisation of German asylums had proceeded so far that a lot of written paper was produced; but the progress of psychiatry and neurology on its way toward hard science was still in its beginnings. In that situation, it was precisely the aim of becoming an exact science that at first led to a certain agnosticism. Intelligent doctors knew best that they did not know very much and that they had to listen to their patients. Many records are testifying that awareness. In many cases, it seems that the patients could speak more or less frankly and tell their own nervous experience without being influenced too much by medical questions.

As a result, we get from the patient records an abundance of personal stories that are often touching and even exciting. But is it possible to make history out of these stories? That is the big question; and one should not answer it with a clear 'yes' too quickly. By reading these records, one can again and again be overwhelmed by a feeling of agnosticism with regard to the historical truth within these documents. Surely, one should be cautious with major theories about the historical evolution of mental illness and the connections between society and nervous disease. But in the end, looking over the mass of records, it seems to be feasible – though with some caution – to formulate a series of positive results. I will briefly outline a dozen points.

The patients' role in the formation of the neurasthenia concept

It seems to be of special interest for the history of medicine that these records point to the decisive role of the patients' experiences in the construction and further development of the concepts of neurasthenia. To be sure, manuals on nervous diseases usually start

204

with a neurological introduction; but analysed from close up, the neurasthenia construct does not seem to be really deduced from scientific paradigms of that time. On the whole, the researcher gets the impression that neurasthenia stems much more from the medical consultation room than from neurological theory. Experience much more than science is at the roots of neurasthenia, though science is not without importance. But the endeavours to localise neurasthenia according to the question of the famous Virchow '*Ubi est morbus?*' were thwarted by the plethora of patients' experiences. As the records frequently point out, the medical diagnosis is directly derived from the patient's anamnesis. To be sure, in many cases the patient's experience is itself influenced by medical terms and concepts; but the patients made their own choice, whereby they often irritated their physicians. One record from Bellevue remarks: 'Patient gained comprehensive knowledge of neurasthenology [sic] by communication with doctors and from medical books... For each statement of the attending physician he quotes another medical authority who said the exact opposite.' Previously, the patient – a well-to-do lawyer from Vienna – had been analysed by Freud, but the effect had been a 'complete breakdown'.[18]

In typical cases, the transition from the rest cure toward more active methods of therapy seems to have been influenced by patients who often were bored to death by the calmness of the asylum. A teacher who spent seventy-one days in Otto Binswanger's clinical hospital at Jena grumbled afterwards: 'I was very stupid to go to a clinic for nervous diseases. Not in Jena was I healed, but only by my will have I improved my condition, which I strengthened by systematic training.'[19] Then as now, teachers were not easy patients.

The impact of modern acceleration

Starting from the history of technology, I have paid special attention to the significance of new technologies and industrial developments as the presumed origins of nervousness in the light of the patient records. I was somewhat disappointed: these factors appeared relatively seldom as direct factors of nervous diseases, at least not so frequently as in the contemporary literature, which especially since the 1890s liked to stress the *Hetzen und Jagen* (haste and hurry), the acceleration of a lot of processes due to the modern economy and technology, as the main cause of 'modern nervousness'. At first, this acceleration often caused euphoria, not a feeling of illness and a demand for therapy. As a rule, people went to the doctor only if they felt their professional or sexual 'energy' to be at risk. The complaint

Figure 9.1: 'Our Nerves.'
Poem and caricature from the *Fliegende Blätter*, 1888.

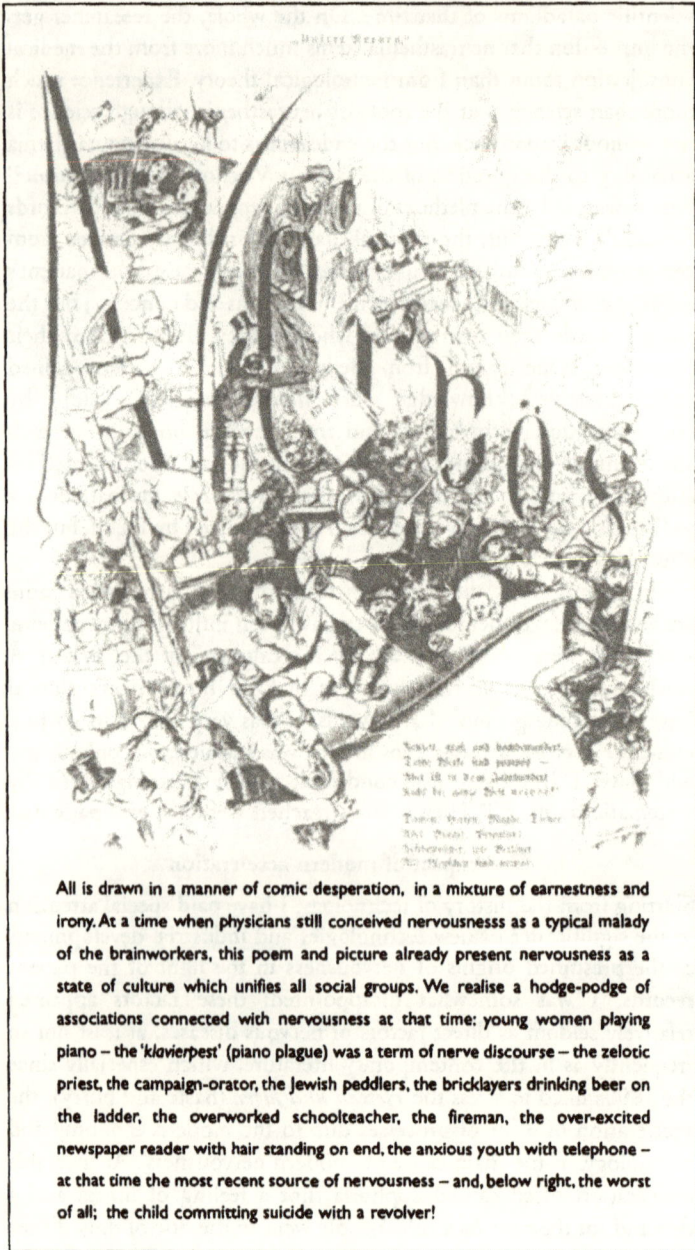

All is drawn in a manner of comic desperation, in a mixture of earnestness and irony. At a time when physicians still conceived nervousnesss as a typical malady of the brainworkers, this poem and picture already present nervousness as a state of culture which unifies all social groups. We realise a hodge-podge of associations connected with nervousness at that time: young women playing piano – the '*klavierpest*' (piano plague) was a term of nerve discourse – the zelotic priest, the campaign-orator, the Jewish peddlers, the bricklayers drinking beer on the ladder, the overworked schoolteacher, the fireman, the over-excited newspaper reader with hair standing on end, the anxious youth with telephone – at that time the most recent source of nervousness – and, below right, the worst of all; the child committing suicide with a revolver!

206

about the loss of energy is typical for the neurasthenic confessions of that time. A slowing down of working energy and sexual misfortune: both seemed to be signs of loss of energy and caused panic. In 1906, a butcher's journeyman was taken to the Eichberg asylum. He had slaughtered bulls in piecework and had tried to commit suicide. 'What is wrong with you ?' he was asked. 'The energy', he answered, 'the nerves'.[20] 'Energy' was at that time a relatively new term in everyday language; it was often associated with nerves. A working man, asked about his condition in the Charité in 1909, replied: 'Quite well, only my energy and nerves are failing.' The suggestive power of the term 'energy' in patient records is one of the main points where one feels the influence of the 'energetic age' (*Eugen Diesel*) and perceives a close affinity between the history of neurasthenia and technological change.[21]

The main issue: sex

The role of sexual frustrations in the patients' experience of neurasthenia is immense; it is clearly the most important point. Contrary to Freudian assumptions, in many cases sexual desires and fears were in no way suppressed by the mechanisms of memory; on the contrary, they dominated medical histories. Admittedly, this holds true mainly for male and not for female patients; but nevertheless, it is very hard to believe what Peter Gay asserts – in contradiction to much of his material – that female sexuality had to be rediscovered by Freud.[22] The patient records demonstrate as clearly as possible the fact that, although sex was taboo in social conversation, it was not absent from thoughts! A man of private means, thirty-six years old, who entered the Ahrweiler Kuranstalt in 1896, seemed to have no other thoughts in his mind than sex. He was no exception among neurasthenics. 'He says the bed is the genuine battleground of the neurasthenic' (*Er sagt, das Bett ist der eigentliche Kampfplatz des Neurasthenikers*).[23] Many patient records seem to point to the truth of Foucault's assertion that the worst modern problem with sex is not the suppression of sexual thought, but the permanent discourse – maybe more or less hidden – about sex ! The diary of Franziska Gräfin zu Reventlow (1871-1918) who was notorious for her tireless search for manifold sexual experiences 'from Paul to Pedro' is full of vehement complaints of agonising nervousness; perhaps it is the most exciting neurasthenic confession of that time in the German language at all.

The great fear: onanism

Of all sexual anxieties, the fear of having destroyed their nervous and sexual energy by masturbation is clearly dominant among male patients. Reading the papers of the neurasthenics, one can get the impression that onanism was a much bigger problem at that time than militarism or socialism! From the perspective of many patients, there is a very intimate connection between neurasthenia and masturbation. This is documented by an immense mass of records. The nervous autobiography, which is so often presented by the life stories of neurasthenic patients, frequently gets its dramatic highlights from masturbation and the heroic fight against it.

In 1904, a college student of twenty arrived at Bellevue, where he stayed for one year. Binswanger gave the diagnosis 'neurasthenia' whereas the student himself had apparently worse suspicions. He was continuously afraid of losing his sexual potency; he seems to have masturbated in order to assure himself of his potency and at the same time he was afraid to destroy his potency by masturbation.

> The sensual instinct cried for satisfaction, like a hungry tiger... The whole day, I played with my male member... and the more enormous was the superhuman energy required not to masturbate! Whispering I cried 'No!' and stopped myself with all my power. My head was red-hot, my lips were burning. But the victory was won.[24]

What shall we do with confessions of this kind? Were they merely the reflection of medical warnings? But German medical literature around 1900 was deeply ambiguous about the presumed dangers of masturbation. On the whole, it presented a mixture of alarm and all-clear signals. Perhaps it was just this alternation which fostered neurasthenia: this characteristic pell-mell of desire and fear. The patients' role in this story is not merely a passive one; often fears of masturbation were maintained even if the physician tried to calm the patient. On the other hand, medical warnings of nervous diseases caused by coitus interruptus made a much weaker impression upon patients. People did not believe every medical lesson! A 40-year-old farmer when told of the purported dangers of coitus interruptus coolly replied, 'I don't believe that. Otherwise everybody would be sick.'[25] A kind of practical Malthusianism had a tradition among peasants.

A nervous musician staying in the Affenstein asylum at Frankfurt praised the outbreak of war as being the only effective therapy for masturbation: 'I masturbated till the war, until July 31, 1914. Afterwards came the enthusiasm, and now I found it beneath my dignity to yield to bestial desires' (*mich tierischen Gelüsten hinzugeben*).[26] At times, the euphoria of August 1914 arose out of the shortcomings of psychiatric therapy!

Women, sex and neurasthenia

What about female sexuality from the viewpoint of neurasthenic experience? Generally – and not astonishingly – female patient records are more reserved with regard to sex than the testimonies of the men. In the *Autobiography of a Neurasthene* (1910), written by the American physician Margaret Cleaves, we read much about energy – personal and cosmic – but nothing about sex.[27] Does the scarcity of the records about feminine sexuality testify to the suppression of the women's bodies? At least as to Germany and Austria, I am not sure. In the records of Ahrweiler we encounter the case of a young woman who had been confined in a lunatic asylum for eight years after a series of thefts and love affairs. She frankly declared that 'she could not live without sexual intercourse'. When she was transferred to Ahrweiler and worked well in the kitchen, von Ehrenwall found her quite normal, and with a medical report of eighteen pages he destroyed all the medical opinions which had led to her long confinement.[28] At that time, there was no general consensus about what is normal and abnormal with regard to female sexual behaviour.

Notwithstanding, the whole concept of male sexual neurasthenia was based upon the – explicit or implicit – conviction that the woman has a natural right of full sexual joy and that it is not enough for a healthy man to generate children, but that he must also give this pleasure to his wife. Frequently the premature ejaculation appears to be at the core of neurasthenia. Male patient records are full of fear of sexual overexcitement causing *ejaculatio praecox*. Georg Hirth, the editor of the influential journal *Jugend* and an authority in sexual matters, exhorted the man to concentrate all his self-control in order to secure the '*Juhschro*' (a Bavarian term for orgasm) of the woman.[29] But Hirth's own son was a prototype of all forms of neurasthenia, and he believed to have inherited his nervousness from his parents![30]

Intestinal hardships

The Ahrweiler records tell about a corpulent clergyman who spent half the day resting upon the chaise longue where all his thought circulated 'around his stool'.[31] Digestion is perhaps the most neglected major theme of psychohistory. It seems to have been a main topic of neurasthenic experience, as well, though it was not a new issue at that time. Probably digestion problems are a typical outcome of a general crisis in early modern lifestyles generated by the combination of a sedentary way of life and meals which were too heavy. The era of healthy food and fitness training was still in its infancy. The water cure was the usual therapy for constipation. When Richard Wagner became an enthusiast of hydrotherapy, he developed a real philosophy of digestion in a letter to Franz Liszt (1852):

> Unhappy people, care for a sound digestion, and suddenly life appears totally different than you saw it when you were tormented by your abdomen! Truly, all our politics, diplomacy, ambition, weakness and science have no other foundation than our ruined abdomens (*Unterleibe*)![32]

The *Nervenheilstätten* arose in many cases out of Wasserheilstätten, hydrotherapeutical sanatoriums.[33]

The class-crossing fear of bad air

In 1909, a skilled tailor of fifty-three who worked as a barkeeper in Berlin was examined at Charité Hospital, where he was given the diagnosis 'hypochondriac neurasthenic'. He had grown up in the north German heath country (*Lüneburger Heide*), and the bad air of Berlin was discomfortable to him. 'Are you ill?' he was asked.

> Yes, so I think (*Na mein ich*). So hard a life and nothing to show for it (*man hat nichts davon*). If I am together with people, I am always afraid of their bad odours (*Ausdünstungen*). You always have to breathe the odours of others. They spit so much. Nowadays I have to run for air; formerly, it used to be for money.[34]

Apparently he was afraid of being infected with tuberculosis; and presumably this fear was justified, as later on he was transferred to a tubercular sanatorium.

We encounter an early kind of environmental awareness here, which has been – then as now – strongly influenced by the care for health. The environmental historian Ulrike Gilhaus believes that at the turn of the century, the longing for good air was limited to the middle and upper-classes.[35] The tailor-barkeeper offers a counter-example. And this does not seem to be totally unique. On the whole, the patient records give the impression that the class differences in mentality were not so sharp at that time as is often assumed. In the same year, 1909, a 24-year-old shoemaker came to the Charité with the same diagnosis 'hypochondriac neurasthenia'. He was terrified by the Berlin street noise and by a bad conscience because of masturbation. He had often tried homeopathic remedies.[36] These were anxieties and hopes of regeneration that crossed the class boundaries of nineteenth century. Then as now, environmental awareness and desire for nature had something to do with nerve experience!

Neurasthenia: a malady of a patriarchal society?

In 1886 a Prussian professor of law who consulted Robert Binswanger was concerned because his seven-year-old son asked his permission for everything. The father believed the patriarchal behaviour of his little son to be pathological![37] In the light of numerous patient records, the German society of that time does not appear so overwhelmingly authoritarian and patriarchal as is often imagined today. If one takes this imagination for granted, the following story appears incredible: when a very successful businessman from the Rhineland returned home to discover that his wife had separated their bedrooms and had probably had an affair with a Frenchman, he did not react with an outburst of patriarchy and chauvinism, but with anxious reflections as to whether he provided sufficient sexual joy for his wife. And when during a row at lunch his wife spilled over him a dish of asparagus he felt a strong demand of therapy for himself, not for his wife![38]

Nationalism as a cure for the nerves?

The Viennese lawyer mentioned above inveighed against his physician at Bellevue: 'He neglected the only efficient remedy: opium. Instead of that, I had to read Treitschke's *Politik*: an insufferable book.'[39] To my surprise I did not find a single case where nationalism was an efficient remedy against nervousness: a remarkable phenomenon at the peak of the chauvinist age! The feeling of regeneration which overcame many people at first after the outbreak of war was so overwhelming because it was unexpected. Up to 1914 neurasthenia was a decidedly anti-Darwinist experience in which the 'struggle for existence' appeared as a cause of illness, not as a force for racial progress.[40] In 1911, a Charité physician ordered a nervous tailor to write a paper on the topic 'Does even war have advantages?' But the tailor described only the dark sides of war; and he concluded his paper with the remark, 'We will pray to the good Lord that He will give us the blessings of peace.'[41]

Anti-Semitism in the neurasthenia discourse?

In September 1914, one week after the outbreak of war, a 31-year-old businessman of German-Jewish origin arrived at Ahrweiler, where he confessed that he had escaped mobilization by simulating deep melancholy. 'I said to myself: The farther away from the enemy, the better for you.' Or was he a real melancholic – had he simulated simulation? He called himself a 'dégénéré, not worth the bullet it would take to kill him' (*keinen Schuß Pulver wert*); useless people like him should 'disappear from the earth'. His speech was partly a lament, sometimes obscene. But the Ahrweiler physician refrained from any deprecatory commentary, diagnosed 'neurasthenia' and saved the businessman from the war.[42] If the physician had had any hidden anti-Semitic feeling, this would have been an occasion for outing them. But though Jews were asserted to be predestined for neurasthenia, I found anti-Jewish undertones only very rarely in the whole German discourse on neurasthenia. With regard to publications, one could explain this absence as tactical;[43] but even in the patient records and medical commentaries I found hardly any indication of anti-Semitism. George Mosse asserted that the discourse on nervousness fostered the stigmatisation of the Jews;[44] I got rather the contrary impression for the time before the First World War. Ursula Link-Heer thinks she perceives a kind of German nerve nationalism;[45] but for me, the evidence to the contrary is overwhelming. Innumerable documents testify that there was a general feeling that nervousness was not only a Jewish, but as well a German malady. Sometimes Beard flattered the Germans to be a people with strong nerves; but as far as I see, no German author picked up this compliment! One should not jump too quickly to conclusions about direct continuities between the neurasthenia discourse before 1914 and the Nazi rule, even though apparently certain connections – I would say of a 'dialectical' kind – do exist.[46]

Travelling: a key element of neurasthenic culture

A 35-year-old businessman who had formerly lived at Frankfurt and finally at Buenos Aires, told at Bellevue, that in the capital of Argentina he had had too much sex with a mistress and at the same time very much distress in business. 'I have been nervous for a long time. I was well-known as the nervous man at Buenos Aires.'[47] He seems to have gained a kind of nervous self-consciousness. His life story consisted of continuous travelling, always with much work and with much sex. The secret of the attractiveness of exotic travels usually was the chance for sexual escapades. By travelling one frequently tried to cure nervousness, but travels were usually the source of new nervous excitement. Travelling was a method to transform neurasthenia from a malady to a modern lifestyle. Emperor William II, sometimes nicknamed the '*Reise-Kaiser*' (William the Traveller), set an example for many other contemporaries.

•

'The awful to and fro'

The most significant change within the aspects of neurasthenic disease during the decades around 1900 is probably the evolution from a malady of prevalent weakness – as is indicated by the term 'neurasthenia' – toward a malady of over-excitement. In this regard, the story of neurasthenia in Germany is a mirror of its time. At first neurasthenia was conceived as a state of extreme weakness. The Swiss alienist Paul Dubois told about nervous patients who 'during the consultation were sliding from the chair'.[48] But a more hectic and hyperactive type of neurasthenic was advancing. Perhaps the best German example is the inventor Rudolf Diesel as he has been described by his philosophical son Eugen Diesel. He portrayed his famous father as a 'high-pressure man' who tried to apply the principles of his high-pressure engine upon himself and became by this way a prototype of his 'neurasthenic age'. Most disastrous for his nerves was the fact that frequently he did not have a single clear aim for his life and work, but was driven by an 'awful to and fro' (*schreckliches Hin und Her*).[49] This *Hin und Her* was apparently a new type of stress at the turn of the century. The neurologist Willy Hellpach, who wrote a series of publications about nervousness, observed that since the 1890s dissipation of activities had become a widespread stress phenomenon.[50] At the same time, many Germans began to observe very critically the permanent *Hin und Her* of the Imperial 'zigzag policy'. The neurasthenic experience shaped the political consciousness. But the therapy of 'political neurasthenia' turned out to be much worse than the malady itself.

The First World War was hailed as a *Stahlbad* (chalybeate spa) for the nerves by several physicians, mostly by those who were far from the front. But even the lance-corporal Adolf Hitler wrote on 5 February 1915 from the western front: 'Now I am very nervous. Day after day we are in extremely hard artillery fire from eight in the morning till five in the afternoon; over time that ruins even the strongest nerves' (*das macht mit der Zeit die stärksten Nerven kaputt*).[51] Against that, Chancellor Hitler proclaimed at the Reichsparteitag of 1934: 'We have finished definitely the nervous nineteenth century.'[52] But when the tourist propaganda of Kraft durch Freude praised the *Salzkammergut* as '*Gau der guten Nerven*',[53] it revealed that in fact weak nerves were a problem of Nazi time, too. But at that time, it was no longer fashionable to admit neurasthenia! Nervousness, however, continued to exist even without a discourse on neurasthenia: it was more than a mere product of discourse!

In order to draw a conclusion: the whole story of German nervousness – is it after all a good story or a bad one, or is it simply naïve to put a question of this kind? From the retrospective one could perhaps state that wherever the nerve discourse had to do with real suffering, it had at least on the whole a 'soft', humane tendency, in contrast to the polemical use or rather abuse of 'nervousness' as a reproach. One should remind that the German public social insurance system was an outgrowth of the age of neurasthenia being based upon the philosophy that in order to work well you have to sleep well, and that therefore people should not be stressed too much by the Darwinist struggle for existence. It was a philosophy with long-range effects, lasting until the present time. When the French economist Michel Albert prophesies that after the downfall of socialism the great intellectual struggle of the future will be fought between American and 'Rhenish' capitalism (which might be called 'Prussian' or 'Scandinavian' capitalism as well), that could mean that the big alternative of the future will be the denial of nervousness or the respect of nervousness!

Neurasthenia and culture: can we realise a peculiar path of German-speaking countries in international comparison? Though with some caution, I would give an affirmative answer. At the turn of the century, neurasthenia appeared in Central Europe more than in England or France as an acute and urgent mass phenomenon and as a sign of contemporary time. In the general perception, it had more to do with sex than in England and more with modern industrial stress than in France. Perhaps the closest nervous affinity existed at that time between Germany and the United States; but the German perception of nervousness was on the whole more earnest and less optimistic than the American. But, most important from the view of general history: in Germany existed probably more than in other countries an intimate connection between the neurasthenia boom and characteristic political and cultural trends of the time, such as the politics of social insurance, the sanatorium movement, the extensive spread of nature cures (*Naturheilbewegung*) and further modes of life reform. In many cases, these trends were inconsistent with the chauvinist and militarist mainstream.[34] Again: neurasthenia was in its core no outgrowth of dominant ideologies, but of vivid experience!

But there are further cultural contexts of neurasthenia. Particularly the history of German exotic desires - from the Samoa imperialism of 1900 until the present boom of tourism and of eastern religions and therapies - has much to do with nerve experience: with the quest of exotic quietness.[35] Whether this will be a good story in the end, we cannot say. Apparently there is more than one single story of neurasthenia. Perhaps we need a new style of historical writing – telling a plurality of possible stories – in order to give a true picture of nervous experience.

Notes

1. J. Radkau, 'Zum historischen Quellenwert von Patientenakten – Erfahrungen aus Recherchen zur Geschichte der Nervosität', in D. Meyer and B. Hey (eds), *Akten betreuter Personen als archivische Aufgabe* (Neustadt an der Aisch: Degener, 1997), 73–101; the volume contains further contributions on the juridical discussion.

2. G. B. Risse and J. H. Warner, 'Reconstructing Clinical Activities: Patient Records in Medical History', *Social History of Medicine*, 5 (1992), 183–205: 196.

3. S. Damm and N. Emmerich, 'Die Irrenanstalt Dalldorf-Wittenau bis 1933', in *Totgeschwiegen 1933 – 1945. Zur Geschichte der Wittenauer Heilstätten. Seit 1957 Karl-Bonhoeffer-Nervenklinik* (Berlin: Hentrich, 1989), 11 ff.

4. K. Leonhard, 'Über die Geschichte der Nervenklinik der Charité', in *250 Jahre Charité Berlin* (Jena: Gustav Fischer, 1960), 492 ff.

5. R. Snell, 'Landes- Heil- und Pflege-Anstalt Eichberg im Rheingau', in *Deutsche Heil- und Pflegeanstalten für Psychischkranke in Wort und Bild* (Halle: Marhold, 1910), 181 ff.

6. H. Hoffmann, *Lebenserinnerungen* (Frankfurt: Insel, 1985), 181 ff. Lynn Payer: *Medicine and Culture. Varieties of Treatment in the United States, England, West Germany, and France* (New York: Henry Holt, 1988), 91 ff.

7. 'Dr. von Ehrenwall'sche Kuranstalt zu Ahrweiler', in *Deutsche Heil- und Pflegeanstalten, op. cit.* (note 5), 499-520.

8. O. Binswanger, *Die Pathologie und Therapie der Neurasthenie* (Jena: Gustav Fischer, 1896). For documents about the history of Bellevue see Universitätsarchiv Tübingen, Zentrales Krankenblattdepot 443/125.

9. I am indebted to Professor Gerhard Fichtner (Tübingen) for putting these statistics at my disposal.

10. T. Lutz, *American Nervousness 1903 – An Anecdotal History* (Ithaca: Cornell University Press, 1991), 31.

11. J. Radkau, 'Die Männer als schwaches Geschlecht. Die wilhelminische Nervosität, die Politisierung der Therapie und der mißglückte Geschlechterrollentausch', in Th. Kornbichler and W. Maaz (eds): *Variationen der Liebe. Historische Psychologie der Geschlechterbeziehung* (Tübingen: Edition Discord, 1995), 249–93.

12. *Bericht über die erste Konferenz deutscher evangelischer Irrenfürsorger* (Münster, 1889), 6.

13. D. Rössler, 'Pfarrhaus und Medizin', in M. Greiffenhagen (ed.): *Das evangelische Pfarrhaus* (Stuttgart: Kreuz Verlag, 1984), 231 ff.

14. J. Radkau, *Das Zeitalter der Nervosität* (München: Hanser, 1998), 112.

15. A. Baumgarten, *Neurasthenie – Wesen, Heilung, Vorbeugung* (Wörishofen: Verlags-Anstalt Wörishofen, 1905), 119.

16. K. Stockhecke, *Marie Schmalenbach – Pfarrersfrau und Schriftstellerin aus Westfalen* (Bielefeld: Verlag für Regionalgeschichte, 1993), 146.

17. R. Hughes, *Political Correctness oder die Kunst, sich selbst das Denken zu verbieten* (München: Droemer, 1994), 166 ff.

18. Radkau, *op. cit.* (note 14), 105.

19. *Ibid.*, 360.

20. *Ibid.*, 241.

21. *Ibid.*, 232–46.

22. P. Gay, *Erziehung der Sinne. Sexualität im bürgerlichen Zeitalter* (München: Beck, 1986), 184.

23. Radkau, *Ibid.* (note 14), 146.

24. *Ibid.*, 159.

25. A. McLaren, *A History of Contraception* (Oxford: Blackwell, 1990), 189.

26. J. Radkau, 'Die wilhelminische Ära als nervöses Zeitalter, oder: Die Nerven als Netz zwischen Tempo- und Körpergeschichte', *Geschichte und Gesellschaft*, 20 (1994), 211–241: 240.

27. M. A. Cleaves, *The Autobiography of a Neurasthene, as Told by One of Them* (Boston: Adger, 1910).

28. J. Radkau, 'Zwischen freier Liebe und Koitus interruptus: Sexualität in Psychiatrie und Patientenerfahrung um 1900', in K. Tebben (ed.): *Frauen – Körper – Kunst. Literarische Inszenierungen weiblicher Sexualität* (Göttingen: Vandenhoeck, 2000) 53–70.

29. G. Hirth, *Wege zur Liebe* (München: Verlag der Jugend, 1917), 569 ff.

30. Radkau, *op. cit.* (note 14), 144.

31. *Ibid.*, 26.

32. J. Radkau, 'Nationalismus und Nervosität', in W. Hardtwig and H.-U. Wehler (eds): *Kulturgeschichte heute* (Göttingen: Vandenhoeck, 1996), 284-315, 312.

33. E. Shorter, 'Private Clinics in Central Europe 1850 – 1933', in: *Social History of Medicine*, 3 (1990), 159–195: 159.

34. Radkau, *op. cit.* (note 1), 87 ff.

35. U. Gilhaus, *'Schmerzenskinder der Industrie': Umweltverschmutzung,*

*Umweltpolitik und sozialer Protest im Industriezeitalter in Westfalen,
1845 – 1914* (Paderborn: Schöningh, 1995), 488.

36. Radkau, *op. cit.* (note 14), 150 ff.
37. *Ibid.*, 143.
38. Radkau, *op. cit.* (note 26).
39. Radkau, *op. cit.* (note 30), 308.
40. J. Radkau, 'Das Stahlbad als Nervenkur ? Nervöse Ursprünge des
    Ersten Weltkrieges', in Arbeitskreis Militärgeschichte (ed.):
    Newsletter, 10 (Oct. 1999), 6–8.
41. Radkau, *op. cit.* (note 14), 401.
42. Radkau, *op. cit.* (note 1), 97.
43. So does E. Shorter, *From the Mind to the Body. The Cultural Origins
    of Psychosomatic Symptoms* (New York: Free Press, 1994), 100.
44. G. L. Mosse, *Nationalismus und Sexualität* (Reinbek: Rowohlt,
    1987), 173.
45. U. Link-Heer, '"Männliche Hysterie" – Eine Diskursanalyse', in U.
    A. J. Becher and J. Rüsen (eds), *Weiblichkeit in geschichtlicher
    Perspektive* (Frankfurt: Suhrkamp, 1988), 364–396: 385 ff.
46. Radkau, *op. cit.* (note 14), 374, 449 ff.
47. *Ibid.*, 250.
48. P. Dubois, *Die Psychoneurosen und ihre psychische Behandlung* (Bern:
    Francke, 1905), 157.
49. E. Diesel, *Jahrhundertwende. Gesehen im Schicksal meines Vaters*
    (Stuttgart: Reclam, 1949), 184.
50. W. Hellpach, *Universitas Litterarum. Gesammelte Aufsätze* (Stuttgart:
    Enke, 1948), 348.
51. B. Ulrich, 'Krieg als Nervensache: Skizzierung einer verhängnisvollen
    Beziehung', *Die Zeit*, (22. 11. 1991), 54.
52. M. Domarus, *Hitler - Reden und Proklamationen 1942 - 1945*, vol.
    1/I (Wiesbaden: R. Löwit, 1973), 448.
53. Th. Hellmuth, 'Von der Sommerfrische zum Massentourismus', in J.
    Stehrer (ed.), *Strobl am Wolfgangsee* (Strobl: Eigenverlag, 1998),
    490–499: 495.
54. J. Radkau, 'Die Verheißungen der Morgenfrühe. Die Lebensreform
    in der neuen Modern', Institut Mathildenhühe Darmstadt (ed.), *Die
    Lebensreform* (Darmstadt, 2001).
55. J. Radkau, 'Aloha – Vom Abheben deutscher Eliten. Die
    verborgenen Inseln der Insider und die Demokratisierung der
    Nervosität', *Kursbuch*, 139 (March 2000), 45–58.

10

The Public's View of Neurasthenia in Germany:
Looking for a New Rhythm of Life

Heinz-Peter Schmiedebach

Introduction

Around 1900, neurasthenia was not only a widely accepted medical
entity, but it also represented particular social and cultural features of
the 'nervous age'. This phenomenon was found in all modern
industrialised countries, although there were some differences
according to national and cultural peculiarities.[1] Not surprisingly,
authors paid a lot of attention to nervousness and neurasthenia.

In some cases they themselves became afflicted with the very
disorder they were writing about. Two famous German examples of
such an affliction are the brothers Thomas and Heinrich Mann. In
1890, Heinrich wrote the short novel *Haltlos* in which he worked out
the nature of a neurasthenic male person. Thomas Mann followed his
brother. In 1897, he made some self-observational reflections in his
diary and diagnosed himself with a lack of sufficient 'nerve-power'.[2]
There is no doubt that these and many other literary works and
personal speculations reflect the mood and the cultural attitude of
the age, and that they, to some extent, convey an impression of the
public's view of neurasthenia. However, this chapter aims to focus on
another kind of public source that probably offers a more trivial view
on nervousness and neurasthenia, far away from literary erudition.

Reading through the two most important contemporary German
weekly magazines, *Gartenlaube* and *Simplicissimus*, one can find
articles and advertisements dealing with neurasthenia and
nervousness, hysteria and hypochondriasis. The articles in
Gartenlaube were written by doctors and it is the doctor's view that
we find in these articles. So the question is raised whether those
articles provide us with evidence of the public's view. It is obvious
that the doctor's articles influenced the reader's view on that theme.
So we have to question whether we actually can assess the public's
view independently of the doctor's opinion on this topic.

Another point must be considered: who or what is or was the public. The magazines read through were more-or-less middle-class oriented. Therefore we find an emphasis on brain-work as an important cause for the emergence of neurasthenia. Brain-work is connected with middle-class culture and work. Therefore it is only a confined middle-class view considered in this chapter.

Despite the fact that both magazines were middle-class oriented they showed a totally different nature concerning contents and rhetorical style. While *Gartenlaube* emphasised a more cultural, academic, and literary side, and provided information on health care,[3] hygiene and scientific progress, *Simplicissimus* was more politically and satirically-oriented. These two magazines were the most widespread of their kind. *Gartenlaube* was founded in 1853 and reached its peak circulation with 382,000 in 1875. Similar contemporary magazines could not achieve that high a circulation. The magazine *Die Welt der Frau* which was founded in 1904 was aimed primarily at a female reading public. Only a few years after 1904 it became a supplement to *Gartenlaube* and in 1920 it was entirely integrated into *Gartenlaube*. *Simplicissimus* became very soon after its foundation in 1896 the leading magazine in the field of the few satirically-oriented magazines. It reached a circulation of between 80,000 and 100,000. Its biting derision of authority-oriented mentality and its mockery of the Kaiser which brought a charge of *lèse majesté* against *Simplicissimus*[4] resulted in a circulation figure of 100,000. Both magazines existed until 1944, but underwent some political shifts. From their inception on they showed a national orientation,[5] but more or less as a kind of liberal patriotism without aggressive hostility towards other nations. *Simplicissimus* argued against chauvinism, imperialism and militarism that were seen as the main dangers of European peace.[6] But after the beginning of World War I, both *Simplicissimus* and *Gartenlaube* struggled for the national affair and supported the German warfare.

Issues of *Gartenlaube* from 1880 to 1919 and of *Simplicissimus* from 1896 to 1919, including the time covering World War I, shall be concentrated on here. In the years previous to the war *Gartenlaube* presented two to four articles a year on nervousness and neurasthenia in an educational and enlightening tone. During the wartime, from 1914 to 1918 *Gartenlaube* published only one article on nervousness. *Simplicissimus* published only a very few short remarks referring to the nerves or nervousness. The majority of the articles published in *Gartenlaube* were written by doctors specialising in the field of psychiatry or neurology. In their articles they avoided a professional style. They wrote to an educated reader and always ended with advice which mainly was concerned with living conditions, life-style, food and rest, not forgetting to exhort the reader to go to a doctor and get professional care if the disorder became uncontrollable. In several articles Beard was mentioned as the first doctor who had described neurasthenia. In contrast to *Gartenlaube, Simplicissimus* included a few pages every week filled with advertisements. Some of these pages showed at times up to five advertisements concerned with *Nervenschwäche,* or neurasthenia.

Despite the very different nature of these two sources, there are some similarities:

1. According to both magazines, nervousness or neurasthenia was seen primarily as a product of modern times, over-excitedness and the special requirements of brain-work, etc. which led to an exhaustion of the nerves and the brain. Due to these causes the disorder was widespread and on the increase.

2. The disorder was said to have a somatic correlation: the performance of the nervous system was impaired because of nutritional problems or a hereditary condition. The spectrum of the different metaphors the magazines referred to embraced the nervous system as a 'battery', or as a mechanically structured framework.

3. Both the advertisements and the articles written by the professional experts conveyed the belief that there was a rich variety of remedies, measures, and other ways available for coping with nervousness as well as for improving individual performance.

With respect to these similarities between the two magazines, one can argue that the view on neurasthenia, derived from the above-mentioned sources, reflects a double nature of neurasthenia. On the one hand the neurasthenic person was a modern person; he or she was in accordance with the modern way of living and with the modes of brainwork. The neurasthenic stood at the head of social and cultural progressive development. On the other hand, it was this very development, with its severe social and cultural changes, which led to exhaustion, a suffering from pain and other complaints.

Thus, the progress of the modern world became threatened by its own features. This problem raised questions from how to cope with neurasthenia on up to the problem how to handle modernity. Neurasthenia became a challenge to search for new ways in dealing with the social and cultural effects of modernity. The public discussion on this disorder fostered reform projects in society and led to a review of individual living conditions.

Fig 10.1

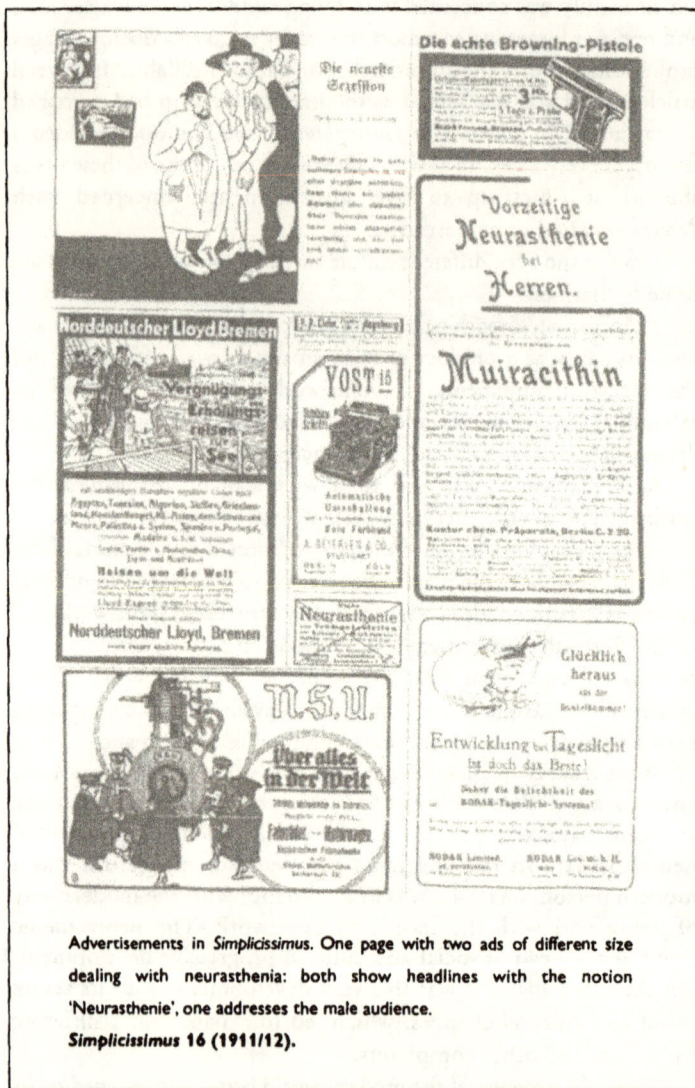

Advertisements in *Simplicissimus*. One page with two ads of different size dealing with neurasthenia: both show headlines with the notion 'Neurasthenie', one addresses the male audience.
Simplicissimus 16 (1911/12).

This chapter is divided into two main parts, according to the two different types of sources. The first part discusses the articles in *Gartenlaube*, and the second part focuses on the analysis of the advertisements in *Simplicissimus*. The short third and last attempts to draw a conclusion.

Neurasthenia in *Gartenlaube*: enlightenment and reforms

In *Gartenlaube* a group of contemporary physicians qualified in psychiatry and neurology wrote articles on all types of psychosomatic disturbances. But, different from the medical discourse in the professional periodicals, all medical authors avoided sophisticated discussions about exact definitions of the particular psychic disorders. Nervousness or neurasthenia was used in a broader and more general sense. The authors focused on the explanation of the cause of 'nervousness', on the description of the wide spectrum of symptoms, and on therapeutic advice.

There were many other articles that did not emphasise neurasthenia, yet referred to the nerves and the nervous system. Father and son Dornblüth were two important contributors to *Gartenlaube*. In 1886, Dornblüth senior maintained that a shortage of blood could lead to insufficient nutrition of the nerves and the brain that would cause, particularly in the case of mental strain, a long-lasting exhaustion of the whole nervous system.[7] Other themes in this context were the 'stutter', which son Otto Dornblüth[8] connected to a nervous nature and a nervous disposition[9] in 1900. E. Heinrich Kisch, professor in Marienbad, discussed 'emaciation' which he saw as a result of a negative influence on the nervous system,[10] along with other causes.

It is not surprising that in the context of superstition and suggestion, Falkenhorst referred to a nervous disposition.[11] According to a widespread opinion of contemporary physicians, the emergence of 'false' ideas and the susceptibility to suggestion were caused by disarranged functions of the nervous system. In another article the influence of light was seen as a positive factor that activated the function of the nerves.[12] Yet, tropical light was said to be too strong a stimulus for European nerves, which reacted to this stimulus by producing a nervous irritability, typical for Europeans living in Africa.[13]

Other articles dealt with drug addiction and alcoholism. The consumption of morphine and cocaine was seen as caused by the desire to overcome the tormenting character of nervous complaints.[14] In 1899, Hugo Hoppe contributed to the question of the curability of alcoholism. He hypothesised that a nervous nature, inferiority, moral deficiency or weak will were due to hereditary flaws. Therapeutic intervention should aim at a restoration of one's physical power, and at a regeneration of the shattered nerves in order to activate energy and to strengthen power of resistance.[15] Albert

Eulenburg, who was one of the contemporary medical professors and founder of a private ambulatory clinic for patients suffering from neurological diseases, also contributed articles dealing with the problem of alcoholism. He, too, supposed a nervous nature of the concerned individuals and a particular structure and function of the nerve apparatus led to alcoholism. He explicitly spoke of neurasthenic persons, using the synonyms 'degenerated' and 'persons of inferior value' (*minderwertig*), and maintained that a physical intolerance towards alcohol, which he said was responsible for alcoholism, was typical in neurasthenic persons.[16]

All of the aforementioned articles made arguments with reference to the nerves. Their authors constituted a nerve-oriented explanatory model and applied this to several cultural phenomena and problems of health care. In addition to those articles, we find several others dealing with neurasthenia and nervousness. One could analyse this central discussion and to answer the following questions: what was seen as the cause of neurasthenia or nervousness? Was there a gender or a social-class-related approach? Which suggestions were made to overcome the disorder?

All authors who discussed neurasthenia and looked for its causes referred to the modern struggle for life, urban living conditions, the one-sided burden on the nerves and brain through mental strain, etc. Yet besides those considerations, one's individual nature and hereditary disposition played a more or less crucial role. Most of the authors saw no difficulties in combining these two approaches;[17] in 1881 Paul Hasse, director of the Königslutter lunatic asylum, gave the impression that acquired weakness of the nerves could be transmitted to off-spring.[18] In the articles of *Gartenlaube*, degeneration did not play such an important role. Other authors, such as Emil Kraepelin, emphasised the theory of degeneration and maintained a more pessimistic view with regard to insanity and nervous illness in a broader sense.[19] Kraepelin was much more engaged in the investigation of the severe forms of insanity than the doctors who wrote their articles in *Gartenlaube*. The latter group focused mainly on less severe disturbances of the nervous system, and because they could avoid an intensive confrontation with those patients suffering from almost untreatable forms of insanity, this group of doctors did not acquire the pessimistic mood which affected several other doctors and psychiatrists. The large majority of the authors of *Gartenlaube* did not have a university appointment. They mostly ran a private practice or worked in public health institutions. They attempted to convince their patients and the reading audience of *Gartenlaube* of a new way of life and therefore had to avoid a pessimistic attitude that was expressed through the theory of degeneration.

Three articles dealt with the so-called '*Schulnervosität*' (school nervousness). Joachim Radkau recently published a chapter on this topic in his book.[20] The problem of real or alleged overburdening of school children became a very important topic from the 1870s onwards. The newly-established academic societies of psychiatrists raised this problem. This discussion fitted into the general debate on nervous weakness or neurasthenia very well. It is interesting that the very common cultural techniques of reading and writing became a point of discussion. Falkenhorst maintained that extensive reading and writing were a real strain for the brain, the eyes and the spine, and caused an increase in the number of short-sighted people, curvature of the spine and an increase of the nervous complaints.[21] Albert Eulenburg presented some statistical accounts on the ratio of pupils with nervous complaints. According to those numbers, about one half of the children studied suffered from nervous disturbances. Eulenburg attacked the school on the basis of two main issues: First, school lessons and homework absorbed too much time which led to a lack of time for recreation and rest; second, the school curriculum only emphasised one-sided brain work and neglected 'muscle' work.[22]

This debate on the overburdening of children underlines the fact that an external factor, the mental strain caused by school requirements, was seen as responsible for the increase of nervous exhaustion. Moreover, it shows that in this context there was no gender-oriented interpretation. Children of both sexes who were forced to go to school ran the risk of acquiring a neurasthenic disorder.[23] The main reference was mental strain. It was said explicitly that working class people who were not exposed to brain work, and the rural population in general, did not suffer from neurasthenia. This opinion was certainly not generally accepted in the medical community. Nervous exhaustion was also considered with regard to working class poeple.[24]

None of the authors in *Gartenlaube* maintained the view that neurasthenia only affected females. Eulenburg equated both sexes and mentioned 'male and female neurasthenia' without pointing out differences with regard to the symptoms or to the conditions of origin.[25] Yet this does not mean that the authors avoided discussing the different natures of males and females. Women were considered more sensitive, and Dornblüth held that, because the female temper was unpredictable and capricious, women were more prone to

225

nervousness than the rugged man. Yet Dornblüth also pointed out that it was impossible to draw a distinct line between the two sexes.[26] In contrast to the articles in *Gartenlaube*, many of the advertisements in *Simplicissimus* were obviously addressed to male persons.

Almost all of the authors accepted that a special individual nervous disposition existed, sometimes acquired through other serious diseases in childhood, or sometimes transmitted genetically by the parents. But this irreversible flaw was not seen as an argument for a pessimistic attitude or resignation to an evil fate. On the contrary, this particular disposition was seen as a need to increase efforts that could overcome the effect of this particular nature of the concerned individual. A rich variety of options that would strengthen the individual's nerves and prevent further deterioration were considered. The suggested measures dealt not only with the individual's life style, but also demanded reforms concerning school, working conditions, urban structure and an elevation of the moral condition. The last aspect in particular provides evidence of the above-mentioned thesis that neurasthenia functioned as a legitimate medical argument for bringing about social and cultural changes.

The medical advice touching the individual's life concerned the balancing of mental and physical activities;[27] an adequate time for rest and recreation was to be secured, and work on Sunday was to be avoided.[28] Most of the authors condemned hedonism and excessive stimulus of the nerves. Reasonable nutrition, particularly in the case of nervous pain of the stomach,[29] with special ingredients for the blood and the nerves, as well as personal hygiene, were also recommended. In some cases electrotherapeutic applications, hydrotherapy and massage were considered very helpful.[30] Other measures were a stay in a spa or a sanatorium;[31] recreation leaves fostered good results,[32] but very nervous persons needed to avoid travelling by train because of the shaking ride and the noisy and overcrowded stations. For those persons, a journey with a steamboat was the best way to travel.[33] Most of these recommendations had one single goal in mind – to take a break. They encouraged a limited break out of the daily grind and provided a resistance against acceleration of life in modern society. Coping with neurasthenia led to the discovery of a deliberately slow-paced withdrawal from daily life, legitimated by medical arguments.

These newly-discovered and demanded relaxation periods were to be used for a renewal of inner moral and cultural attitudes. They provided the chance to develop a self-referential strengthening of body and mind.[34] Albert Eulenburg saw an inner emptiness and solitude of the individual, a lack of ideals, faith, authority, and conviction. The modern mood of 'decadence' corresponded to the nature of the neurasthenic person. But in an optimistic tone and emphasising a pedagogical approach, Eulenburg called for an education of the character, training of thinking, understanding, and power of judgement. These faculties were to provide the base for a robust and independent volition. This was a very important protection against the flood of nervousness.[35] Another article encouraged a similar concept and wrote about the physician's role as educator.[36]

Yet neurasthenia also functioned as an argument in the debate on social and cultural reforms by addressing the administration of the state and communities. In the context of the discussion on the overburdening of school children we found several suggestions for a reform of school education. Paul Hasse called for a reduction of the school curriculum and for the establishment of regular times with games and physical training in order to overcome the mental strain of brain work. This careful treatment of youth would lead to higher performance later.[37] Eulenburg made a similar statement and demanded an abolishment of afternoon lessons, a decrease in time spent on single lessons, a prolongation of the recess and an arrangement of the lesson plan that would meet the children's needs for sleeping and eating.[38] In an article about the harm that writing and reading does to the brain and nerves, Falkenhorst called for a reform of the script used. He argued for short words because short words were much easier to conceive than longer ones, and advocated simple rules of orthography. Such changes would be a relief for the overburdened brain of nervous humankind.[39]

In 1885, *Gartenlaube* came out with a short article upon the publication of Krafft-Ebing's book on sick and healthy nerves. The article focused on statements of Krafft-Ebing which maintained that brain workers should receive a leave entitlement of four weeks a year and that teachers be given a higher salary so that they were not forced to give lessons on Sundays and holidays. Moreover, the state should provide a subsidy for necessary stays in a spa. The application of these suggestions would enhance the performance of the individual brain worker and prevent premature and forced retirements.[40] Obviously *Gartenlaube* supported the demand for organised breaks and called for a reform in order to take part in deliberately slow-paced recess.

One last public demand in the context of the debate on neurasthenia must be mentioned. It was said that one crucial cause of the origin of nervous weakness was urban noise. To a large extent this noise originated from the horse carts which rumbled over the stone pavement, accompanied by the cracks of the whips of the drivers. In order to diminish this source of noise, it was necessary to call for a new street covering and to prohibit the drivers' unnecessary cracks. In 1896, these demands were fostered by an article in *Gartenlaube*,[41] with a reference to an article in the *Lancet*. All the mentioned examples give evidence that the public debate on neurasthenia was used to call for reforms and other improvements. Thus neurasthenia also initiated a discussion on how to cope with life's modern strains and how to find ways to handle the requirements of modern life.

During the wartime, the articles dealing with medical problems were concerned with the rehabilitation of casualties or with hygienic or nutritional topics. Only one single article on nervousness was published. The author, Artaria, who was not a medical doctor, welcomed the war that was said to have swept away unhealthy attitudes and nervous behaviour.[42] The author obviously felt bothered by the discussion on nervousness and by the complaints of nervous people. But his jubilation was a little bit premature. In 1919 there were again two articles dealing with that problem. Carl Pototzky, doctor of a children's outpatient clinic in Berlin, wrote about the nervous child.[43] Helenefriederike Stelzner, educated in psychiatry and who in 1905 became the first appointed physician responsible for schools in Charlottenburg (Berlin), published an article on the nerves of women in bad times.[44] Both authors explicitly mentioned a hereditary disposition of neurasthenia but did not refer to degeneration. The post-war situation was expressed in these articles. It was characterised by enlarged strain of the nerves, combined with insufficient nutrition. The authors referred to the well-known measures: avoiding of over-excitedness of nerves and brain, taking breaks with sufficient long periods of recreation, and strengthening of the body through physical exercises.

The reading public was exhorted to be careful with its energetic resources in order to save and enlarge the 'capital' of nerves and energy of the German nation. This was a reference to nationalism, but it was the only one and it avoided any aggressive attitude towards other nations. Like the articles on neurasthenia of the pre-war time, the post-war ones did not show a particular nationalistic bent. This is not surprising, because neurasthenia was seen as a product of the modern way of life, typical for all civilised societies and nations. Therefore neurasthenia could not be cited to discriminate against other nations. After the war, when nervousness and neurasthenia were revisited, *Gartenlaube* aimed to point out ways of how to overcome the detrimental situation, and to give helpful advice. In order to demonstrate medical competence it was best to concentrate on medical explanations, to avoid political incitement, and to use an optimistic tone. Particularly the last point made it necessary to keep distance from degeneration because this pessimistic concept with its negative predetermination of decline did not give way for a real improvement of one's personal situation.

Neurasthenia in *Simplicissimus*: the marketplace of remedies

Simplicissimus published a large amount of advertisements referring to neurasthenia or weakness of the nerves. The average number is two to three advertisements per week. These ads had to address the customer's needs; yet it was also necessary, particularly in the case of a disease or the sale of remedies, to meet the patient's knowledge about the disease and the coping-habits of the individual involved. The text also had to diminish possible anxieties of the potential customer and to legitimate the effectiveness of the product. A good advertisement had to be in accordance with the images and metaphors of neurasthenia that the public audience was already familiar with. In analysing the different types of advertisements we have to deal with the different metaphorical models of neurasthenia, and to ask which group of patients the advertisements were mainly addressed to. In this context it is necessary to refer to the gender perspective.

The advertisements are of different sizes. Some of them fill half a page; others are much smaller. They all are arranged on pages that consist only of other advertisements. Only a few of the ads concerned were illustrated. Two ads show an apparatus providing galvanic current against head-neurasthenia applied to a person. Yet those advertisements are the exception; the majority consist primarily of text, and very often we find full phrases, similar to a small article. Very common is a large and prominent headline. Some headlines addressed a special group of patients, for example males (*Männer-Nervenschwäche*). Some advertisements, especially during war-time, did not refer to the nervous system alone but also mentioned other parts or fluids of the body. Very often we found the connection between '*Blut und Nerven*' (blood and nerves). According to the special demands of the battlefield, these advertisements aimed at a strengthening of the whole individual, including the body and the mental sphere. About half of all advertisements included the names of the inventors in the text, most of who were highly educated persons with a doctoral or a professorial title. Academic authority was seen as conducive to the sale of the product.

Fig. 10.2

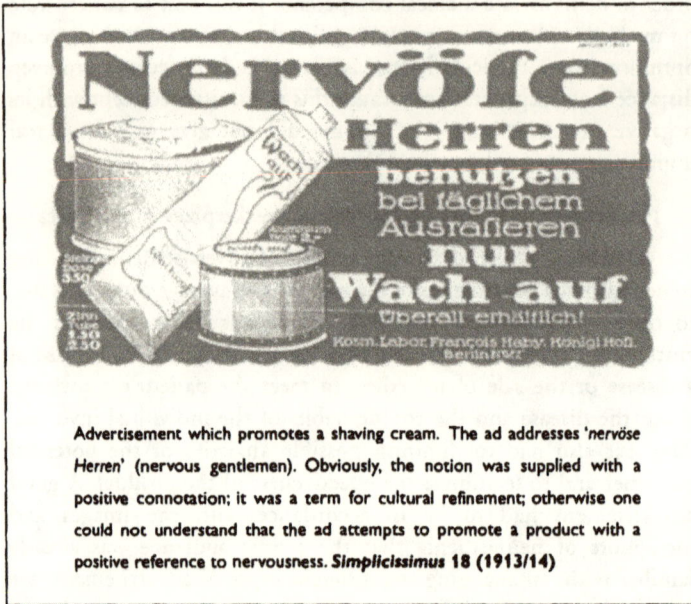

Advertisement which promotes a shaving cream. The ad addresses '*nervöse Herren*' (nervous gentlemen). Obviously, the notion was supplied with a positive connotation; it was a term for cultural refinement; otherwise one could not understand that the ad attempts to promote a product with a positive reference to nervousness. *Simplicissimus* **18** (1913/14)

Most of the advertisements did not give an elaborate statement on the nature of neurasthenia. Yet a large number of ads provide us with more information; they render an account of the effectiveness and offer some kind of simple physiological explanations. We can discern two different models:

1. The anatomical-mechanistic approach. The nervous system was seen as something like a framework consisting of ropes and cables; their function depended on sufficient nutrition. This metaphor of the nervous system as a living framework was connected with the promotion of remedies that were synthesised on the basis of lecithin. This substance, a chemical compound that contains phosphorous acid, was seen as the basic building block of the nervous system. In the 1830s, it was proved that phosphorous acid was an agent of the nervous system. This evidence had become the basis of widely endorsed therapies by the 1880s.[45] The advertisement which promoted 'Biocitin', which was said to consist of ten per cent biologically pure lecithin, referred to nerve nutrition. According to this text, 'modern times' required the full power of mind and nerves daily. This process could lead to a deterioration of the 'nerves'; within the weak, tired or sick nerve the 'nerve matter' would dwindle, which could be seen through a microscope. The nerves would lose their normal tension. By applying the substance that was lacking, the re-creation process could be initiated. The nerves would grow stronger, normal tension would be restored and soon, full function would be available.[46]

2. The other model of nerve function which was implicitly seen in some of the advertisements referred to a more energetic approach, based on the idea of the electric nature of nerve-force.[47] In the early decades of the nineteenth century, some physiologists had linked electricity with the nervous function and around the middle of the nineteenth century, electro-therapy became a crucial therapeutic remedy with regard to all kinds of nervous diseases, particularly in France and Germany. Beard had also recommended galvanism and general faradisation for patients with nervous complaints. The application of any kind of current required electric devices that the doctor was obliged to purchase. Therefore advertisements that promoted electric therapies for neurasthenia did not aim to sell such an apparatus to patients, but offered a therapeutic service provided by a special institute which was established for this purpose.

Again, modern life with its increased 'struggle for life' was seen as the cause of strain that would lead to a strong over-excitement of the psychic functions. Very soon after this over-excitement, neurasthenia would emerge. A repetitive application of galvanic current with the '*Kopfgalvanisator*' (galvanic apparatus for the head) could bring about positive results and thus help to avoid expensive care in a sanatorium. Those advertisements that announced therapeutic services based on the application of galvanic current subscribed to this energetic and dynamic model of the nervous systems.[48]

As we have seen, the advertisements referred to two models of the nervous system and accordingly derived two different explanatory metaphors for neurasthenia: 1) a more mechanically based model of the nervous system, and 2) an electric and energetic model. The brain and the nervous system worked like batteries that lost their power in the case of 'over-excitement' and serious strain. Both models co-existed at the same time in the same magazine. The question of which metaphor was maintained by which type of advertisement is easy to answer: the type of metaphor used depended on the nature of the product that was for sale. If the product was a remedy that was seen as a nutritive substance for the nerves, then the mechanical framework metaphor was used; if the product was a therapeutic service offering the application of galvanic current, then the battery-metaphor was applied. Both models represent two different sides of one single system. The mechanistic approach refers to the anatomical basis of the nervous system; it is concerned with the matter and form of nerves and brain. This approach corresponds to the anatomical view of a bodily structure. The energetic approach is concerned with the functions of an organic system. In order to investigate these functions one needs the methods of physiology; accordingly, this approach goes in the direction of physiology. The combination of the anatomical with the physiological view leads to an elaborate consideration. The use of only one of these two approaches in the previously mentioned advertisements, according to the character of the product which was promoted, means a reduction of the complex problem. This reduction is advantageous to the promotion of the concerned remedy, because it more easily met the level of medical knowledge of the average laymen who were to be persuaded to buy the product.

We have to state that the same models of the nervous system and neurasthenia which dominated the medical discourse were also prevalent in the advertisements, though of course somewhat simplified. Modern life and the increased struggle for life were seen as the causes of neurasthenia. There were no hints at other aetiological factors such as endocrinological dysfunction of the glands or anything of the sort. Yet, apart from the articles in *Gartenlaube*, an individual hereditary disposition was not mentioned. This is not surprising. The customer only buys the product when he or she is convinced that the product will produce results. However, in the case of a hereditary determination, the effect of the product was extremely questionable. To bring up heredity is to risk a pessimistic attitude. This seems to be one crucial reason why the designation of a hereditary flaw in an advertisement was avoided.

The text in most of the ads does not address a special group. The frequent complaints listed in these advertisements are: general exhaustion, tiredness, weakness, nervousness, headache, insomnia, restlessness, weakness of memory, irritability, etc. However some ads show particular phrases and formulations which were directed to special complaints and therefore addressed selected groups of persons. The advertisement announcing 'Biocitin' explicitly mentioned feeble children who had difficulties in school. For those children 'Biocitin' should be suitable for enhancing their mental forces by increasing the patient's nerve matter.[49]

Another type of advertisement used the headline to address male customers: '*Männer Nervenschwäche*'. With this headline there was no doubt which group of persons was being targeted. [50] There were some other types of advertisements that primarily addressed the male audience. Some of those notices did not hesitate to point out which problem they wanted to deal with: the weakness of sexual organs or impaired potency. One of these remedies, 'Rubiacitol', did not only strengthen the whole nervous system but particularly the brain, spinal cord, and the sexual organs.[51]

The notion 'male neurasthenia' was a metaphor for sexual weakness or impotence. Another term which denoted the same kind of weakness was '*vorzeitige Nervenschwäche*' (premature neurasthenia). Especially the remedy 'Muiracithin' was recommended in the case of 'premature male neurasthenia'. The text of the advertisement said that this remedy combined lecithin as a drug for strengthening the nerve-force with 'Muirapuama' that was in one advertisement characterised as stimulating.[52] Another ad promoting the same drug used more direct words. 'Muirapuama' was described as a Brazilian '*Potenzholz*' (wood for affecting potency). This advertisement showed the headline '*Neurastheniker aller Länder verwenden mit bestem Erfolg Muiracithin*' (Neurasthenic persons from all countries are using Muiracithin very succesfully) and presented six professors who testified the surprising results of therapy with 'Muiracithin'. Two of those six professors lived abroad, one in Italy (Naples) and the other in France: the international success of the drug could be praised in this advertisement. One of the professorial witnesses also referred to 'female neurasthenia' that he was able to treat successfully with this drug while all other remedies failed.[53] Despite the fact that this witness focused on 'female neurasthenia', the main point of those advertisements was the 'male' or 'premature neurasthenia'.

Another rare type of advertisement addressed the male consumer by propagating 'Kola-Dultz' which was something like a cocaine-pill.[54] With respect to the well-known effect of cocaine on sexual potency, it is most likely that this advertisement also addressed the problem of 'premature male neurasthenia'. The advertisement of 'Tamulecon', which helped fight 'premature neurasthenia of gentlemen', quoted four doctors from different towns who witnessed successful therapies. Two of those doctors were military physicians,[55] which means that this advertisement suggested a widespread 'male neurasthenia', even among military persons who were a crucial pillar of imperial Germany.

The male consumers became the main group of interest for the producers of treatments during the wartime. A large number of advertisements recommended different remedies against weakness of nerves and against physical exhaustion. An example of such a drug is 'Sanatogen' that was said to restore body and nerve-force.[56] Although those remedies did not particularly aim at 'male neurasthenia' they emphasised the male customer, because a large number of potential male consumers at the front suffer from general exhaustion. The advertisement addresses the family members at home who were encouraged to buy the product and send it to the husband or son on the battlefield.

One advertisement directly addresses female customers. It has the headline: '*kluge Hausfrauen*' (clever housewives) always have 'Leciferrin' at hand. It was recommended to heal nervous exhaustion as well as anaemia. There was no reference to female neurasthenia. The advertisement addressed women in their role as housewives because the housewife was seen as the crucial person who provides a sufficient supply of remedies against all common disturbances and diseases.[57] This advertisement did not reveal a gender-related aspect of female neurasthenia, but emphasised the traditional role of the housewife as a family doctor.

Conclusion

The sources of the two magazines are only a small segment out of the huge amount of books and articles dealing with neurasthenia. These magazines give the impression that neurasthenia was a very common and widespread nervous disorder. With regard to cause, symptoms, remedies, and metaphors of neurasthenia, we find the well-known descriptions often in accordance with medical discourse. The notion 'premature male neurasthenia' made it possible to deal publicly with male impotency. With the exception of these advertisements, a special gender-related preference could not be found. Neurasthenia afflicted children, male and female persons.

Contrary to discussion within the medical community, hereditary conditions did not play such an important role. To some extent this was due to the special nature of the source (advertisement), as already pointed out above. Yet, even in articles that referred to a hereditary flaw, we can find an optimistic tone. All authors in *Gartenlaube* were engaged to persuade the concerned reader to follow their advice and to change his life in order to overcome the detrimental weakness.

This optimistic mood was rooted in the conviction that the effects of modern pressure that harmed the nerves and brain could be successfully dealt with by the establishment of longer restorative periods. The newly-discovered slower pace of those recreation times was to be used for a restoring of the nerve-force. This was particularly important for the brain-workers of the middle-class. Therefore we find the call for several social and cultural reforms which were intended to bring those persons the pleasure of a summer resort. It was felt that government funding should enable the middle class brain-worker to copy an aristocratic life-style in a spa, at least for four weeks a year.

Neurasthenia was the essential signum of exhaustion caused by modern life-style and by modern mental strain. Yet this disorder, the incarnation of weakness, played a central enough role in society to result in a productive tension that fostered an intensive discussion of the problem of how the human individual was to adapt to the requirements of modern work and life. Neurasthenia was simultaneously a symbol for the attainments of the modern age and for the detrimental consequences of modern features. This productive ambiguity initiated the search for a new rhythm of life.

Notes

1. For Germany see Volker Roelcke, *Krankheit und Kulturkritik. Psychiatrische Gesellschaftsdeutungen im bürgerlichen Zeitalter (1790-1914)* (Frankfurt am Main and New York: Campus, 1999); *idem*, 'Biologising Social Facts: An Early 20th Century Debate on Kraepelin's Concepts of Culture, Neurasthenia, and Degeneration', *Culture, Medicine and Psychiatry*, 21 (1997), 383–403; Joachim Radkau, *Das Zeitalter der Nervosität. Deutschland zwischen Bismarck und Hitler* (München and Wien: Carl Hanser Verlag, 1998); Wolfgang U. Eckart, 'Die wachsende Nervosität unserer Zeit – Medizin und Kultur um 1900 am Beispiel einer Modekrankheit', in Gangolf Hübinger, Rüdiger v. Bruch und Friedrich W. Graf (eds), *Kultur und Kulturwissenschaften um 1900, Vol.II. Idealismus und Positivismus* (Stuttgart: Franz Steiner, 1997), 207–26.

2. See Manfred Dierks, 'Krankheit und Tod im frühen Werk Thomas Manns', in Thomas Sprecher (ed.), *Auf dem Weg zum 'Zauberberg'. Die Davoser Literaturtage 1996* (Frankfurt am Main: Vittorio Klostermann, 1997), 11–32: 13–14 (Thomas–Mann–Studien, 16).

3. See Cora Guddat, *Wie erziehe ich ein Kind zu einem gesunden Menschen? Gesundheitsaufklärung in der Gartenlaube und in Hand- und Lehrbüchern von 1885-1914* (Diss. med. Köln, 1999).

4. See Helga Abret and Aldo Keel, *Die Majestätsbeleidigungsaffaire des 'Simplicissimus'-Verlegers Albert Langen. Briefe und Dokumente zu Exil und Begnadigung 1898-1903* (Frankfurt am Main, Bern and New York: Peter Lang, 1985).

5. On the political bent of the two magazines see Kirsten Belgum,

Popularising the Nation: Audience, Representation, and the Production of Identity in Die Gartenlaube, 1853-1900 (Lincoln etc: University of Nebraska Press, 1998) (Modern German culture and literature); Ruprecht Konrad, *Nationale und internationale Tendenzen im 'Simplicissimus' (1896-1933): der Wandel künstlerisch-politischer Bewußtseinsstrukturen im Spiegel von Satire und Karikatur in Bayern* (Diss. phil. München, 1975). See also Ann Taylor Allen, *Satire and Society in Wilhelmine Germany: Kladderadatsch and Simplicissimus; 1890-1914* (Lexington, Kentucky: University Press of Kentucky, 1984); Gertrud Maria Rösch (ed.), *Simplicissimus. Glanz und Elend der Satire in Deutschland* (Regensburg: Universitätsverlag, 1996) (Schriftenreihe der Universität Regensburg, 23).

6. Ruprecht, Konrad, 'Politische Zielsetzungen und Selbstverständnis des "*Simplicissimus*"', in *Simplicissimus. Eine satirische Zeitschrift München 1896-1944* (München: Haus der Kunst München e.V., 1978), 88-109.

7. F. Dornblüth, 'Blutarmuth und Bleichsucht', *Gartenlaube* (1886), 690-2.

8. Otto Dornblüth worked as psychiater and neurologist and published Otto Dornblüth, *Die Psychoneurosen Neurasthenie, Hysterie und Psychasthenie* (Leipzig: Veit und Comp, 1911) .

9. Otto Dornblüth, 'Ueber das Stottern', *Gartenlaube* (1900), 591-2.

10. E. Heinrich Kisch, 'Wie bekämpft man die Abmagerung?', *Gartenlaube* (1896), 7-8.

11. E. Falkenhorst, 'Die Suggestion im Dienste des Aberglaubens', *Gartenlaube* (1895), 312-15.

12. J. H. Baas, 'Mehr Licht', *Gartenlaube* (1891), 568-71.

13. Steudel, 'Die Kraft der tropischen Sonne und ihre Wirkung auf den menschlichen Körper', *Gartenlaube* (1907), 242-5.

14. Landenberger, 'Die Morphiumsucht', *Gartenlaube* (1886), 90-1; H. Otto; 'Morphium- und Cocainsucht', *Gartenlaube* (1891), 191-2.

15. Hugo Hoppe, 'Die Heilbarkeit der Trunksucht', *Gartenlaube* (1899), 472-5.

16. Albert Eulenburg, 'Noch einmal zur Frage der Alkoholenthaltung ('Alkoholabstinenz')', *Gartenlaube* (1901), 876-9.

17. Enoch Heinrich Kisch, 'Nervöse Magenleiden', *Gartenlaube* (1886), 160-3; Enoch Heinrich Kisch, 'Das nervöse Herz', *Gartenlaube* (1889), 16-18; A. Eulenburg, 'Ueber Schulnervosität und Schulüberbürdung', *Gartenlaube* (1896), 192-6; Otto Dornblüth, 'Nervöse Angstzustände', *Gartenlaube* (1897), 444-7.

18. Paul Hasse, 'Schule und Nervosität. Zur Beleuchtung der Ueberbürdungsfrage vom irrenärztlichen Standpunkte', *Gartenlaube*

(1881), 7–9.

19. See the article of Volker Roelcke in this book.

20. On that theme see Radkau, *op. cit.* (note 1), 315–22.

21. E. Falkenhorst, 'Buchstaben und Nerven', *Gartenlaube* (1894), 399–402.

22. Albert Eulenburg, *op. cit.* (note 17), 192–6.

23. In his book Otto Dornblüth wrote a special chapter on 'Neurasthenie des Kindes', see Dornblüth, *op. cit.* (note 8), 210–31.

24. See G. Heilig, Fabrikarbeit und Nervenleiden. Beiträge zur Ätiologie der Arbeiterneurosen (Diss. Med. Berlin, 1908). On neurasthenia and health insurance see Felix Boenheim, 'Ueber Neurasthenie', *Soziale Medizin* (1929), 433–6; a more psychologic approach has Hans Lehmann, ' Neurasthenie und soziale Lage', *Soziale Medizin* (1929), 481–94.

25. Albert Eulenburg, 'Ueber Nervenschutz und Nervenstärkung', *Gartenlaube* (1899), I. 860–4, II.891–5.

26. Dornblüth, *op. cit.* (note 8), 13–14.

27. Otto Dornblüth, 'Ueber den Schwindel', *Gartenlaube* (1899), 154–6.

28. Anonymous, 'Ueber kranke und gesunde Nerven', *Gartenlaube* (1885), 627–8.

29. E. Heinrich Kisch, *op. cit.* (note 17), 160–3.

30. Otto Dornblüth, *op. cit.* (note 17), 444–7.

31. E. Heinrich Kisch, 'Brunnen- und Badekuren', *Gartenlaube* (1898), 190–1.

32. P. Meißner, 'Erholungsreisen', *Gartenlaube* (1909), 378–9.

33. A. Hübner, 'Mehr Ruhe!', *Gartenlaube* (1896), 808–11.

34. Hermann Baas, 'Das Herzklopfen', *Gartenlaube* (1897), 560–3.

35. Eulenburg, *op. cit.* (note 25), 891.

36. C.F., 'Der Arzt als Erzieher des Kindes', *Gartenlaube* (1909), 188–90.

37. Hasse, *op. cit.* (note 18), 9.

38. Eulenburg, *op. cit.* (note 17), 195–6.

39. Falkenhorst, *op. cit.* (note 21), 402.

40. Anonymous, 'Ueber kranke und gesunde Nerven', *Gartenlaube* (1885), 628.

41. Hübner, *op. cit.* (note 33), 810–11.

42. A. Artaria, 'Die Nervösen', *Gartenlaube. Supplement Die Welt der Frau*, Nr. 36 (1915), 572–3.

43. Carl Pototzky, 'Das nervöse Kind. Briefe eines Arztes', *Gartenlaube* (1919), 595–7, 624–5, 682–3.

44. H. Stelzner, 'Das Nervenleben der Frau in ernster Zeit', *Gartenlaube.*

Supplement Die Welt der Frau, Nr. 52 (1919), 409–10.

45. See David Walker, 'Modern nerves, nervous moderns: Notes on male neurasthenia', *Australian cultural history*, 6 (1982), 49–63.

46. See Anonymous, 'Nervenarbeit und Nervensubstanz (Lecithin)', *Simplicissimus*, 17 (1912/13), 547; advertisement 'Biocitin', *Simplicissimus*, 17 (1912/13), 126; advertisement 'Biocitin', *Simplicissimus*, 17 (1912/13), 46; anonymous 'Ich bin so nervös!', *Simplicissimus*, 17 (1912/13), 514.

47. See Roelcke, *op. cit.* (note 1), 101–11.

48. Advertisement 'Neurasthenie des Gehirns', *Simplicissimus*, 16 (1911/12), 410; advertisement 'Die Behandlung der Kopfnervosität', Simplicissimuüs, 16 (1911/12), 498.

49. Anonymous 'Ich bin so nervös!', *Simplicissimus*, 17 (1912/13), 514.

50. Advertisement 'Männer Nervenschwäche', *Simplicissimus*, 15 (1910/11), 742.

51. Advertisement 'Rubiacitol', *Simplicissimus*, 17 (1912/13), 789.

52. Advertisement 'Muiracithin', *Simplicissimus*, 17 (1912/13), 401.

53. Advertisement 'Neurastheniker aller Länder', *Simplicissimus*, 15 (1910/11), 841.

54. Advertisement 'Kola-Dultz', *Simplicissimus*, 17 (1912/13), 48.

55. Advertisement 'Neurasthenie bei Herren', *Simplicissimus*, 16 (1911/12), 96.

56. Advertisement 'Sanatogen', *Simplicissimus*, 20 (1915/16), 450.

57. Advertisement 'Kluge Hausfrauen', *Simplicissimus*, 21 (1916/17), 612.

11

Neurasthenia in the Netherlands

Joost Vijselaar

> The importance of functional neurosis needs no further
> demonstration nowadays. Every layman knows that the number of
> neurasthenics is increasing alarmingly. A large number of ill people
> looking for treatment is actually suffering from neurasthenia directly
> or indirectly....[1]

wrote Gerbrandus Jelgersma, the future professor at Leiden
University and one of the foremost Dutch psychiatrists of his day, in
1897. His judgement echoed general ideas of the European/
American medical community. But apart from evident similarities
between the history of neurasthenia in Holland and other European
countries, the ideas about this 'modern' illness and the societal and
cultural functions it had, took on a distinct characteristic in the
Netherlands, owing to the specific social and cultural developments
in this country. This distinctness is closely intertwined with the
question of the nature of the *fin-de-siècle* in the Netherlands, which
is generally thought of as having been more optimistic than
pessimistic in tone. This chapter will discuss three domains in which
neurasthenia played a significant role, to know: politics, literature
and medicine. The order of subjects is intentional because of the
chronology of the developments.

Neurasthenia in politics

Already in the late seventies of the nineteenth century, even before
the concept of neurasthenia was coined and made popular by Beard,
Dutch political commentators complained about a 'loss of nerve'
among the Dutch population, especially among the male part of it.
The nation had been 'weakened' and 'wearied', it was 'adrift' and had
lost its moral orientation. Especially men showed a conspicuous lack
of character, strength and willpower. They had become 'unnerved'
and 'effeminate'. This weakness, which would in the long run
endanger the international position of the Netherlands, was

attributed to both a sickening 'over-civilisation', which was accompanied by hedonism, materialism and scepticism, and a disintegration of community.[2] During the 1880s the concept of neurasthenia of Beard with its strong ring of social and cultural criticism was taken over by these Dutch commentators.[3]

The political and cultural background to this pessimistic view of Dutch society has been thoroughly analysed by the historian Henk te Velde, among others in his thesis *A sense of community and responsibility. Liberalism and nationalism in the Netherlands, 1870-1918*. As Te Velde made clear the aforementioned commentators were mostly representatives of the governing liberal elite, that dominated politics in the Netherlands since 1848. The position of liberal government remained unchallenged until the seventies of the nineteenth century, when different developments weakened its control of power. First of all liberalism itself fell apart into a conservative faction, upholding orthodox principles like laissez-faire, and a grouping of 'young liberals', that advocated mild social reform and government intervention. At the same time different emancipatory movements made their appearance on the political scene. First of all orthodox Calvinists organised themselves into the first political party. A step that is often regarded as the first symptom of the advent of mass democracy in the Netherlands and – together with the rift between the liberals and the Roman Catholics – the beginning of the phenomenon of denominational 'pillarisation' that was to characterise Dutch society for almost a century. The seventies also saw the first upsurge of the labour movement and political radicalism in the Netherlands.[4]

The appearance of overt dissension and strife in politics as well as the participation of the first lower-class elements in the political debate (e.g. the orthodox protestant party had a strong lower-class constituency) shattered liberal certainties. The idea of the Dutch society as a harmonious community governed by a paternal, altruistic and congenial group of bourgeois citizens, that legitimised liberal control of government, received a fatal blow. It was against this background that the reigning elite started to doubt the future of the nation, feared for the disintegration of society and the loss of moral. Especially the growth of a pluralistic code of ethics, one of the results of the emancipation of labour, religious groups and women, fuelled the old-liberal worries about the 'weakening' of Dutch society. It was in this context that the said political commentators talked about a fatal 'loss of nerve' and adopted the ideas on neurasthenia.[5]

To redress this situation the old-liberals did not think, of course, in terms of healing and individual medicine, but of a programme of (individual) moral regeneration that stressed the importance of character building and creating a sense of patriotism. They put forward ideas about the introduction of general conscription, voluntary military exercise and a reform of education that would stress will, emotion and physical exercise as against purely intellectual development. Around 1880, the time of the occupation of the autonomous state of Transvaal (in South Africa) by the British, these critics contrasted the flaccid Dutch with the stern, heroic, unspoiled and God-fearing Dutch speaking Boers, their far off relatives. They propagated a return to these values of old as a remedy against 'morbid over-civilisation' and the loss of a moral anchor in Western society. However, the old-liberals fought a losing battle, as they had to leave government to a younger generation and their pessimistic prophecies about an uprooted society did not come about.[6]

Literary neurasthenia

Over and against this old-liberal faction a group of progressive radicals and 'young liberals' manifested itself during the eighties in the arts and especially in literature. The group comprised young intellectuals, journalists, lawyers and doctors, an occasional psychiatrist amongst them (e.g. Frederik van Eeden, A. Aletrino). Like elsewhere in Europe, this new generation of writers (the 'Movement of the Eighties'), many of them belonging to the bourgeoisie and the higher middle-classes, criticised the materialism, complacency and the stifling mores of the 'bourgeois satisfait'. In their literary work they turned on the one hand to a new, highly individualised Romanticism inspired by English poets (Shelley, Keats), and on the other hand to French Naturalism. Inspired by Taine and Zola and contemporary medical and psychological science, they made the novel into a 'scientific experiment' with heredity and social environment or 'milieu'. The 'neurasthenic', the 'hysteric' and the 'dégénéré' became the chief protagonists of their novels. By their stories of unavoidable fate, thwarted expectations and misery these writers attacked the lifestyle of the middle classes. It was the rigid sexual morality and narrow-minded conventions of the bourgeoisie together with the tainted blood of old settled families that according to these novelists were the mainspring of neurasthenia and depression in their literary characters. At the same time they in a way hailed nervousness as a sign of higher 'artistic' sensibility and some of them posed as degenerate dandies, standing aloof from the philistine culture of the establishment. All this mirrored in a rather faint way the literary trends in for example Paris or Vienna.[7]

The naturalistic novel did not reap much appreciation among the Dutch reading public and literary critics. It was regarded as being unaesthetic in its 'scientific objectivity'. It lacked the uplifting aims of the traditional 'idealistic' novels. On the contrary it stressed the gloomy, pathological aspects of life and society. More outspoken commentators vilified it as 'pornography' that unjustly emphasised lust and animality. However, the brunt of criticism was levelled against the overt determinism of Naturalism. The idea of inexorable fate and heredity eroded the dogma of the autonomous soul, central to the Calvinist ethos pervading Dutch culture. For the same reason the original theory of degeneration, so important in French literature and (psychological) medicine, was hardly accepted in intellectual circles in the Netherlands.[8]

During the last decade of the nineteenth century – the (real) *fin-de-siècle* – Dutch literature slowly turned away from pessimistic Naturalism and the cult of extreme subjectivity. As art in general novelists and poets embraced mysticism and esotericism or on the other hand committed themselves to 'higher' humanitarian or socialist aims of reform. The arts, especially in their applied form, were now thought of as instruments for the creation of a real community and the improvement of life and society. Artists should devote themselves by vocation to the common cause, their chief means of expression being the '*Gesamtkunstwerk*'. In literature this tendency expressed itself both in the genre of 'social naturalism' dealing with the life of the lower classes and a more positive, optimistic plot of the stories. Degeneration, heredity and neurasthenia did not disappear from literature, but figured less prominent among the subjects.[9]

This change of the cultural atmosphere towards hope, optimism and trust marked Dutch society as a whole around the turn of the century and must be seen in context of major social and political developments. The Netherlands went at the time through a process of rapid economic expansion, industrialisation took off, the population and its prosperity grew. Social and political strife abated as the most important public debate – that about equal rights for education along denominational lines (*de 'Schoolstrijd'*) – was resolved. At the same time a new role of the state in creating social justice and security and in adjusting socio-economic development was accepted by the young-liberal and confessional parties that came into power in a broader democratic constituency. Social and cultural policy by the national and local government and communal action – young-liberals taking the initiative - eased the strains of modernisation and stimulated societal and national integration. This initiated a process of integration of state and nation that countered centrifugal tendencies of modernisation. The apprehensions of the seventies and eighties about a disintegration and decline of Dutch society and culture did not come about. Just the opposite was true: Dutch society witnessed a wave of moderate nationalism at the occasion of the ascension of the young Queen Wilhelmina (in 1898) and in answer to the successful 'imperialistic' campaigns in the Dutch Indies. So the proverbial gloom, nihilism and decadence did not mark the *fin-de-siècle* in the Netherlands. Its is almost a matter of communis opinio among Dutch historians to regard the decade around 1900 as one of expectancy and promise.[10]

These cultural conditions coloured the 'discours' on neurasthenia in the Netherlands. Apart from the medical community, only small and specific groups seem to have taken up the idea of neurasthenia with its concomitant critical concept of social and cultural aetiology, and that only for a short spell of time mainly during the 1880s. Both old-liberals and paradoxically the opposite group of dissatisfied radical authors of a younger generation, used the theory of neurasthenia to demonstrate the pathological consequences on respectively the decline and moral rigidity of bourgeois 'civilised' society. In the nineties a change of political and social climate occurred that took away many of the worries that had fostered the theory of neurasthenia. The old-liberals ended up as a conservative political minority whereas radicals and young-liberals acquired positions that gave them a chance to work towards their social and humanitarian ideals. Apart from its medical meaning, 'neurasthenia' seems to have lost its political and moral usefulness around 1900.

Owing to different cultural circumstances, a strong aversion to determinism among them, the talk about neurasthenia never gained the pessimistic, even fatalistic overtones of the French debate. In the Netherlands it did not have the strong biological perspective of degeneration, but it was maybe distinguished by moral views. It was less about telephone, trains and traffic, in general the speed of modern life, and more about character, education or sexual conventions.

Dutch psychiatry

The 'neurasthenia' old-liberals and naturalist novelists wrote about or described in their political or moral 'discours', did not refer directly to actual patients suffering from nervousness, fatigue, headaches or tics. Although many writers and poets had personal experience of nervous symptoms, it was doctors who dealt with people whose concrete complaints could be diagnosed as neurasthenia. Before discussing the place of neurasthenia in the Dutch medical domain, a brief outline of Dutch psychiatry will be given.

In the Netherlands the care for the insane had been reformed on a modest scale only around 1845 as a result of the introduction of the first nation-wide lunacy act in 1841. Private madhouses were systematically suppressed, old madhouses were closed down or slowly converted into public asylums. Around 1884, when a new legislation was enacted, there existed sixteen asylums providing for some 4800 patients. At the time psychiatry as a 'profession' was restricted to those doctors working within asylums, having their own society and journal since 1871.[11]

The law of 1884 in itself did not change the major principles of lunacy legislation in the Netherlands. As hitherto involuntary confinement with judiciary consent remained the rule, no provisions were made for voluntary admission to an asylum. The authority of the national inspectorate (the equivalent of the English commissioners in lunacy) was in 1884 made to include all dwellings that housed three or more insane people. These houses were officially to be regarded as asylums. This last measure would in the long run have some influence on the treatment of neurasthenia, as we will see.[12]

With hindsight the lunacy act of 1884 can been seen as a turning point. During the years between 1884 and 1916 Dutch psychiatry changed in character. First of all it was a period of rapid expansion: apart from the flourishing of the 'neurasthenia-business' (that is to be described) and the establishment of specialised institutions for e.g. mentally retarded and epileptics, the traditional asylum system almost doubled in size. In 1910 there were twenty-eight asylums taking care for some 12,000 inmates. In the process Dutch psychiatry became rigidly compartmentalised along denominational lines as did society as a whole. For almost seventy-five years protestant, Roman Catholic, Jewish and public institutions would coexist in mental health care.[13]

During the last decade of the nineteenth century Dutch psychiatry also 'professionalised'. The Dutch Psychiatric Association and a number of asylums inaugurated in 1892 an official training of psychiatric nurses.[14] A year later the first academic chair in psychiatry and neurology – the two disciplines being combined – was created at the University of Utrecht. Soon the universities in Amsterdam (1896), Leiden (1899) and Groningen (1903) followed this example. At the beginning of the new century academic psychiatry was rounded off with the construction of specialist clinics for psychiatry and neurology in the college hospitals.[15] Whereas Dutch alienists at mid century still had been open to French influences (Esquirol chief among them), around 1900 academic psychiatry was almost exclusively oriented towards German medicine. The German *'Gehirnpathologie'*, the empirical nosology of Kraepelin and German therapeutic developments (e.g. the *'Dauerbad'* and bedtreatment) were the frame of reference for psychiatrists in the Netherlands. An author like the American father of neurasthenia Beard was read in a German translation.

Neurasthenia or *'het zenuwlijden'*

Neurasthenia surfaced sporadically as a subject in medical circles during the last two decades of the nineteenth century. In this respect doctors seemed to lag behind the critical commentators and Naturalist novelists mentioned above, that were the first to adopt Beards diagnosis in the eighties. It was only in 1897 that the first, and in some respects the only major Dutch treatise on neurasthenia was published by the later professor of psychiatry at Leiden, Gerbrandus Jelgersma. The first volume of Jelgersma's *Handboek der functioneele neurosen; Pathologie and therapie der neurasthenie* (*Handbook of functional neuroses; pathology and therapy of neurasthenia*)[16] amounted to a veritable compendium of the causes and symptoms of *'zenuwlijden'*, as neurasthenia was colloquially called in the Netherlands.

In his work Jelgersma, who combined a talent as a clinical anatomist and neurologist with genuine interest in dynamic psychiatry (he was the first to introduce the work of Janet in the Netherlands),[17] did not deny the importance of heredity and the advance of technology as factors in the 'undeniable increase' of neurasthenics in contemporary society.[18] Nevertheless Jelgersma stressed the decisive contribution made by moral causes. 'The chief reason why modern civilisation works to the detriment of our nervous system must be sought in the overwhelming emotions it generates. Only to be followed by the intensified intellectual effort it demands.'[19] According to Jelgersma there had developed a discrepancy between the fast evolution of knowledge and the refinement of morality that lagged behind. Religious doubt, wrong educational practices, the new demands of feminism and the emotional agitation caused by democracy compounded the problem.[20] Even Darwinism itself troubled the modern mind and nerves: 'The principles of Darwin offer explanations former generations could not even dream of. It has created unprecedented turmoil and conflict by its application on the human sciences and in the spiritual sphere.'[21] Whether this strong moral flavour permeated the Dutch medical debate on neurasthenia remains as yet a matter for further study. It would certainly be consistent with our analysis of the political and literary use made of the concept of neurasthenia and the general moral overtones in the Dutch public and political debate.

'Neurasthenia-business'

Whereas the discussion of neurasthenia among the medical profession remained limited in scope in comparison with Germany or France, neurasthenia as an object of care and cure was nevertheless of concrete significance. As in Germany a new type of institution came into existence around 1890 providing for the needs of those said to be suffering from neurasthenia.[22] The traditional asylum was ill suited to the reception of neurasthenics. The Netherlands did not have any private asylums. The public asylums were crowded with pauper lunatics paid for by the poor law authorities, while the lunacy act only permitted the involuntary committal of certified madmen. The loss of civil rights and liberties that was implicated by this procedure made those suffering from nervousness refrain from entering a psychiatric hospital. In the literature of the day there are occasional references to well to do neurasthenics who sought relief in foreign sanatoria and private asylums, because of the lack of facilities at home. It was also the stigma associated with being mad and internment in an asylum that made people go abroad.[23]

From the mid-1880s onwards private institutions for the care of the neurasthenics came into being. Around 1900 there were at least twenty-three of these.[24] Among these new institutions three main types can be discerned: the medical sanatorium, the specialised therapeutic institution and thirdly the nursing or rest home. The first of these, the real sanatoria, were often amongst the largest and offered rest and recreation, a mild regime of occupation and therapeutics mostly by medical doctors. The specialised therapeutic institutions did not offer any accommodation like the sanatoria, but catered for ambulatory patients. Unlike most of the sanatoria and nursing homes they were situated in larger cities like Amsterdam, Haarlem or The Hague. Physical therapies, like hydropathics, electrotherapy or physiotherapy, seem to have been the most popular. The renowned

Fig. 11.1

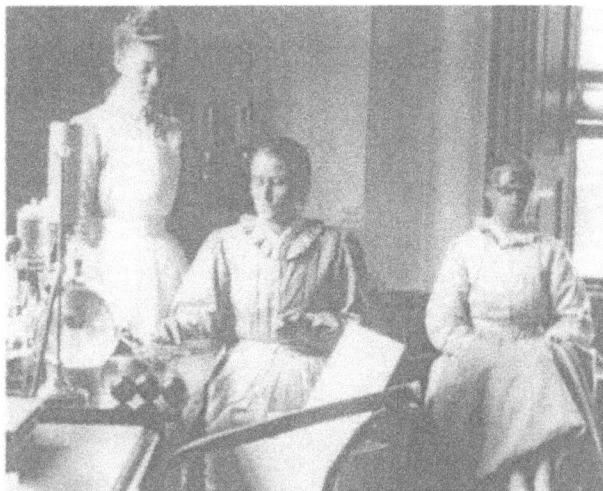

A demonstration of electrotherapy in the psychiatric asylum of Deventer (the Netherlands) in 1907. The patient on the right is seated on an isolated chair, while an electrode is attached to her head. As elsewhere, electrotherapy was part of the standard treatment in the Netherlands around 1900. *Adhesie Deventer.*

'Physiatric Institute Natura Sanat' in Scheveningen near The Hague for example combined all of these therapeutic approaches together with colour and light-therapy, gymnastics, massage and dietetics. Rather exceptional among these institutions was the first institute for psychotherapy founded by A.W. van Renthergem MD and the doctor and novelist Frederik van Eeden. In 1887 they were amongst the first to introduce hypnotism from the School of Nancy to the Netherlands. The majority of the new institutions were of the rest house type. Many of them were very small, taking care of only a few guests or patients, and located in wooded or coastal villages at some distance of 'civilisation'.[25] Why were these institutions created, who were their clients?

The majority of the 'institutions' that came into existence during these decades had a private character. As said private asylums had been dissolved as a result of the 1841 Lunacy Act. Nevertheless home nursing for insane not belonging to the own family continued as a quite common practice in the nineteenth century, although being frowned upon by the psychiatric profession. Under the provisions of the 1884 mental health legislation houses where more than two

247

Fig. 11.2

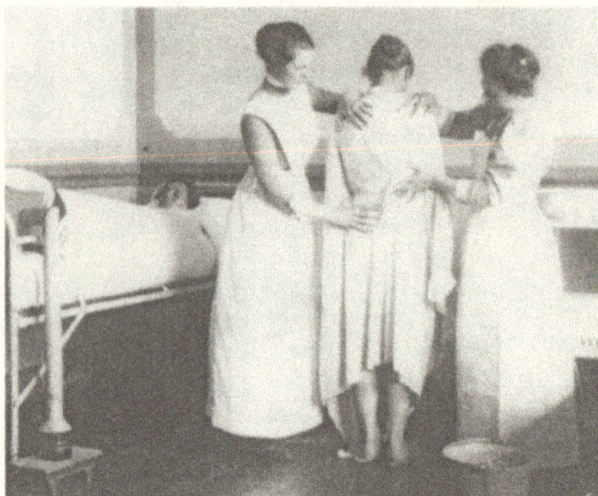

The application of steam and of cold (wet) rubbings, both regarded as a form of hydrotherapy in psychiatric asylum of Deventer (the Netherlands) in 1907. **Adhesie Deventer.**

psychiatric patients were kept had to be regarded as an asylum. Their owners were obliged to apply for a licence by the government and were subjected to inspection by the commissioners in lunacy. As private citizens could hardly meet the criteria for official recognition, it is likely that some of them started looking for a new clientele. Insane patients were exchanged for neurasthenics. In a way it was old business under a new fashionable cloak.

More so, as many of those staying in sanatoria and rest houses should be regarded as psychiatric patients, as the commissioners soon found out. In practice it was hard to distinguish between the milder forms of insanity and cases of 'severe' neurasthenia. As it seemed, well-to-do families used the label of neurasthenia as a cover to send their insane family members to rather expensive institutes, save in name being private asylums. By doing so they could escape the stigma of becoming a certified madman and losing their civil rights. As the commissioners wrote:

According to this view a wealthy disturbed person suffering from hallucinations and delusion... who can not be kept at home but who can be taken care of without too much trouble in a sanatorium for nervous disease – apart from being isolated every now and then – is officially to be regarded as a neurasthenic. When suddenly robbed of his wealth the same man, who can not afford the expenses of the private institution any longer, will become a psychiatric patient and will be transferred to a public asylum.[26]

There even seems to have existed an informal co-operation amongst public asylums and some of the sanatoria and nursing homes for 'neurasthenics'. Sometimes convalescent psychiatric patients discharged from an asylum were sent to a sanatorium to prepare for the return to their homes. On the other hand sanatoria occasionally served as an intermediate stage between society and admission to an asylum, apparently with the consent of the superintendent of the asylum. In The Hague for example their existed a lively traffic between the two local asylums (a neutral and a Calvinist one) and some of the nursing homes that could be found in this polite city and the adjacent bathing resort Scheveningen. So the establishments for neurasthenics at least partly played a role as 'halfway houses' *avant la lettre*.[27]

The development of the sanatoria as intermediaries had everything to do with the background of their owners and staff. A considerable number of these institutions were set up by representatives of the new generation of trained psychiatric nurses. They sought new respectful careers outside the 'stigmatised' public asylum, which offered only meagre prospects to its personnel. The same holds true for psychiatrists that seem to have been looking for an employment with more esteem and professional satisfaction than the asylums, that were said to have become overcrowded nursing homes for chronic cases. Maybe it was the wish to work with curable patients and to experiment with new therapies that brought some doctors to work as a consultant or a part-time staff member in a sanatorium.[28] It was also against the background of the appearance of a well-to-do 'neurasthenic' clientele that the phenomenon of the private specialist consultant was introduced in Dutch psychiatry around the turn of the century.[29] Individual psychiatrists set up practice in the larger cities, combining private practice with a job in an asylum. As such the growth of the 'neurasthenia-business' was a consequence of the professionalisation and the growth in numbers of both nurses and psychiatrists and signified a widening of the medical market. Psychiatry claimed neurasthenia as its professional domain as is amply born out by the new university clinics that explicitly provided for both psychiatric patients and neurasthenics. The position of psychiatry (still being integrated with neurology) in this matter seems hardly to have been contested by other medical disciplines in the Netherlands, notwithstanding an exceptional skirmish with gynaecology.

Neurasthenia, being treated in private practice and private institutions, offered an opportunity to doctors to experiment with new therapies that could not be introduced in public (pauper) asylums because of financial reasons or the character of the asylum population. The new hydropathics, electrotherapy as well as psychotherapy (hypnotism, early psychoanalysis, persuasive psychotherapy *à la* Dubois) started off (sometimes anew) in the domain of neurasthenia only to be imported in the world of the asylum at a later date. As hopes about the asylum being an effective means in healing the mad were being shattered in the second half of the nineteenth century, neurasthenia seems to have provided the alienist with a 'helpful' alternative. In the Netherlands prominent psychiatrists, the commissioners amongst them, even worried about the consequences, the asylum becoming a stagnant backwater inhabited by hopeless, untreatable cases left aside by the majority of professional psychiatry.[30]

Apart from its meaning for the nursing and psychiatric professions, the 'neurasthenia-business' may have had a very different social function. As Professor Jelgersma wrote 'The general urge for vacation that is so manifest in our time, is doubtlessly a result of a light nervousness...'[31] And indeed the late nineteenth century saw the beginning of mass tourism, sports and gymnastics. The need to travel, to exercise, to disport or recreate was at the time also legitimised by an appeal to medical arguments, that is to prevent or to cope with neurasthenia. Looking to the geographical distribution of sanatoria and the nursing homes there is a striking congruence between their location and the newly established holiday resorts near the coast and in the wooded 'inland'.[32] The spas, again popular at the end of the century, had always been characterised by this double culture of everyday amusement and therapeutic intentions. Likewise there was not always a sharp distinction between medically prescribed rest and general relaxation, or for that matter between 'fitness' and physiotherapy. The 'neurasthenia-business' was at least to some extent mingled with recreational and relaxational demands.

The 'disappearance' of neurasthenia

After 1910 interest in the subject of neurasthenia seems to have abated. As a subject of medical inquiry it did not seem to receive special attention any longer. It seems as if some of the institutions for neurasthenics disappeared and others changed their function. The emphasis shifted from the neurasthenic (or the quiet insane in disguise) towards the (somatic) convalescent, those who needed rest and 'mild neurasthenics'. New rest houses for the 'overstrained' and the 'overworked' were established at the beginning of the century by organisations of employers as well as by trade unions.[33] In all it looked as if at least in appearance a process of de-medicalisation took place. At first sanatoria and nursing houses had been conceived of as medical or therapeutic institutions, now they were being stylised more as rest homes *per se*.

One of the reasons for this change is to be found in the amendment of the lunacy legislation in 1904. This created the option of voluntary admission to special institutions that were licensed to receive both psychiatric patients and neurasthenics. This change of legislation had been enacted with an eye on the creation of university clinics for psychiatry that were to attend to both the insane and the neurotic. In 1916 the traditional public asylum was opened up to voluntary patients, a measure that inaugurated the psychiatric institution or hospital combining the 'asylum' (involuntary admissions) and the special ward for voluntary patients.[34] This move was amongst others inspired by a desire to change the old asylum into a therapeutic institution, preventing the gap between the therapeutic 'neurasthenia-business' and the asylum system to widen. Around the same time the first outpatient services were founded in the Netherlands, for example in Amsterdam.[35] Both developments, voluntary admission to psychiatric hospitals and the creation of official outpatient clinics, obviated the need for intermediary institutions as some of the sanatoria had been.

As for the milder neurasthenic complaints the private practice of the psychiatrist or the psychotherapist (mostly a psychoanalyst) may have become the therapeutic setting of choice among the wealthier strata of society. From 1910 onwards psychoanalysis made headway in Dutch mental health, especially in the cities in the west of the country (Amsterdam, Leiden, The Hague).[36] Simultaneously the interpretation of neurasthenia as primarily a disturbance of the nerves gave way to a more psychological or psychoanalytical explanation of these complaints, now diagnosed as (psycho)neurosis. Electrotherapeutic or hydrotherapeutic institutions slowly disappeared, whereas in 1941 the first modern Institute for Medical Psychotherapy opened its doors to welcome those from the lower-classes that needed psychotherapeutic assistance.

As a consequence of this development the map of mental health care was redrawn in the long run. What had been 'neurasthenia' was distributed over three areas: broadly speaking those suffering from fatigue, surménage and 'overwork' went to the rest homes, patients with milder forms of psychosis could be found at the outpatient services or in the voluntary wards of the psychiatric hospital, whereas the neurotics sometimes had access to a psychoanalyst or a psychotherapist. As the diagnostic criteria for these categories were rather vague there were in reality no sharp boundaries between these domains. Neurasthenia as a diagnosis almost disappeared and was reserved for a small category of patients. The complaints remained but were rearranged into other diagnoses or approached with other means.

Conclusion

The Dutch history of the concept and theory of neurasthenia shows that it could have different and even contradictory meanings and functions depending on the context it was used in. Old liberal commentators in the 1880s adopted it to reformulate their previous complaints about the weakening and the moral breakdown of the nation as a whole. For them the values of liberal bourgeois society were at stake. On the other hand Naturalist authors applied the modern 'scientific theories' of neurasthenia and hysteria as a critical argument to castigate bourgeois culture. They saw it as a means to destruct 'Victorian' moral and to liberate their own generation from oppressive convention. It was not the patient but the cultural and political meaning of the diagnosis that mattered most to them.

Neurasthenia seems to have played this role within quite restricted socio-political groups and within a short period of time. The cultural and social developments of the Netherlands during the 1890s were not very conducive to the pessimism and the decadence that characterised the *fin-de-siècle* in France. A slow but unmistakable process of integration of state and nation mitigated political contention and social strife. Revitalised nationalism, humanitarian aspirations and a sense of community building, in the arts as well as in politics, typified the atmosphere in the Netherlands around 1900. Together with a deep-rooted Calvinist and also humanist ethos that left no room for overt determinism and materialism, these conditions worked against the acceptance of the darker versions of the concepts of degeneration and neurasthenia.

In psychiatry the concept of neurasthenia was instrumental in expanding the profession and creating a new domain outside the asylum. It offered opportunities to introduce new therapies, new institutions and new careers both for doctors and nurses. It created a welcome alternative alongside the public asylum. At the same time it was not all about neurasthenics but about psychiatric patients as well. The 'neurasthenia-business' functioned, at least for some of its clientele, as an intermediary between society and the asylum. Once the asylum was opened up for voluntary admissions and outpatient services were established, the 'business' seems to have changed in character, a development that was compounded by the development of the private 'psychotherapeutic' practice. In the Netherlands the 'neurasthenia-business' may have had a transient character.

Notes

1. G. Jelgersma, *Handboek der functioneele neurosen; Pathologie and therapie der neurasthenie* (Amsterdam: Scheltema & Holkema, 1897), 3–4.
2. H. te Velde, *Gemeenschapszin en plichtsbesef; Liberalisme en Nationalisme in Nederland 1870-1919* ('s-Gravenhage: Sdu, 1992), 56–62, 78–82.
3. H. te Velde, '"In onzen verslapten tijd met weeke hoofden"; Neurasthenie, fin de siècle en liberaal Nederland', *De Gids*, 152 (1989), 14–24.
4. Te Velde, *op. cit.* (note 2), chapters II and III, 31–119.
5. *Ibid.*
6. *Ibid.*, 71–82, chapter IV, 89–119.
7. T. Anbeek, *De naturalistische roman in Nederland* (Amsterdam: De Arbeiderspers, 1982), 49–72; M.G. Kemperink, 'Medische theorieën in de Nederlandse naturalistische roman', *De negentiende eeuw*, 17 (1993), 115–71; *idem*, 'Hysterie in de Nederlandse roman van het fin de siècle', *Nederlands Tijdschrift voor Geneeskunde*, 139 (1995), 2194–8; E. H. Kossmann, *De lage landen 1780-1940. Anderhalve eeuw Nederland en België* (Amsterdam/Brussel: Elsevier, 1984), 241–50.
8. J. H. C. Bel, *Nederlandse literatuur in het fin-de-siècle* (Amsterdam: Amsterdam University Press, 1993), 280–90; J. Fontijn, '16 december 1887: Een liefde van Lodewijk van Deyssel wordt gepubliceerd; Van Deyssels roman en de mentaliteit van de bourgeoisie', in M. A. Schenckeveld-van der Dussen (ed.), *Nederlandse Literatuur, een geschiedenis* (Groningen: Martinus Nijhoff, 1993), 530–6.
9. Bel, *op. cit.* (note 8), 291–295; F. van Vree, 'De stad van het betere leven. Cultuur en samenleving in Nederland rond 1900', *Bijdragen en Mededelingen Geschiedenis der Nederlanden* (*BMGN*), 106 (1991),

641–51; W. E. Krul, 'Nederland in het fin-de-siècle. De stijl van een beschaving', *BMGN*, 106 (1991), 581–94.

10. Kossmann, *op. cit.* (note 7), 331–42; N. C. F. van Sas, 'Fin de siècle als nieuw begin. Nationalisme in Nederland rond 1900', *BMGN*, 106 (1991), 595–609; P. de Rooy, 'Een hevig gewarrel. Humanitair idealisme en socialisme in Nederland rond de eeuwwisseling', *BMGN*, 106 (1991), 625–40; S. Stuurman, 'Het einde van de productieve deugd', *BMGN*, 106 (1991), 610–24; Te Velde, *Gemeenschapszin en plichtsbesef*, chapters V, VI, VII (21–206); F. Boterman en P. de Rooy, *Op de grens van twee culturen. Nederland en Duitsland in het fin-de-siècle* (s.l.: Uitgeverij Balans, 1999), 9–85.

11. J.W.M. Binneveld, *Filantropie, repressie en medische zorg. Geschiedenis van de inrichtingspsychiatrie* (Deventer: Van Loghum Slaterus, 1985); J. Vijselaar, 'Van kleine en grote gestichten; Een overzicht van de institutionalisering van de zorg voor krankzinnigen van 1400 tot heden', in *Voor gek gehouden. Geschiedenis van de krankzinnigenzorg in Nederland* (Haarlem/Gouda, 1983), 42–9.

12. J. Vijselaar, *Honderd jaar krankzinnigheid. Geschiedenis van de krankzinnigenwetgeving in Nederland* (Utrecht: NcGv, 1985).

13. Binneveld, *op. cit.* (note 11), 156–87; Vijselaar, *op. cit.* (note 11), 46–8; J.A. van Belzen, *Psychopathologie en religie. Ideeën, behandeling en verzorging in de gereformeerde psychiatrie, 1880-1940* (Kampen: Kok, 1989).

14. G. Boschma, *Creating Nursing Care for the Mentally Ill: Mental Health Nursing in Dutch Asylums, 1890-1920.* University of Philadelphia, 1997, Ph.D. Thesis.

15. P. van der Esch, *Geschiedenis van het staatstoezicht op krankzinnigen*, vol. 3 (Leidschendam: VOMIL, 1980) 88–92; H.G.M. Rooijmans, *99 jaar tussen wal en schip. Geschiedenis van de Leidse Universitaire Psychiatrie (1899-1998)* (Houten en Diegem: Bohn Stafleu Van Loghum, 1998), 1–16.

16. The next volume was dedicated to the subject of hysteria. The promised third volume on the therapy of neurasthenia was never published.

17. See the chapter by Sonu Shamdasani in this volume.

18. Jelgersma, *op. cit.* (note 1), 10–14, 24, 33.

19. *Ibid.*, 30.

20. *Ibid.*, 22-7, 37, 30–2, 48–9, 82.

21. *Ibid.*, 29.

22. For an extensive analysis: A. Kerkhoven and J. Vijselaar, 'De zorg voor zenuwlijders rond 1900', in G. Hutschemaekers en C. Hrachovec (eds), *Heer en heelmeesters. Negentig jaar zorg voor*

zenuwlijders in het christelijk sanatorium te Zeist (Nijmegen: SUN, 1993), 27–58. The rest of this article is primarily based on this study.

23. See a.o.: G. Jelgersma, 'Boekbeschouwing over neurasthenie', *Psychiatrische en Neurologische Bladen* (PNB), 1 (1897), 66–7; *idem*, 'Zenuwinrichtingen', PNB, 1(1897), 186–8; *idem*, *Leerboek der Psychiatrie* (3e edition, Amsterdam: Scheltema&Holkema, 1926), 525; P.E. Abbink Spaink, 'De eerste honderd gevallen der neurologische kliniek te Apeldoorn', *Psychiatrische Bladen*, 14 (1896), 203–10: 203; A.O.H. Tellegen, *Psychiatrische bladen*, 2 (1884), 44; J. Vijselaar, *Krankzinnigen gesticht. Psychiatrische inrichtingen in Nederland, 1880-1910* (Haarlem: Fibula Van Dishoeck, 1982), 25.

24. A.H.van Andel, *Les établissements pour le traitement des maladies mentales et des affections nerveuses des Pays-Bas, des colonies néerlandaises et de la Belgique en 1900* (Leiden, 1901).

25. Kerkhoven and Vijselaar, *op. cit.* (note 22), 32–43.

26. *Verslag van de Inspecteurs van het Staatstoezicht op Krankzinnigen en Krankzinnigengestichten over de jaren 1903-1908* ('s-Gravenhage: Belinfante, 1912), 12. See also: J. Wijsman, *Voorlezingen over psychiatrie* (Amsterdam: Scheltema&Holkema, 1896), 183 (noot 15); Abbink Spaink, *op. cit.* (note 23), 205.

27. Kerkhoven and Vijselaar, *op. cit.* (note 22), 44–5.

28. *Ibid.*, 40–4.

29. M.J. van Erp Taalman Kip, *De behandeling van functioneele neurosen* (Amsterdam: Scheltema&Holkema, 1912), 1.

30. D. de Ridder, 'Psychiatrie tussen asiel en behandelingsinstituut. De geschiedenis van de behandelbaarheid', *Psychologie en Maatschappij*, 8 (1980), 382–99.

31. Jelgersma, *op. cit.* (note 23), 485.

32. Kerkhoven and Vijselaar, *op. cit.* (note 22), 44.

33. W.B. Huddleston Slater, *Gids Nederlandsche sanatoria en herstellingsoorden* (Den Haag: Ten Hagen, 1933), XV–XXIV, XXXXI–XXXXIV.

34. J. Legemaate, *De rechtspositie van vrijwillig opgenomen psychiatrische patiënten* (Arnhem: Gouda Quint, 1991), 42–54; De Ridder, 'Psychiatrie tussen asiel en behandelingsinstituut', 391–7.

35. T. van der Grinten, *De vorming van de ambulante geestelijke gezondheidszorg. Een historisch beleidsonderzoek* (Baarn: Ambo, 1987), 42–56.

36. I.N. Bulhof, *Freud in Nederland. De interpretatie en invloed van zijn ideeën* (Baarn: Ambo, 1983); C. Brinkgreve, *Psychoanalyse in Nederland. Een vestigingsstrijd* (Amsterdam: De Arbeiderspers, 1984).

12

Neurasthenia as Pandora's Box?
'Zenuwachtigheid' and Dutch Psychiatry around 1900[1]

Jessica Slijkhuis

It is 1884, and a small book entitled *De zenuwachtigheid* is available
in Dutch bookstores for NLG 1.25. Written two years earlier by the
German nerve-doctor Paul Julius Möbius, this work had been
revised and translated into Dutch by C.P. ter Kuile, a physician
working in Enschede.[2] It was the first handbook translated into
Dutch that dealt with phenomena also referred to as 'nervousness',
'nervous breakdown', or 'neurasthenia'. This chapter will be
employing the latter term as much as possible, as one can consider it
to be the umbrella medical term for an aggregate of physical and
psychological complaints that were associated with strain and
nervous exhaustion.

Was neurasthenia like Pandora's box,[3] a herald of both individual
suffering and collective doom? The psychiatrists Sigmund Freud, R.
von Krafft-Ebing, and P.J. Möbius and the electrotherapist G. Beard
certainly thought so. They viewed it as one of the greatest individual
and social problems facing people in the late-nineteenth century.
Taking into account the lack of an adequate anatomical and
physiological description and explanation of neurasthenia, let alone a
method of treatment, Möbius felt called – following the example of
his French and American colleagues Bouchut and Beard, respectively
– to inform as large a segment of society as possible about the causes
of this social evil, which was spreading like wildfire.

The translation of Möbius' work, the countless book reviews and
the references to German and French medical practitioners in
particular all bear witness to the fact that this message appealed to the
late-nineteenth century imagination of psychiatrists in the
Netherlands as well. The fact that Dutch doctors in the final decades
of the nineteenth century actually did consider nervousness to be a
great social and medical problem is expressed in the growing number
of both professional and popular (translated) publications about
'nervous phenomena', their cause, prevention and treatment.

This chapter will focus on the Dutch medical discourse on neurasthenia around the turn of the century and on the vision of the psychiatrist Gerbrandus Jelgersma (1859–1942), in particular. This prominent professor of psychiatry will figure centrally, because of all his Dutch medical contemporaries he wrote the most about neurasthenia. His productive writing does not imply that he is representative of Dutch medical thought regarding cause and prevention of neurasthenia. A comparison with other medical practitioners will throw some light on his position.

Using medical handbooks and text books, the contributions to Dutch medical journals such as the *Nederlandsch Tijdschrift voor Geneeskunde, Psychiatrische Bladen, Uit Zenuw- en Zieleleven* and more accessibly written pieces in popular magazines and publications originating in the minds of Dutch doctors like Jelgersma and Albert Willem van Renterghem, here a Dutch medical perspective on neurasthenia will be explored. To keep from going too far afield, impressions will be tested as much as possible by means of comparative secondary literature on the discourse about nervous conditions in Germany and England, making grateful use of the articles of the other contributors to this collection and the extensive historical research that Janet Oppenheim and Joachim Radkau have done on neurasthenia in Victorian England and in the German Reich, respectively.[4]

In the Netherlands, a clearly visible change in the medical approach to neurasthenia took place during the period 1880-1920. Seen from a modern perspective a gradual shift in accent took place, from a somatic-physiological approach, more or less associated with the degeneration theory, to a more psychological view. Here, it will be argued that the ideas about neurasthenia around the turn of the century indeed indicated a shift within Dutch psychiatry, whereby more and more attention was given to psychosocial factors, both in terms of aetiology and treatment. This growing attention for the *psyche* can be clearly observed in the thought of Jelgersma: from a scientific-oriented degenerationist thinker (1897), he changed in less than twenty years into a psychiatrist who, besides his work as an anatomical researcher, championed an explicitly psychodynamic approach to psychological disorders (1919).

The professional status of Dutch psychiatry at the close of the nineteenth century was plainly problematic. This chapter will argue that the increasing attention for psychosocial ailments, as provided in the form of the neurasthenia discourse, might have created a niche, which Jelgersma thought to use to expand the influence of psychiatrists and improve their status as medical experts. Also discussed will be when neurasthenia became 'popular' among members of the medical profession in the Netherlands, which foreign authors they read, cited and translated, how Dutch doctors construed the causes, therapies and prevention of neurasthenia and the extent to which they saw connections between this concept and circumstances like gender, social class, age and type of work. Some attention will also be given here to the demarcation between neurasthenia and other psychological disorders, especially hysteria, and to the distinction the medical profession made between neurasthenia, which it considered to be rather 'innocent', and 'real' insanity.

Neurasthenia according to Jelgersma.

Jelgersma, too, considered neurasthenia to be one of the great social problems of his time. This is evident from his *Leerboek der functioneele neurosen* (1897), the first Dutch medical handbook to give any significant attention to neurasthenia.[5] Like Möbius, Jelgersma was very alarmed about the drastic increase in the number of neurotics since the 1870s. He gave no arguments or figures to support this claim, however, but simply presented the increase as a matter of fact.

Who did produce Dutch statistics on the number of neurasthenics, although on a very small scale, were the physicians Albert Willem van Renterghem and Frederik van Eeden.[6] In 1887, they opened the first Dutch institute for Psychotherapy in Amsterdam, where they concentrated on the treatment of neuroses and related conditions.[7] According to Van Renterghem, psychotherapy, by means of suggestion, hypnosis and talking patients 'into' an improved mental health seemed to be a suitable remedy for neurasthenic and other complaints. Next to *practising* psychotherapy, the voice of this Amsterdam physician was also particularly often *heard* in this regard.[8] He broke a lance for psychological treatment in the Netherlands, having introduced and translated the way of thinking of the French psychiatrist Liébeault there. The 'fashionability' of neurasthenia can also be traced in the foundation of other specialised institutions and sanatoria for nervous diseases from the 1880s onward.[9]

So Jelgersma – who was the Medical Superintendent at the Sanatorium for Nervous Disorders in Arnhem at the time of publication – was not the first or only Dutchman concerned with neurasthenia. The doctors Th. Swart Abrahamsz in 1888 and, four

Fig. 12.1

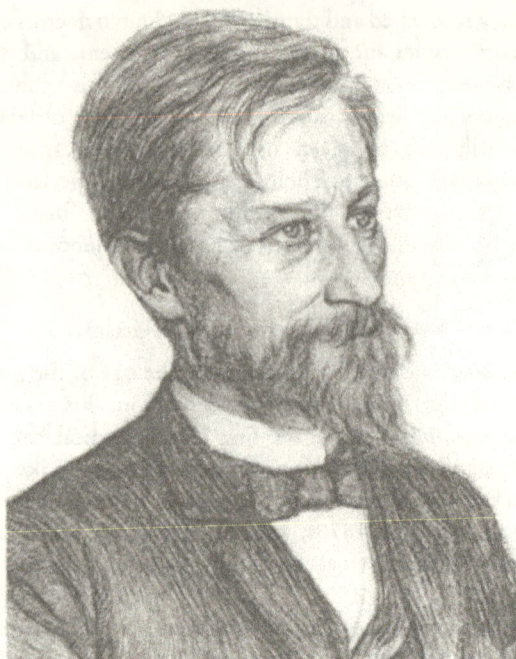

Prof. Dr Gerbrandus Jelgersma (1859-1942) was appointed as the first medical professor of psychiatry at Leiden University in 1899. Before, he had been the medical superintendent of a sanatorium for nervous patients in Arnhem and had published in 1897 the first Dutch treatise on neurasthenia.

Source: Carp, E. A. D. E (1942) *Jelgersma Leven en werken van een verdienstelÿk Nederlander* Lochem: De Tydstroom.

years earlier, A.O.H. Tellegen too, mention an increase in nervous patients, while J. van Deventer was already interested in nervous disorders before Jelgersma started publishing on neurasthenia.[10] Nevertheless, prior to the appearance of Jelgersma's textbook Dutch doctors were almost totally dependent on publications by their foreign colleagues for information on neurasthenia. In particular, Beard and Möbius were often consulted.[11]

For the Arnhem physician, nervousness was the popular term for the symptoms he included within the diagnosis of neurasthenia. He defined this, just as Möbius did, as a state of exhaustion of the nerves. Neurasthenia was a *functional* neurosis: a disorder of the nervous system, whereby no visible deviations as to the form of the organs could be observed. It was a syndrome that could vary from person to person, it could appear in any number of forms and gradations, and it was characterised by an arsenal of psychosomatic symptoms. It could effect a single organ, for example the stomach or the reproductive organs, but it could also concern the organism as a whole. Due to its multiple symptoms, neurasthenia could, at first sight, easily be confused with other psychological disorders. Jelgersma mentions things like epilepsy, hysteria, melancholy and hypochondria, the manifestations of which could be related to neurasthenia.

According to Jelgersma, this meant that it was often extremely difficult for doctors to diagnose neurasthenia. That was all the more reason for him to take a systematic look at this functional neurosis. Not only because the number of mental patients was increasing, but also because he believed there to be insufficient medical knowledge about functional neuroses in general, as a result of inadequate psychiatric training in the Netherlands.[12]

At the turn of the century, there was general and widespread concern about the supposed increase in nervous ailments. Countless socially-concerned doctors, schoolmasters, educators and ministers raised their respective cautionary fingers within popularising brochures, informing the public about the detrimental social causes of neurasthenia and the possible ways of treating or – better yet – preventing it.

Möbius' book was much imitated in the process. In 1903, the Dutch schoolmaster Bosma referred to Möbius and his colleague Hellpach in pointing out the importance of a good upbringing in preventing nervousness among children, for example, and the popularising work of the Amsterdam physician Juda (1905) is essentially a word-for-word copy of the Dutch translation of Möbius', *De zenuwachtigheid*. Some years later, but likewise, the 'self-help' book by the German physician Schilling, translated into Dutch by C. Bredee in 1910 as *Hoe bevrijd ik mij van mijne zenuwachtigheid?*, shows a remarkable similarity with Möbius' book.[13]

What was the background of this medical perception of the increase of neurasthenia? Contemporary historians explain it by means of the rapid processes of modernisation in nineteenth-century society. Jelgersma experienced his era as an angst-ridden and uncertain period of revolutionary change. In a chapter dedicated to the causes of neurasthenia he points to one main culprit besides hereditary and predisposing factors: modern society. He was a fervent champion of the then-prevailing doctrine of degeneration, according to which human development was determined by a combination of hereditary and social factors. For Jelgersma, neurasthenia was the first stage of degeneration and decline, an unavoidable consequence of increased 'civilisation', whereby civilisation was synonymous with intellectual progress.

For this view, he refers to the Italian psychiatrist Cesare Lombroso, who claimed that neurasthenia and other typically nineteenth-century ailments were caused by the asynchronous intellectual and moral development of people in the Western world. The emotional life of the individual was unable to keep up with the rapid development of human intellectual abilities, and the victims of this discrepancy were found especially within the more developed social classes, which were held to be on a higher intellectual level than the lower classes. Intellectuals, artists and others who performed mental labour – which he called 'long heads' – started out suffering from mild functional neuroses like neurasthenia, and would later, in the following generations, become insane and idiotic. Eventually, they became infertile and ultimately died out, according to Jelgersma's pessimistic vision of the future, as developed along the lines of the Italian degenerationist thinker.[14]

Such pessimistic voices could be heard in neighbouring Germany and England as well, although the degeneration theory in general was more popular in the former than in the latter. In the Netherlands the doctrine of degeneration was not that widespread. Although more medical practitioners emphasised the possible heredity of neurasthenia they didn't commonly connect it with the degeneration thesis.[15] Jelgersma's degenerationist and pessimistic perspective on neurasthenia was not completely representative of the medical opinion of his contemporaries, as Vijselaar shows in his contribution. A more optimistic cultural atmosphere in the decade around 1900 prevented an overall spread of the pessimistic degeneration theory in Dutch society. So Jelgersma seems to have been an exception in this regard.

The opinions of the foreign physicians Jelgersma mentions were rather varied in terms of the role of heredity in contracting neurasthenia. While Bouveret, Levillain, Möbius and Krafft-Ebing offered no hard figures, Löwenfeld and Binswanger claimed that neurasthenia was determined for seventy-five and forty-nine per cent, respectively. In short, doctors were particularly vague about the origins of neurasthenia. They could not quite agree on an actual cause of nervous disorders which seems to be also the case in Jelgersma's textbook under consideration here. He stated in 1897 that, on the one hand, neurasthenia was acquired over the course of one's life in about half of the cases, while on the other hand, the disorder was often caused by a combination of hereditary and external factors.[16]

By external factors he meant – with reference to the German psychiatrist Binswanger – any circumstances that could damage the 'life force' of the individual concerned, such as instances of 'poisoning' and infection like drunkenness (during procreation), syphilis or tuberculosis, chronic malnutrition, or psychological and physical traumas during one's lifetime. In short, every misfortune that a person might face. All of the above-mentioned factors would not only damage the individual, but were also held to damage the human germinative plasma, causing generation after generation to degenerate, such that a descendant from such a degenerated family would already be 'damaged' upon coming into the world.

The foundation of this Lamarckian idea of degeneration had already been toppled eleven years earlier, in 1886, by the German biologist A. Weissman, who showed that characteristics acquired during life could not be passed down. This scientific dislocation of the degeneration theory would hardly have much effect on its supporters throughout the first decade of the twentieth century, however. Although the popularity of the degeneration thesis differed in Dutch, German, English and French psychiatric circles, the toppling of Lamarckianism hardly made the theory less popular by around 1900.[17]

If, at some point, psychiatrists like Jelgersma considered 'misfortune' to be hereditary, did they believe one could close Pandora's box? Could neurasthenia be treated and cured? Jelgersma seems to have been relatively sombre in that regard. He believed that while the effects of neurasthenia could easily be alleviated, the disease itself could never be completely cured. That was related to the Lamarckian view, still common around the turn of the century, that neurasthenia represented the first stage of the degeneration process, and that it was inheritable and thus impossible to cure.[18]

Not all medical practitioners were that pessimistic. Around 1900 there had been a range of treatments that one could try, depending on the symptoms and taking the individual nature of neurasthenic complaints into account. In imitation of what foreign medical practitioners were doing, typical bodily treatments with electricity, mineral water baths, massages and physical exercise were propagated, and the importance of one's diet, rest, regularity and discipline was emphasised, for example in the Weir-Mitchell-Playfair course of treatment, but attention was also given to homeopathic and more holistic natural methods of healing.[19] The physician B.H. Stephan believed that one could cure neurasthenia with the Weir-Mitchell course of treatment[20] while Van Renterghem and Van Eeden in their Amsterdam practice propagated the beneficiaries of psychological methods and suggestion therapy in particular. With the exception of sedative bromides, medicines hardly seem to have been available. Morphine could also bring some relief, according to doctors, but its effect was only short-lived: due to its addictive effect, the prescription of this drug was to be avoided if at all possible.[21]

Fearing progressive degeneration and the epidemic spread of neurasthenia throughout society as a whole, the Dutch medical profession around the turn of the century emphasised especially the *prevention* of the factors that were thought to lead to neurasthenia, and then as early as possible. Parents should not be over-tired or under the influence of alcohol when conception occurs, and these should especially be free of syphilis or tuberculosis. Prevention should take place from early childhood onwards. Parents and teachers should bring children up to be citizens who hold a lease on truth, justice and duty as the most important values.[22] One must always be on guard against becoming 'overloaded' or 'overstrained' however, since an overdeveloped sense of duty could also lead to overtaxed nerves. Too much tension was bad, but too little was not good either.[23] Too little self-control might well lead to neurasthenia, but too great a sense of duty could also take its toll. The vague and broad concept of neurasthenia offered room for many contradictions of this type.

For Jelgersma, the most plausible explanation for the increase in functional neuroses in general and in neurasthenia cases in particular lay thus in modern society. Besides such 'predestined' factors as hereditary predisposition, sex, age, race and climate, it was one's social position and upbringing, along with industrialisation and urban life that directly influenced whether or not one would develop neurasthenia. Jelgersma considered the latter factors, influenced by processes of modernisation, to be the reason that neurasthenia had taken on epidemic forms by the end of the nineteenth century.[24] Beard and Möbius had made a similar distinction. They, too, blamed the rapid rise of nervousness on the modernisation within Western society.

Beard, for example, held five characteristics of modern society responsible for the growing number of nervous disorders,[25] while Möbius held materialism – and thus also the decline of religion – along with the high pace of life and the growing difference between rich and poor to be directly responsible for the increase in mental illnesses.[26] Modern urban life was likewise seen to play an important role. Its characteristics – agitation, haste, restlessness, the overload of sensory impressions – made humans, but especially males, more susceptible to neurasthenia.

Jelgersma maintained that neurasthenia was more common among men than it was among women, since men took a more active part in public life and thus had to cope with the competition so characteristic of modern capitalism. Their well-developed sense of duty and their sense of responsibility as breadwinner took their toll among these men. Here, too, Jelgersma failed to back up this firm claim with any statistical data. If neurasthenia did occur among women, it usually struck those women who did paid work, such as switchboard operators, schoolteachers and performing artists. Nervousness was also supposed to occur among women with a weakened constitution as a result of pregnancy or gynaecological problems.

Oppenheim notes that English physicians held a similar view. At the end of the nineteenth century neurasthenia among men was usually blamed on external factors, like the pressures of work and the Darwinian 'survival of the fittest' in the fast-paced world of business. In contrast, women, as a result of their reproductive physiology, were by their very nature thought to be much more susceptible to neurasthenia. Here is another example of how the amorphous concept of neurasthenia provided the medical profession with room for ambiguity: on the one hand, women were more prone to develop nervous conditions due to their naturally weaker nerves and intellectual disadvantage, while on the other hand, those women who had paid jobs, thus deviating from their 'natural' role as mother, were more apt to be neurotic.

A lot of foreign physicians generally diagnosed women with similar symptoms as suffering from hysteria rather than neurasthenia.[27] As a result, neurasthenia appeared to be a typically masculine disorder.[28] Radkau claims that, in the event that German women actually were diagnosed as being neurasthenic, it was usually because doctors had wanted to protect them from the stigma that went along with hysteria.[29] As a matter of fact, the boundary between hysteria and neurasthenia appears to have been quite vague.

Although they were sometimes identical in their manifestations and both were included among the functional neuroses, physicians were convinced of a distinction between them. According to Beard, hysteria distinguished itself by means of its acute symptoms and the sudden occurrence of cramps, while Jelgersma posited the difference between neurasthenia and hysteria in the heredity of the latter disorder. This seems inconsistent with his earlier mentioned view that neurasthenia was *partly* hereditary, but it is not. According to Jelgersma, heredity alone could never be the sole or dominant factor in one's susceptibility to neurasthenia, while he considered hysteria to be a clearly degenerative, congenital disorder. Both disorders were congruent with respect to the importance of emotions in their appearance.[30]

The age of the patient was also thought to play a role in the prevalence of neurasthenia. In claiming that neurasthenia was most frequent among people between twenty and fifty years old, Jelgersma referred to the statistical data of the German physician Hösslin. Among those in this age category, the social demands were once again what ultimately did the patients in: the pressures of work, unfulfilled desires and family circumstances facilitated nervous exhaustion, forming a breeding ground for neurasthenia. According to Jelgersma (and, likewise, to Möbius) race and climate had hardly any influence on the cause of neurasthenia – in contrast to what Beard had claimed.

Social status that derived from work also played an important role in the aetiology. Once again basing his claim on Hösslin's figures, Jelgersma ascertained that, besides striking students, soldiers and artists, the disorder was particularly apt to afflict merchants, civil servants and teachers. That was not so much due to their social status itself, according to Jelgersma, but rather to the type of work that these people did. In particular, those who frequently had to make demands upon their intellectual capacity suffered exhaustion of the nerves. That explained directly, in his view, why neurasthenia rarely occurred among labourers: overstrained nerves were generally not the consequence of practical and physical labour.

Although Jelgersma held that there was in fact no more than a gradual distinction between mental illness (neurosis) and insanity (psychosis), there was still one truly practical difference: nervous patients were aware of their disorder, while psychotics lacked such insight. Accordingly, Jelgersma claimed that mental patients usually came on a voluntary basis to the sanatoria and private clinics where they would be treated by neurologists and nerve-doctors, while those who were not aware of their pathological behaviour – and who could thus have been a danger both to themselves and to those around them – were apt to land involuntarily in institutions where they would be treated by psychiatrists. Thus, in terms of the type of treatment provided and the place in which it occurred, there was a big difference as to whether doctors diagnosed someone as neurotic or psychotic.

However, in 1899, the psychiatrist Johannes van Deventer described a case of 'insania neurasthenica' that illustrates quite well how vague the border between insanity and neurosis really was. In this case, the patient, in accordance with his precarious behaviour, was first admitted to a sanatorium specialised in nervous disorders, while three years later he was involuntarily locked up in a mental institution.[31]

Jelgersma held that his colleagues did not always base their diagnoses on purely medical grounds. In an article published in 1909, he argued that both doctors and laymen (both often members of the well-to-do middle-class) had the tendency to label seriously disturbed individuals from the prosperous middle class as nervous patients in order to account for the existing derangement while protecting the patients from being stigmatised and involuntarily admitted to overcrowded insane asylums.[32] This means that the diagnosis of psychosis or neurosis, like the treatment and institutionalisation of patients, depended on the social class of the individuals concerned. While neurologists in sanatoria and private clinics treated patients from bourgeois circles, it was primarily the institutional psychiatrists who had to look after the more serious, incurable cases from the lower classes. The discourse on neurasthenia was therefore not only bound up with class but also with institutional factors.

According to Oppenheim and Radkau, the view that neurasthenia only occurred among the intellectually developed urban well-to-do was not shared by the medical profession in that era. Labourers too, began to suffer from stress and symptoms of fatigue.[33] The difference, however, was that the prosperous burghers were in the privileged position to indulge their neurasthenic complaints. In contrast, labourers ran the risk of losing their jobs if they were to call in sick. Nevertheless, Radkau and Oppenheim both maintain that social differences did in fact play a large role in the medical diagnosis: for the same complaints, middle-class patients were declared nervous, while labourers were labelled insane.[34]

The historian Edward Shorter gives a clear and plausible explanation for the above-mentioned connections between neurasthenia, gender, social class, methods and place of treatment. He indicates that the diagnosis of neurasthenia offered those psychiatrists who worked outside of the asylums the possibility of medicalising stressed groups, which could provide them with money and status but which had previously been beyond their reach. Just like Radkau, Shorter also ascertained that beginning in the 1890s, neurasthenia was increasingly being diagnosed among labourers and had thus undergone a sort of democratisation. In his view, this served a dual purpose: both the improvement of the lot of the likewise stressed labourers and the enlargement of the clientele.[35]

So after all, it was not so much the nature of the disorder as the patient's status that determined where he or she would end up and which diagnosis would be given to his or her symptoms. According to Jelgersma, this worked to the disadvantage of both the psychiatric and the neurological profession: both saw only part of the psychological deviations, with the result that both of them lacked adequate and complete knowledge of nervous disorders and an adequate treatment failed to materialise. For that reason, he pleaded that insane asylums should be connected to sanatoria and institutions, where the patients would not be deprived of their liberty.[36] His desire was realised at the beginning of the twentieth century, with the origin of the so-called 'designated institutions', to which individuals could be admitted on a voluntary basis.

Neurasthenia and the Dutch psychiatric profession.

Jelgersma's plea, in 1897, that neurologists and psychiatrists should work together in the struggle against neurasthenia, had a strategic objective in relation to the poor image that Dutch psychiatrists had towards the end of the nineteenth century. Neurology and psychiatry were young shoots on the medical branch in the second half of the nineteenth century, both aspiring to achieve full medical status. While the professional position of neurology, which had developed out of medical science, was reasonably solid by the close of that century, and while neurologists and nerve-doctors enjoyed quite some respect in their practices, psychiatry, being associated with mental asylums, had a bad name. The asylums were overcrowded with untreatable and chronically sick patients, and a certain therapeutic pessimism was therefore prevalent.

Like their British and German colleagues, Dutch psychiatrists tried to bolster up their image by basing their work, in theory, on the successful scientific biomedical model, in which mental illnesses were considered to be disorders of the brain with an organic substrate, even when the latter could not always be observed.[37] Jelgersma and his famous colleague Cornelis Winkler (1855-1941) – professor of psychiatry and neurology in Utrecht, Amsterdam and Utrecht respectively – were no exception in that regard. In the institutional method of treatment, however, this approach turned out not to make much sense. As mentioned earlier, there were hardly any medical therapies for the often congenital and incurable diseases, and if such therapies did exist, there was no time, space or qualified staff to perform them. The scientific orientation of psychiatrists around the turn of the century was thus highly problematic in day-to-day practice.

This 'practice' was comprised of patients burdened by stress, fatigue and anxiousness in a period of rapid and radical modernisation. At any rate, that is the image presented by the medical profession itself: the extent to which patients experienced it that way themselves is an issue that goes beyond the scope of this chapter. Social and psychological factors certainly received more and more attention in the medical discourse on the cause and treatment of neurasthenia at the fin de siècle. The dominant somatic treatment of neurasthenia was noticeably losing more and more of its authority to - what we might nowadays call - a more psychosocial treatment. Psychiatrists seem to have combined their role as physician more and more with that of moral advisor. Accordingly, the place where the psychiatrist practised his profession changed as well: besides the asylums, he now worked in private clinics, university clinics and sanatoria.

There was, as the Dutch psychiatrist De Waal so rightfully claimed, already an interest in a psychological approach before the turn of the century. While moral treatment – although almost impossible to perform in the overcrowded asylums – had never really left the doctors' nineteenth century arsenal of therapeutic methods, from 1887 onwards, the physicians Van Renterghem and Van Eeden propagated scientific attention to the connection between body and mind and systematically incorporated Liebéault's suggestion cure into their private practice.[38]

Dutch doctors grew more and more sympathetic towards the idea that the specific pattern of symptoms and the psychosocial origin of neurasthenia would be best served by a 'psychological' treatment. The patients' awareness of their illness formed an important factor in the process of 'psychologising' neurasthenia. Only by closely observing the patient as a whole, by talking with him or her and posing questions about the patient's own behaviour could the psychiatrist be capable of judging whether or not the patient had insight into the illness, which distinguished neurasthenia from numerous other diseases, such as hypochondria. In 1909, Jelgersma argued for a more holistic approach, which would focus not merely on the disease itself but also on the diseased person as a whole. In conversing with the patient, the medical practitioner would discover just how much his patient could benefit from a listening ear, advice and understanding.[39]

This sort of impetus for a psychosocial approach can be clearly observed in the development of Jelgersma's ideas about neuroses. His view on the cause and treatment of neurasthenia changed radically as he went along. This is very well illustrated in his second book, the four-volume *Leerboek der Psychiatrie*, published in 1911 and 1912.[40] This work demonstrates how Jelgersma, then Professor of Psychiatry at Leiden and a scientist *par excellence*, had completely discounted heredity as having any role in the aetiology of neurasthenia: neurasthenia was now considered to be one of the so-called intoxication psychoses and defined as a state of exhaustion of the nervous system, affected by a foreign substance and thus acquired during the lifetime of the patient. Jelgersma was clearly no longer looking for the causes of mental illness on the level of a Lamarckian combination of hereditary and social factors, of nature and nurture, but more and more on the social and individual level.

The syndrome, Jelgersma now argued, was always characterised by psychological fatigue, although the symptoms could vary from individual to individual and include such things as hypersensitive senses, palpitations of the heart, sexual problems, melancholy or a loss of appetite. He no longer considered neurasthenia to be a functional neurosis – the object of study in neurology – but included the diagnosis within the group of *psychoses*, thereby turning it, at least in theory, into an object for psychiatry.[41]

Although the Leiden Professor still acknowledged that neurasthenia was a nervous disorder, and originally belonged to the field of neurology, psychiatrists were much better equipped than neurologists to diagnose and treat the disease effectively, due to their expert insight into the psychological functions of humans, as Jelgersma declared in 1912. Van Erp Taalman Kip, medical superintendent at the Sanatorium for Nervous Disorders in Arnhem who wrote a textbook about functional neuroses in that same year, supported him in this view.[42] The latter and L. Bouman, Professor of Psychiatry at the Free University of Amsterdam, did not go as far as Jelgersma in their classification of neurasthenia. Echoing Krafft-Ebing, they labelled neurasthenia rather as psychoneurosis in order to emphasise that it was a chiefly psychological illness, albeit it one with a hidden organic substrate.[43]

In his second textbook Jelgersma maintained that the therapy for neurasthenia should focus primarily on removing the social causes of the disease as much as possible. In his view, thus, those causes lay outside the individual. Neurasthenia could, for example, be caused by the pressures of work or an excess of sensory impressions. The disease could be treated, according to him, by adapting our values and standards to those environmental factors, such as by getting enough relaxation before it is too late, by not demanding so much from ourselves or by working in an orderly and disciplined fashion.[44] At his home practice or at a private clinic, the psychiatrist could provide his patients with advice to that effect, according to the Leiden professor. In more serious cases, the neurasthenic would need to be removed from his familiar surroundings and admitted to an institution for mental patients, where the medical treatment would consist of bed rest and good nutrition.[45]

From 1912 onwards the Dutch medical community could gain extensive familiarity with Freud's psychoanalysis. *Psychiatrische en Neurologische Bladen* devoted two papers by the neurologist A. Stärcke and Prof. Bouman to psychoanalysis, and the physician J.G. van Emden translated Freud's *Fünf Vorlesungen über die Psychoanalyse* (originally published in 1909). In the series *Uit zenuw- en zieleleven. Uitkomsten van psychologisch onderzoek* too, medical practitioners could get acquainted with Freud's theory. Van Renterghem, for example, described Freud's way of working along with his own experience in working with the psychoanalytical method. He agreed with Freud's view that neuroses are caused by the contemporary moral, which forces us to repress our sexual urges.[46]

Jelgersma, who two decades before was one of the most important Dutch champions of the degeneration theory, was extremely interested in the ideas of the Viennese psychiatrist and was now opening up to Freud's psychoanalysis. He became more and more convinced about the idea that neurasthenia was caused by a discrepancy between the individual's personal desires and his social environment. In acting on his fascination for the ideas of the Austrian psychiatrist, he was setting a trend, which many Dutch psychiatrists, albeit years later, would follow.[47]

The memorable rectoral address Jelgersma gave in 1914, *Ongeweten Geestesleven*, is a striking tribute to Freud's psychoanalytical method and to the latter's attention to the unconscious. It is striking, because his earlier scientific preoccupation did not in the least fit in with this 'profession of faith' in the unconscious part of the human mind. In 1915, he related how he had been diligently trying for three years already to absorb the psychoanalytical principles in an unbiased way. In his new vision, complaints like neurasthenia were no longer blamed on external factors, but could be attributed to *internal* and unconscious secret and repressed desires, which, once made visible by means of psychoanalysis, could also be dispelled.⁴⁸ The small group of Dutch psychoanalytic-oriented psychiatrists conceived his address as a great victory for their pioneering – until 1917 unofficial – movement: an academic of prestige converting himself to the Freudian doctrine!⁴⁹

Winkler who, like Jelgersma twenty years earlier, interpreted mental illnesses as brain diseases and considered psychiatry to be a natural science, was a great opponent of Freudian psychoanalysis. According to him, hypnosis and psychoanalysis did not make any sense. Unlike Freud and Jelgersma, Winkler found the idea that there would be something like an unconscious mind absurd. In 1917 he wrote a polemic article against psychoanalysis, in which he considered Freud's theory to be a house of cards.⁵⁰ Winkler considered man to act mechanically, without freedom of will, without an unconscious. The psychiatrist should engage in anatomical research and microchemistry instead of dealing with hypnosis, 'soul' and 'psychology', Winkler said.

Jelgersma held the opposite view. There was a clear task in store for the psychiatrist in this *psychodynamic* approach to mental disorders, as Jelgersma declared in 1919, during a pioneering lecture on the occasion of the commencement of Psychiatry classes for the 1919–1920 academic year.⁵¹ Looking back on thirty-five years of professional experience, the innovative professor called for a 'new style' of psychiatry, in which there would be room for a hermeneutic, humanities-based approach beside the scientific objectifying method still so common at that time.

Psychoses like neurasthenia did not stand to benefit from a thoroughly natural scientific approach. That is what Jelgersma's years of experience had taught him in the end. A psychiatrist trained exclusively in neurology would be unable to explain and cure a disorder like, for example, agoraphobia, because he would not recognise that this fear of open spaces was due to life experiences. He could only stand there with empty hands. As an objective scientist, the neurological psychiatrist could never see more in the human individual than a 'machine' with a disturbed nervous function, since nothing that is characteristic of humans – the subjective, inspiration, feeling and thinking – is ever objective. If psychiatry wanted to cure psychological disorders, it will have to exist as a science independent from neurology, while remaining in close cooperation with it. Jelgersma literally reinforced this intended turnaround from 'soma' to 'psyche' by declaring that, from that moment onward, he would no longer be giving any classes or laboratory sessions in neurology, but would be dedicating himself entirely to this 'new style' psychiatry.[52]

Conclusion

By way of conclusion one could say that the medical discourse on neurasthenia shows an increasing psychiatric attention for psychosocial factors that came to be expressed first of all in the emphasis on the social causes and their prevention. From the turn of the century onwards, the conviction grew that, besides prevention, neurasthenia would benefit most from a 'psychological treatment', a humanities-based approach to psychological problems that demanded the expert view of a psychiatrist. In accordance with this new way of looking at mental illnesses, complaints that had once been labelled as neurasthenic were, from the first decade of the twentieth century onwards, more and more often being called psychoneuroses, as if to emphasise their psychological character.[53] Nevertheless, even in a 1964 textbook for psychiatric nurses, the diagnosis neurasthenia can still be found.[54]

The individual and collectively experienced psychosomatic problem known by the medical name of neurasthenia formed a niche in which psychiatrists were able to find a way out from their problematic scientific frame of thought. An example of how this took shape in practice can be observed in the turnaround in the way Jelgersma saw things. From 1914 onwards, he visibly took the initiative in the Dutch humanities-based approach to psychosocial problems and can therefore be referred to as a trendsetter. A clear development in his thought can be observed, from an explanation of neurasthenia based on the doctrine of degeneration – whereby the emphasis shifted over time ever more from hereditary to social and psychological factors – to a psychodynamic explanation and treatment of the phenomenon. One needs to keep in mind, though, that Jelgersma never completely abandoned the scientific laboratory: although he 'confessed' to psychoanalysis, he still kept working as an anatomical researcher.[55] And, although being very progressive as a member of the psychiatric profession, he was not the first and only one to proclaim a psychosocial approach to mental problems: the physicians Van Eeden and Van Renterghem already did so in the late 1880s.

One could say that Jelgersma's eclectic attitude towards a new psychiatric approach emanated from the wish and ambition to extend the role of psychiatrists in the treatment of the growing number of people with neurotic problems and to improve the scientific status of his profession. It offered disillusioned psychiatrists a way out of the overcrowded asylums. Jelgersma didn't completely succeed in this ambition: neurologists and psychiatrists remained closely related professions in the first half of the twentieth century and the psychoanalytic perspective did not gain much respect of the Dutch medical establishment till after the Second World War.

While contemporary psychiatry still moves back and forth like a sort of Foucaultian pendulum between a scientific-biological approach and a humanities-based social-psychological approach, the discourse on nervous conditions around the turn of the century in no way functioned as Pandora's box for the psychiatric profession. On the contrary! Jelgersma's view of neurasthenia was forward-looking, focused on the twentieth-century future in which the psychotherapeutic treatment of the older 'nervous' complaints in their modern garb – e.g. stress, nervous exhaustion, burn out, RSI and ME – would reach a pace unknown in earlier times.

Notes

1. With many thanks to Tom Johnston for translating this paper and Harry Oosterhuis and Stine Jensen for their helpful comments on earlier drafts.
2. P. J. Möbius, *De zenuwachtigheid* (Groningen: Noordhoff & Smit, 1884).
3. The comparison is from R. von Krafft-Ebing, who, according to J. Radkau, considered neurasthenia to be a source of danger and misfortune. J. Radkau, *Das Zeitalter der Nervosität* (München and Wien: Carl Hanser Verlag, 1998), 68.
4. J. Oppenheim, *'Shattered Nerves'. Doctors, Patients and Depression in Victorian England* (New York and Oxford: Oxford University Press, 1991); J. Radkau, *op. cit.* (note 3).
5. G. Jelgersma, *Leerboek der functioneele neurosen* (Amsterdam: Scheltema & Holkema, 1897).
6. See Marijke Gijswijt-Hofstra's contribution.
7. A.W. van der Chijs, 'Dr. A.W. van Renterghem', *Psychiatrische en Neurologische Bladen*, 20 (1916), 279–91.

8. See A.W. van Renterghem, 'Bespreking van "Die Suggestionstherapie bei krankhaften Erscheinungen der Geslechtssinnes, mit besonderer Berücksichtigung der conträren Sexual-Empfindung" door Dr. A. von Schrenck-Notzings', *Nederlandsch Tijdschrift voor Geneeskunde*, 36, II (1892), 585–8. *Idem*, Kort begrip der psychische geneeswijze (Amsterdam: F. van Rossen, 1904). *Idem*, 'Freud en zijn school. Nieuwe banen der psychologie', Uit zenuw- en zieleleven. Uitkomsten van psychologisch onderzoek, II, 9 (1913), 1–40. The latter wrote a preface to H. Zbinden, *Raadgevingen aan zenuwlijders* (Amsterdam: F. Van Rossen, 1907). Van Renterghem also translated S. Freud, *Inleiding tot de studie der psychoanalyse. Academische voorlezingen van Prof. dr. S. Freud. Uit het Duitsch vertaald en met een voorwoord voorzien door Dr. A.W. van Renterghem* (Amsterdam: Maatschappij voor goede en goedkope lectuur, 1918).

9. See Joost Vijselaar's contribution.

10. See also Marijke Gijswijt-Hofstra's contribution.

11. G. M. Beard, *American Nervousness. Its Causes and Consequences* (New York: Putnam, 1881). *Idem, A Practical Treatise on Nervous Exhaustion (Neurasthenia): Its Symptoms, Nature, Sequences, Treatment* (London: Lewis, 1890).

12. Jelgersma, *op. cit.* (note 5), 3.

13. Among the titles appearing in the period 1880–1920 were: J. Holland, *Nette menschen* (Deventer: W. Hulscher G.J. Zn, 1879). H. Bosma, *Zenuwachtige kinderen. Medische, paedagogische en algemeene opmerkingen* (Almelo: Wilarius Wzn, 1903). M. Juda, *Hoe moeten wij zenuwziekten en zenuwachtigheid voorkomen? Wat is er tegen te doen?* (Amsterdam: Meulenhoff, 1905). The already mentioned Zbinden also treated the subject in *Raadgevingen aan zenuwlijders, op. cit.* (note 8). But also by the German nerve doctor Hoppe, 'Hoe behoeden wij onze kinderen voor nervositeit', *De vrouw; weekblad voor de vrouw in en buiten het gezin (1909)*, 170–3. Dr. Schilling, *Hoe bevrijd ik mij van mijne zenuwachtigheid? Kenteekenen, oorzaken en nieuwe raadgevingen, op geneeskundige gronden berustend, tot vlugge beoordeling en zelfgenezing* (Den Haag: C. Bredee, 1910). F.J. Soesman, *De geestelijke draagkracht der jeugd* ('s-Gravenhage: [s.n], 1904).

14. Jelgersma, *op. cit.* (note 5), 30.

15. That this is also the case in Great Britain can be read in Chandak Sengoopta's contribution.

16. Jelgersma, *op. cit.* (note 5), 8–14.

17. See also Oppenheim, *op. cit.* (note 4) 271–92. And Radkau, *op. cit.* (note 3), 179–83.

18. Jelgersma, *op. cit.* (note 5), 189.
19. Among others F. Halmar, 'Het hypnotisme in de geneeskunde', *Vragen van den dag: maandschrift voor Nederland en koloniën*, 4 (1890), 432–46. J.V., 'Neurasthenie' *Homoeopathisch maandblad*, 12 (1901), 267–70. A. Gorter, 'De natuurgeneeswijze en Eykmans physiatrische inrichting "natura sanat"', *Vragen van den dag: maandschrift voor Nederland en koloniën*, 15 (1900), 37–50. This 'holistic' approach, in which the whole person is taken into consideration, including his somatic and psychological condition, enjoyed considerable popularity and was also propagated outside of homeopathic circles. See e.g. Juda, *Hoe moeten wij zenuwziekten en zenuwachtigheid voorkomen? op. cit.* (note 13) and Zbinden, *op. cit.* (note 8).
20. In the Netherlands, this course of treatment was also known as the mestkuur ('fattening cure'). The therapy consisted of completely isolating the patient by removing him from his familiar surroundings and placing him under the supervision of a friendly nurse who would be present round the clock and make sure that the patient regularly ate copious amounts of food. B.H. Stephan, *De behandeling van sommige vormen van zenuwlijden met mestkuren* (Amsterdam: W. Versluys, 1896).
21. G. D. L. Huet, 'Over functioneele neurosen', *Nederlandsch Tijdschrift voor Geneeskunde*, 30, II (1886), 53–70. J. Hanlo, 'Bespreking van "De Weir-Mitchell-Playfairsche behandelingsmethode der neurasthenie" ', *Nederlandsch Tijdschrift voor Geneeskunde*, 30, I (1886), 595–6. T. Broes van Dort, 'Een geval van vasomotorische neurose, genezen na het gebruik van broomkali' *Nederlandsch Tijdschrift voor Geneeskunde*, 15, (1876), 213–19.
22. This underlines Vijselaar's statement elsewhere in this volume that the Dutch neurasthenia discourse was more distinguished by moral views than that it held a strong biological degenerationist perspective.
23. Bosma, *op. cit.* (note 13), 81.
24. Jelgersma, *op. cit.* (note 5), 18–29.
25. Beard, *op. cit.* (note 11), vi.
26. Möbius, *op. cit.* (note 1), 82.
27. As Hilary Marland shows in her contribution the English physician W.S. Playfair is an extraordinary exception!
28. Oppenheim, *op. cit.* (note 4) 142–53.
29. Radkau, *op. cit.* (note 3) 133.
30. Jelgersma, *op. cit.* (note 5) 193–4.
31. J. van Deventer, 'Bijdrage tot het begrip der insania neurasthenica',

Psychiatrische en Neurologische Bladen, 3 (1899), 487–92.

32. G. Jelgersma, 'Wat is een psychose?', *Nederlandsch Tijdschrift voor Geneeskunde,* 14, II (1909), 1–11.

33. Radkau, *op. cit.* (note 3) 231.

34. *Ibid.,* 32, 128. Oppenheim, *op. cit.* (note 4), 107.

35. E. Shorter, *From Paralysis to Fatigue. A History of Psychosomatic Illness in the Modern Era* (New York: Free Press, 1992), 223–6.

36. Jelgersma, *op. cit.* (note 5), 3.

37. Oppenheim, *op. cit.* (note 4), 36–8.

38. W. J. de Waal, *De geschiedenis van de psychotherapie in Nederland* ('s–Hertogenbosch: De Nijvere Haas, 1992), 29.

39. Jelgersma, *op. cit.* (note 32), 4.

40. G. Jelgersma, *Leerboek der Psychiatrie. Eerste deel specieel gedeelte* (Amsterdam: Scheltema & Holkema, 1911). *Idem, Leerboek der Psychiatrie. Tweede deel specieel gedeelte* (Amsterdam: Scheltema & Holkema, 1912).

41. See also Oppenheim, *op. cit.* (note 4), 312.

42. G. Jelgersma, *De plaats der psychiatrie in de rij der medische wetenschappen. Voordracht ter opening der psychiatrische colleges in den cursus 1919–1920,* (Leiden: S.C. Van Doesburgh, 1919). M. J. van Erp Taalman Kip, *De behandeling van functioneele neurosen* (Amsterdam: Scheltema en Holkema, 1912), 51–2.

43. Idem, *De behandeling van functioneele neurosen ,* 3-14. L. Bouman, 'De beginverschijnselen der organische zenuwziekten' *Nederlandsch Tijdschrift voor Geneeskunde,* 59, II (1915), 1401–16.

44. Jelgersma's view in this regard shows a striking similarity with that of German scientists who, shortly before 1914, considered neurasthenia as a transitional illness, which would disappear after adaptation to the changed environment – as discussed in Radkau, *op. cit.* (note 3), 443.

45. Jelgersma, *op. cit.* (note 40), 365.

46. Van Renterghem, 'Freud en zijn school. Nieuwe banen der psychologie', *Uit zenuw- en zieleleven. Uitkomsten van psychologisch onderzoek,* II, 9 (1913), 3–40. S. Freud, 'De sexueele beschavingsmoraal als oorzaak der moderne zenuwzwakte door Prof. Sigmund Freud', (Authorized translation with a preface by A. Stärcke) *Uit zenuw- en zieleleven. Uitkomsten van psychologisch onderzoek,* III, 5 (1914), 3–43. Also A.W. van der Chijs, 'Inleiding tot de grondbegrippen en techniek der psycho-analyse', *Uit zenuw- en zieleleven. Uitkomsten van psychologisch onderzoek,* III, 8 (1914), 3–48.

47. For the reception of psychoanalysis in the Netherlands see also I.

Bulhof, *Freud en Nederland* (Baarn: Amboboeken, 1983). And C.
Brinkgreve, *Psychoanalyse in Nederland* (Amsterdam: De
Arbeiderspers, 1984).

48. G. Jelgersma, *Ongeweten geestesleven. Rede uitgesproken op den
    339sten verjaardag der Leidsche hoogeschool op 9 februari 1914*
    (Leiden: S.C. Van Doesburgh, 1914). *Idem, Een geval van hysterie.
    Psychoanalytisch behandeld* (Leiden: S.C. Van Doesburgh, 1915).

49. Brinkgreve, *op. cit.* (note 47), 62.

50. C. Winkler, 'Het stelsel van Professor Freud', *Geneeskundige Bladen
    uit kliniek en laboratorium,* 19, VIII (1917), 1–31.

51. Jelgersma, *op. cit.* (note 42).

52. *Ibid.,* 5–27.

53. See L. Bouman & B. Brouwer, *Leerboek der zenuwziekten* (Haarlem:
    de Erven F. Bohn, 1922).

54. B. Hamer & F. Tolsma, *et al, Algemeen leerboek voor het verplegen van
    geestes- en zenuwzieken* (Leiden: Spruyt, Van Mantsem & De Does
    N.V.).

55. Bulhof, *op. cit.* (note 47), 131.

13

In Search of Dutch Neurasthenics
from the 1880s to the early-1920s

Marijke Gijswijt-Hofstra

If neurasthenia was a cultural product of the *fin-de-siècle*, then it is to be expected that the initial distribution and appropriation of this product varied according to the particular nature of the *fin-de-siècle* in different countries. The more pessimism about modern civilisation, the more neurasthenia, so it would seem, at least in Europe. As will be shown, the Netherlands kept a fairly low profile in both respects.

Besides, the turn of the century did not mark the end of neurasthenia. On the contrary, after 1900 it would last another decade or two, if not more. Neurasthenia's 'popularity' and incidence rates, however hard to come by, not only varied through time and per country. They also varied, or were at least supposed to vary, for the different social strata and age groups, and between the sexes. At any rate, the Netherlands seem to have been less 'infected' with neurasthenia than Germany. Where Britain should be positioned remains to be seen. The outcome may well be that the Netherlands held a middle position between Germany and Britain.

Of course, the incidence of neurasthenia is one thing, the experience of suffering from neurasthenic complaints and trying to be cured is another. What exactly were the complaints of Dutch patients, to what extent were they informed about neurasthenia, and what did their therapeutical career look like? These and related questions will be the central concern of the second part of this contribution, while the first part will concentrate on the incidence of neurasthenia in the Netherlands. Ultimately the Dutch incidence and experience of neurasthenia will be interpreted in terms of broader developments within Dutch society and culture, including the specific nature of the Dutch *fin-de-siècle*.

Marijke Gijswijt-Hofstra

The incidence of neurasthenia in the Netherlands

According to the already cited Leiden professor of psychiatry, G. Jelgersma,[1] neurasthenia had without any doubt gained in importance during the past years. He wrote this in his handbook on functional neuroses of 1897, two years before his appointment at Leiden University.[2] Citing Beard in German[3] Jelgersma agreed with his American colleague that many cases of neurasthenia had until then been disposed of as imagination or hypochondria. 'These are golden words, which still completely bear on our country...',[4] Jelgersma commented. He furthermore observed that not only neurasthenia was being misunderstood and misjudged, but that the same applied to most functional nervous diseases. Jelgersma asked special attention for the lighter cases of neurasthenia,

> those persons, who keep their capacity for work, although they often have to exert themselves beyond their power in order to remain what they are and who in the end are glad when they have reached their last destination... This widespread disease condition is to a large extent the cause of the present general weariness of life, of that pessimistic world view, that is increasingly taking root.[5]

So it was, according to Jelgersma, not the pessimistic world-view that caused neurasthenia, but the other way round. The medical view clearly prevailed. Jelgersma ascribed neurasthenia itself to heredity and/or the restlesness of modern life. He further stated that neurasthenia was more prevalent amongst men than amongst women, but that the number of female sufferers was on the increase too, and that, according to German statistics, most neurasthenics were between twenty and fifty years of age, while neurasthenia is especially widespread amongst businessmen, employees and teachers.[6] To this Jelgersma added that 'it is a well-known fact that neurasthenia hardly occurs amongst the working-classes'.[7]

Jelgersma's observations suggest that by 1897 neurasthenia had become widespread in the Netherlands, but that it was still largely unrecognised as such. But were his observations correct, what was their factual basis? Had neurasthenia left the Netherlands untouched until the early-1890s, had the disease then taken the Dutch by storm, and had its true nature and name remained hidden at the same time? Jelgersma did not provide Dutch statistics, but he could draw from his personal experience as medical superintendent of an institution for mental patients at Arnhem from 1894 onwards. He may have underrated the incidence of neurasthenia before the early-1890s, and

280

exaggerated its prevalence in and shortly before 1897, thereby as it were creating an extension of the medical market for himself and his colleagues.

However this may be, a look at earlier publications shows that neurasthenia was certainly recognised before the 1890s. In 1884 a Dutch translation of P.J. Möbius' book on nervousness/neurasthenia had been published, in 1886 the *Nederlandsch tijdschrift voor geneeskunde* (Dutch journal of medicine) had included an article by G.D.L. Huet on functional neuroses which explicitly mentioned neurasthenia, in 1886-87 the *Psychiatrische bladen,* the journal of the Dutch Association for Psychiatry, had paid attention to Weir Mitchell's treatment of neuroses, and in 1888 a Dutch translation of Paul Mantegazza's book on 'Our nervous century' had been published.[8] From that year onwards neurasthenia had also entered the realm of the non-medical journals, to start with an essay by the Dutch physician Th. Swart Abrahamsz on the neurasthenic case history of his nephew, the Dutch writer Eduard Douwes Dekker (*Multatuli*).[9] Moreover, in 1890 a first popular manual for mental patients had been published, a Dutch translation from E. Schneckenberg's book on nervousness or neurasthenia.[10]

This list is by no means impressive as it contains only a fairly limited number of titles, while most of them are Dutch translations of foreign work. It nevertheless demonstrates that information on neurasthenia was made available in Dutch during the 1880s. Moreover, the Dutch medical and educated public was not dependent on publications in the Dutch language. They could easily have read more widely on neurasthenia if they had wanted to. Indeed, the library of the Dutch Medical Association (*Nederlandsche Maatschappij tot Bevordering der Geneeskunst*) contains some twelve foreign books and brochures on neurasthenia from the 1880s, from the 1881 German translation of Beard to H. von Ziemsen's book on neurasthenia and its treatment.[11]

What then did the Dutch authors of the 1880s have to say about neurasthenia amongst the Dutch? Not much. Huet discussed eleven patients with fears and obsessions, but he labelled only one of them as a neurasthenic. Being familiar with Beard's work – he called America the 'land of neurasthenia and Beard her godfather' – he made no mention at all of growing numbers of neurasthenics in the Netherlands.[12] Swart Abrahamsz was the first to do so in 1888, but he did not offer any statistics.

Interestingly, four years earlier the Dutch physician A.O.H. Tellegen had made a similar observation about the increasing

Fig. 13.1

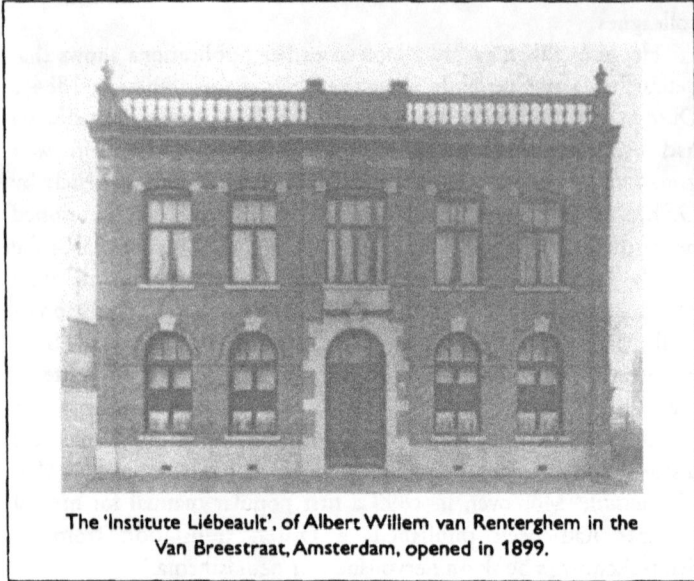

The 'Institute Liébeault', of Albert Willem van Renterghem in the Van Breestraat, Amsterdam, opened in 1899.

numbers of the mad in Dutch society. Although Tellegen did not mention neurasthenia, he came very close to it when he observed that madness was caused by 'the overexertion of body and mind'.

> One may call it the misfortune of this century that one is forced to live at a rapid pace. The present time with its craving for pleasure, its exaggerated demands and excessively high needs, with its railways and trams, its coffee- and beerhouses does not allow a human being any rest.[14]

Tellegen also mentioned that people who had the money went to a German institution for nervous diseases. Being called nervous or ill was not felt to be a problem, but one did not want to be labelled as mad. According to Tellegen there was a great need for such institutions in our country.[14] These would indeed make their appearance from the late 1880s onwards.[15]

The only statistics available for this early period have been produced by the physicians Albert Willem van Renterghem and Frederik van Eeden. In 1887 they had established a psycho-therapeutic institute in Amsterdam, offering hypnotic treatment *à la* Liébeault for both nervous and rheumatic complaints. Their co-operation would last for six years, after which Van Renterghem continued the practice, either with or without a partner, until well into the 1920s if not later.[16] In August 1889 Van Renterghem presented the results of their first two years at the international conference for experimental and therapeutic hypnotism in Paris.[17] He and Van Eeden had classified neurasthenia (*névrasthénie*) under *Affections névropathiques*, next to *nervosisme* and a great many more specific diseases or complaints like chorea, nervous asthma, urine incontinence, insomnia, onanism, impotence, nervous dyspepsia and migraine. The list contains 40 cases of neurasthenia, the majority of which, 35, concerned men. The *nervosisme* cases, 24 in all, show the reverse, but slightly less uneven, distribution with 17 women and 7 men. Van Renterghem and Van Eeden reported more fully on a number of their cases. The only observation of a neurasthenia case regards a 37-year-old businessman for whom intellectual work had become too much.[18]

In 1894 Van Renterghem and Van Eeden published a second report, this time on the years 1889-1893.[19] During these four years they had treated seventy-six cases of neurasthenia of one sort or another.[20] Whereas the Amsterdam physicians had not provided additional information about the types of neurasthenia in their first report, they now refined their presentation after having gained experience over the years. Although the majority of these patients (58) were again men, the share of women had increased (17). To these neurasthenia cases can be added the separately presented group of *troubles nevrasthéniques*, obsessions which counted 25 patients (16 men and 9 women). Added together this makes 101 neurasthenics, one quarter of who were women. In this second report Van Renterghem and Van Eeden offered observations on four male and two female neurasthenics: a 20-year-old student, a 33-year-old country physician, a 40-year-old businessman, a navy physician, and two unmarried women in their early-twenties. Two more observations concerned unmarried woman in their mid-twenties with a mixture of hysteria and neurasthenia, a man with constipation and neurasthenical symptoms, and a young man with neurasthenical hypochondria.[21]

In 1898 Van Renterghem published another report in the *Psychiatrische en neurologische bladen*.[22] This report, which would be the last of its kind, covered the period from 1893 to 1897, after Van Eeden had left. It includes 118 cases of neurasthenia, which means a slight increase compared to the previous period. With 86 men and 32 women the sex ratio had not changed much either.

Thus it would seem that Jelgersma's observations from 1897 do not hold. Dutch physicians were or could have been informed about neurasthenia from the early-1880s onwards. The small number of publications in the 1880s by Dutch writers on the subject may, however, point to a relative lack of interest. On the other hand, the actual diagnoses of neurasthenia in the 1880s could hardly have been as seldom as Jelgersma assumed, for at least Van Renterghem and Van Eeden diagnosed neurasthenia from the very beginning of their practice. Nor did their, or later Van Renterghem's, practice show a remarkable increase of neurasthenia cases. Moreover, in their publications both Van Renterghem and Van Eeden refrained from making observations about supposedly growing numbers of neurasthenics. Unlike Jelgersma they were general physicians in the first place, albeit that they specialised in a particular type of therapy and attracted a large percentage of nervous patients. Indeed, they will have considered themselves also as psychiatrists, for they both became a member of the Dutch Association of Psychiatry as early as 1889.[23]

Of course, an increase of neurasthenics during the 1890s may be traced in yet other ways, for example by looking at the establishment of sanatoria, specialised therapeutical institutes and rest homes.[24] From the late 1880s to the late 1890s some four sanatoria were established: Rustoord in Ermelo (1888-1895), Boschrust in Apeldoorn (1891-1960s), the Sanatorium voor zenuwlijders in Arnhem (1894 or earlier-1920s or later), and Veldzicht and Bornia in Driebergen (1899-1908). Two of them would close down within ten years after their opening, while the other two were more successful. Boschrust in Apeldoorn, belonging to this last category, took ten to twelve patients at a time. During the first five years of its existence, from 1891-1896, about 100 patients had been staying there, 59 of who were neurasthenics. Only 12 neurasthenics were women.[25] The best represented occupations amongst all male patients were salesmen (20), office workers (9), and teachers or civil servants (9). The rentiers came next (6), followed by manufacturers, students and military (4 each).[26] From the 100 patients 74 were cured, according to Boschrust's owner and medical superintendent Dr. P.F. Spaink, whose report is cited here.

Although information about these early Dutch sanatoria is scarce, this much is clear: they were mostly small-scale institutions which were only open to the unhappy few, to those nervous sufferers who could afford to pay the sanatorium fees. However, it appears that nervous patients could also be treated in general hospitals like the Burgerziekenhuis in Amsterdam where the medical superindendent B.H. Stephan booked good results with Weir Mitchell's fattening cure, as he reported in the mid-1890s.[27]

The establishment of Dutch sanatoria during the late 1880s and the 1890s was not necessarily an indication of or an answer to a significant increase of neurasthenics, for the capacity of these sanatoria was fairly modest, and Dutch nervous patients had anyhow been finding their way to German sanatoria. However, the Dutch sanatoria may have been instrumental in stimulating the demand, and to some extent the 'creation' of neurasthenics. Moreover, medical bathing establishments were greatly in demand, also on the part of neurasthenics. Institutes for physical therapy or psychotherapy also had their part of nervous patients. And rest homes for the nervous experienced a period of booming business stretching well into the twentieth century.

Looking at medical and other publications from the 1890s, it appears that the subject of neurasthenia was enjoying an increasing popularity. Except for Van Renterghem and Van Eeden, Spaink and Jelgersma at least two other physicians published in medical journals on neurasthenia. J. van Deventer, medical superintendent of the asylum Meerenberg, had for example already developed a special interest in neurasthenia before Jelgersma started publishing on this disease.[28] The subject also received increasing attention in non-medical journals,[29] and it became quite popular in literature. Although the term neurasthenia was seldom mentioned, the symptoms were prominently there, for example in novels by Louis Couperus, Lodewijk van Deyssel, Marcellus Emants, and the writer/physicians Arnold Aletrino and Frederik van Eeden.[30] Between them they created the image of an all-pervading nervousness, which was especially widespread in the better circles. Whereas the medical publications presented the group of neurasthenics as predominantly male, these novels seem to be peopled with at least as many, if not more, female neurasthenics.[31] It remains to be seen to what extent the novelists' image of Dutch nervousness reflected the actual spread of neurasthenics through Dutch society.[32] It certainly reflects their own preoccupation with nervous complaints, a preoccupation which they may well have shared with or passed on to the better part of their reading public. Altogether neurasthenia's popularity as a subject was certainly growing in the 1890s, neurasthenia's actual incidence may still have been relatively modest, even among the higher and educated circles.

During the early-twentieth century neurasthenia's popularity further increased. Except for a fairly limited number of medical publications for a medical public,[33] an impressive number of popular manuals were printed in Dutch, both from Dutch and foreign sources.[34] The prevention of nervous problems, especially with children, was gradually receiving more attention,[35] while neurasthenia also became a matter of concern in homoeopathic circles.[36] In most of these publications the readers were warned that neurasthenia or nervous diseases in general were widespread and that they would spread even further if nothing was done to prevent this. In 1901 the homoeopathic physician J. Voorhoeve even pointed out that the common people were by no means free from neurasthenia, 'as every physician knows who gets to treat maid servants and labourers with all sorts of nervous complaints'.[37]

Around that time a few more sanatoria were established: Jelgersma's creation, the Leiden municipal Sanatorium Rhijngeest in Oegstgeest (1903), the Christelijk Sanatorium voor Zenuwlijders in Zeist (1903), and Sanatorium Berkenoord in Nijmegen (1904).[38] The first two sanatoria employed a less exclusive formula than other sanatoria, also admitting less well-to-do middle-class patients, something Jelgersma and a few other physicians had been advocating. The care for neurasthenics thus became 'democratised' to a certain extent.

Rhijngeest had 74 beds for second class care in the main building, as well as 8 to 9 beds for first class care in a separate Villa for patients from the upper classes.[39] Initial plans to realise a building for third class patients failed to happen. During the first five years the average occupancy was only 50, but advertising campaigns began to pay off from 1908 onwards. Yearly about 200 patients were admitted, usually more women than men. More than half of the patients belonged to the middle class, called 'burgerlijke stand'. About 30 to 40% of the patients were quiet psychotics whose eventual admission in an asylum could thus be postponed. Some 40% of the patients were diagnosed under the category of neuroses. Initially most of them were neurasthenia patients, but there was a gradual increase of hysteria patients, and, from 1908 onwards, the diagnosis psychasthenia was also used.

In the Christelijk Sanatorium in Zeist more than half of the patients was diagnosed as neurasthenic before 1910.[40] As Giel Hutschemaekers has demonstrated, from then on this score dropped to under 40% in 1920, under 30% in 1925, under 20% in 1930, just over 10% in 1935 and under 10% in 1940. Until World War II the diagnosis of neurasthenia was mainly reserved for men: nearly 70% of the neurasthenics in the Christelijk Sanatorium were men. Before 1910 the diagnosis of neurasthenia was given to 64% of the male patients compared to only 30% of the female patients. Neurasthenia was chiefly diagnosed with patients who had well-paid work, who lived in urban areas, and who were married.

Compared to the joint scores of eight other Dutch sanatoria and mental hospitals,[41] the Christelijk Sanatorium had a relatively large number of neurasthenic patients before World War II. The other eight institutions jointly show the same general trend of dropping neurasthenia diagnoses as the Christelijk Sanatorium, but obviously at a lower level. On the basis of 5450 patient's records from the period 1900-1985 Hutschemaekers has confirmed that the decline of the neurasthenia diagnosis cannot be exclusively attributed to changes in the population of patients or changes in the complaint patterns (fewer somatic complaints, more mental and social problems).[42] The decline of the neurasthenia diagnosis should also be understood in terms of the historical context-boundedness of diagnostics as such: like all others, physicians and psychiatrists were children of their time and society.

A similar conclusion was already in 1921 hinted at by the Dutch physician H. van der Hoeven. According to him 'neurasthenia is no "disease" at all, and even less a fatigue disease, but lack of guts and self-confidence.'[43] Van der Hoeven concludes his article with the following revelation.

> I am very much inclined to think that the ominous increase in 'nervous diseases' of our days (if it really exists) is not a consequence of the overexertion of our modern life, but of the medical views which, since Beard in 1880 has 'invented' neurasthenia, have propagated the fear of 'the nerves'. If this is correct... than only one treatment is the right one, namely... be up and doing, and have guts.[44]

Van der Hoeven may have been somewhat ahead of his time, his views at any rate reflect the medical distancing from neurasthenia. That this process would take a fairly long time is clearly demonstrated by the actual practice of diagnosing neurasthenia in sanatoria and mental hospitals. Neurasthenia may not have swept through the Netherlands but by the early-twentieth century its position was firm enough to withstand attacks during the years to come.

•

Dutch neurasthenics and their experience of suffering

While the preceding search for Dutch neurasthenics was by no means easy for lack of sufficient data, it is even harder to get close to the sufferers, to find out what they suffered from, how they experienced their illness, and how they tried to get cured. Even if their diaries or letters have been preserved, the information on these matters tends to be scanty. Indirect, but potentially valuable sources like correspondence between the family and the physician or patient's records are scarcely available for the period discussed here.[45] The following will therefore be mainly based on data from medical publications.

First some of Van Renterghem's and Van Eeden's neurasthenic patients will be presented as they figure in their medical publications, in Van Renterghem's autobiography from the 1920s, and in case notes by Van Eeden. Then the doctor's filter will be shoved aside in order to listen to the voices of two professed neurasthenics, the Dutch author Lodewijk van Deyssel, a friend of Van Eeden, and Ernst Heldring, director of a big shipping company in Amsterdam. Finally a small selection of neurasthenic patients will be discussed as they appear in other medical publications or letters from the 1890s to the early-1920s.

Neurasthenic patients in Van Renterghem's and Van Eeden's practice

As mentioned before, Van Renterghem (1845-1939) and Van Eeden (1860-1932) published observations on a small number of their neurasthenic patients in their Amsterdam practice. The earliest observation on a neurasthenia case concerns a man of thirty-seven, who entered treatment in August 1887. Intellectual work had become too much for him. His disease dated from seven to eight years back and had been caused by an overload of work due to serious business problems. He had tried all sorts of therapies. He suffered from insomnia, oppression in his head, melancholia, apathy, the inability to work, dyspepsia, and a few other things. Van Renterghem and/or Van Eeden treated him with suggestion therapy (under hypnosis), first daily during three months, then somewhat less frequently. The major symptoms had been suppressed. The patient, whose father was also a neurotic, had had setbacks, but the periods of well-being had become ever longer. His stools had been regulated by suggestion, his impotence had been cured, and he had gone back to work on a daily basis. Reading and corresponding were still somewhat difficult. In the morning he was very slow in getting up, and sometimes he still had slight digestive problems. Van Renterghem and Van Eeden concluded that the improvement had been very remarkable.[46]

Similar observations, this time also on a few women, were offered in their second report from 1894. The patient's family used to count one or more neurasthenics, a difficult situation (business problems, an exam, etc.) had triggered the men's neurasthenical complaints, while the (young) women had been weak for most of their life, several other therapies had been tried before Van Renterghem and/or Van Eeden had been consulted, and the often fairly prolonged suggestion treatment was of course successful. Thus a twenty-year-old student had developed neurasthenic complaints, being in great fear that he would fail his exams. He hoped that suggestion therapy could cure him, but he also doubted if he would be sufficiently suggestible. He had presented himself on the stage when Donato was in Amsterdam, but had then been insensible to hypnotism. However, Van Renterghem was more successful: the student was both hypnotised and completely cured. This took altogether nearly two years. The student passed his exams and afterwards became an army physician in the Dutch East Indies.[47] A physician, thirty-three, with serious neurasthenical complaints was also completely cured. His treatment lasted about one year.[48]

Much longer, well over three years, was the still ongoing treatment of a businessman, born in 1850, with '*neurasthénie grave*'.[49] When he first consulted Van Renterghem in 1889, he had been suffering from nervous complaints (migraine, fatigue, inertia, paralysing apathy) for some ten years, from just after he had been married to the daughter of his boss and had become his associate. Having tried all the usual treatments and having stayed abroad for a long time without benefiting at all, he had developed an absolute disbelief towards physicians and medicine. He had retired from business, stayed in the countryside and refrained from consulting a doctor for over a year. After having heard about 'une cure merveilleuse faite par l'hypnotisme sur un homme connu de lui', a man who had been suffering from similar nervous complaints, he had decided to consult Van Renterghem.[50] The treatment had helped straightaway: the patient had felt better and started walking again. After six weeks he had experienced a first setback, after which several other setbacks would follow. However, as his condition improved, the patient had gradually been able to resume his work.

A retired navy physician with similarly serious complaints, labelled as 'neurasthénie grave', eventually committed suicide. From the time he was fourteen, il contracta l'habitude de se masturber et s'adonna avec passion à ce vice. Le début des accidents nerveux datent de ce temps, se manifestant par de crises alternantes de mélancholie et de gaieté exubérante.[51]

During a voyage to the Indian archipelago he had attempted to kill himself. After another attack of gloominess in Batavia he had been sent to hospital and then back to Europe. There he had consulted several foreign medical professors, had been treated with electrotherapy in Vienna, and had then returned to the Netherlands for a hydrotherapy cure of ten months. As his condition had not improved he had been discharged by the navy. According to Van Eeden, who had treated him at that time, a temporary improvement had been followed by a severe setback and another suicide attempt. Afterwards, in August 1890, the patient had switched to Van Renterghem. During nine months he had stayed at Van Renterghem's house and been looked after like a member of the family, as the doctor wrote. Suggestion therapy had been effective and the patient had left for Paris to specialise in dermatology. There his old problems started all over again. Van Renterghem went to fetch him and again put him up in his home, but to no avail. This time the man killed himself.

The retired navy physician was by no means the only patient who stayed with Van Renterghem. Especially during the years at the Keizersgracht 258, where Van Renterghem both practised (until 1893 with Van Eeden) and lived with his family from 1888 to 1895, he put up many more patients, both male and female, in 1888 even twelve at a time.[52] But also later on, for example in his house at the Willemsparkweg (1899-1909), he would have a few of his patients staying with him. In his autobiography Van Renterghem describes several of his patients (lodgers and others), including both male and female patients with neurasthenic symptoms. However, by the mid-1920s Van Renterghem was no longer lavish with the label of neurasthenia, using it only once in his autobiography.[53] Among the female patients of the early-1890s were Cato Nieuwenhuis, a singing and piano pupil, twenty-nine years old, of the Amsterdam conservatory, who was scared of her exams, and Henriëtte van Gelderen, the first female dentist in Amsterdam, with neurotic fears.[54] Both of them were cured by Van Renterghem.

After Van Eeden had left his (and Van Renterghem's) Amsterdam practice in 1893, he continued practising in his place of residence Bussum for at least six more years, although on a modest scale.[55] Unpublished notes on nearly eighty of his patients have been kept for the period up to 1899. Nine of them were diagnosed as neurasthenics (seven men, including two teachers, and two women), while a female patient got the diagnosis hysteria minor combined with neurasthenia. One of the two female neurasthenics, a thirty-six years old married lady with genital complaints and neurasthenia with anxiety and insomnia had been relieved from her complaints right after the first treatment. Thereafter she had travelled to Switserland. Back home she wrote to Van Eeden that she had been and still was in perfectly good health.[56]

The other female neurasthenia patient was an unmarried young woman of just over thirty years old. Born on Java, she had first come to consult Van Eeden in Amsterdam, in December 1891, accompanied by her mother. Her father, a retired officer of the Dutch East-Indies army, and her sister were also suffering from neurasthenia. She herself had been nervous from an early age onwards. In Holland she had visited a Roman Catholic convent school. Afterwards she had begun to suffer from suicidal impulses and insomnia. Her physician had prescribed valerian, bromine preparations, chloral as well as dissipation and travelling. In the wake of an attack of influenza her neurasthenic complaints had become much worse and she had lost confidence in her physician. This is where Van Eeden came in. He had managed to win her confidence and to induce hypnotic sleep. Daily treatment had resulted in the stopping of all medication and the restoration of the sleep function. During Van Eeden's holiday in summer 1893 she had experienced a setback, while Van Renterghem had replaced him. Until December 1893, more than two months after he had left the Amsterdam practice, Van Eeden had had to treat her daily. From then on three or four times a week had sufficed. Much company, going out, sudden impressions were still harmful. At about this point Van Eeden's report stops.[57] Time to move on to what neurasthenics themselves reported.

Lodewijk van Deyssel: a professed neurasthenic

Lodewijk van Deyssel (Karel Joan Lodewijk Alberdingk Thijm, 1864-1952) was one of the leading members of the Dutch literary renewal movement of the 1880s, called *Tachtig* (Eighty). From the 1880s to 1901 he was great friends with Frederik van Eeden, who was likewise a prominent author and member of *Tachtig*, as well as a physician.[58] In 1886 Van Deyssel confided to another literary friend, Arnold Ising Jr., that he had been 'suffering from weakened and ill nerves', and that he had done nothing, although actually detesting this. Indeed, 'I now want to create a condition of strength of the nerves and much, very much work.'⁵⁹ Two years later, in a letter to Willem Kloos, another member of the *Tachtig* movement, he called himself an irresponsible neurasthenic.⁶⁰ However, it appears that Van Deyssel was not altogether negative about neurasthenia, for in a letter to his mentor François Erens from a month earlier he had asked the rhetorical question: 'is that other suffering, that nervous exhaustion, not an indispensable factor for superior products?'⁶¹

In his letters to Van Eeden Van Deyssel's tone became more sombre, especially from summer 1891 to early 1893.⁶² To begin with he mentioned several times that his nerves were on edge or weakened. He also asked Van Eeden's advice about his wife's unwanted pregnancies (1887 and 1890) and contraception.⁶³ These concerns may well have worsened Van Deyssel's nervous complaints. In 1889 he contrasted himself in his diary with Van Eeden, 'the non-neurasthenic'.⁶⁴ In the following year he further elaborated on the subject in a letter to Van Eeden, writing: 'A balanced system, to be free of neurosis or neurasthenia or whatever it is called, is the greatest general good fortune, which is perhaps most valued by those who miss it.'⁶⁵

Living a fairly solitary life with his family in Bergen op Zoom, not far from the Belgian border, Van Deyssel had visited Amsterdam for a few days in May 1891, while being not quite recovered from influenza. He wrote to Van Eeden that he would have been pleased to visit him in Amsterdam,

> but I was in such a miserable condition of agitation of my weakened nerves, that I, for example, during a whole day could get nothing, wet nor dry, down my throat, and one of the symptoms of this very abnormal condition was also, that I couldn't face a visit to the Keizersgracht: the waiting room with 'people', who look with their eyes in a certain way and possibly a few of them also whispering, horrible!⁶⁶

Two months later Van Deyssel wrote to Van Eeden that he was working hard, which made him happy. At the same time he was suffering from severe strain, and he had even suffered from some sort of heart disorder.⁶⁷ Van Eeden thereupon reassured his friend: 'The feelings in the heart region which you describe are probably purely nervous symptoms. Practically the same description I hear almost daily from nervous sufferers.'⁶⁸ The best part of Van Eeden's letter consisted of an account of his own way of life: vegetarian, much sleep, early rising, next to nothing alcoholic. However, Van Eeden's example was lost on Van Deyssel:

I couldn't possibly follow the method you describe, because ... the life I wish to live is always based on a very abnormal condition of the nervous system. In other words, your physical peace-happiness-rest is based on relaxation...;   my peace-happiness-rest is based on extreme exertion...[69]

In September 1891 Van Deyssel asked Van Eeden to look up for him in his medical almanac 'if there were perhaps in his neighbourhood, for example in Antwerp, hydrotherapeutical establishments according to the Kneipp-method'.[70] Apparently this was not the case, for in the following spring Van Deyssel took a Kneipp cure in Cleve, Germany, just over the Eastern border near Nijmegen.[71] Shortly before he was to return home from his two months' stay, Van Deyssel wrote to Van Eeden that the cure had not helped him at all and that he was quite desperate. After having read Kneipp's books he had gone to Kleve full of trust, but uncomforted he would now return home in order to resume his former life. Van Deyssel was feeling miserable all the time: 'numb and awful, painful and next to fainting'.[72] Two days later Van Eeden replied that 'Kneipp is indeed too crass for you, but the principle, the principle of hardening is good. I wish I could treat you myself. I believe it would help you. But Amsterdam would oppress you too much.'[73]

In autumn 1892 Van Deyssel was still feeling miserable, calling himself an anaemic neurasthenic. Until the beginning of October, he had been, as he wrote to Van Eeden, in a condition of great weakness of the nerves. He had not been able to travel to 'Holland' because of the accompanying conditions of anxiety. Thereafter, in late October, Van Deyssel had suffered a nervous breakdown, which he attributed to the evil effects of the watercure. 'As soon as I will be feeling a bit better, there is for me only one thing in the world and that is a permanent stay on at least five hundred meters. The high air has always helped me immediately.'[74]

In spring 1893 his wish would come true: he managed to realise a stay in the Ardennes and by June he felt practically cured, as he wrote to Ising.[75] This is as far as we go with Van Deyssel, although his nervous complaints would keep cropping up in the years to come.[76]

Van Deyssel's story underlines once more that neurasthenia was not all that unknown during the 1880s as Jelgersma would have it. The young Van Deyssel certainly knew about it. Already in 1888 he called himself a neurasthenic, considering neurasthenia as the necessary condition for superior creativity. As his complaints got worse and kept him from working, he seems to have distanced himself somewhat from his earlier, fairly positive interpretation of neurasthenia. He even took cures, first an unsuccessful one at a German Kneipp-resort, thereafter, with better results, in the Ardennes. However, this would bring him only temporary relief. Van Eeden had been confident that he could cure or at least help his friend. But apparently Van Deyssel did not want to be treated by Van Eeden. Was Van Eeden perhaps too near, Amsterdam too far, or hypnotic suggestion therapy too strange?

Ernst Heldring and neurasthenia's burden

At the age of twenty-eight, Ernst Heldring (1871-1954) became director of a big Dutch shipping company, the *Koninklijke Nederlandsche Stoomboot-Maatschappij*. He would hold this position from 1899 to 1939, when he became president of the *Nederlandsche Handel-Maatschappij* (Dutch Trading Company). Some time after Heldring had become director of the shipping company he began to suffer from nervous complaints. In his reminiscences, he noted down that his younger brother Alex, while studying chemistry in Delft in the 1890s, had:

> overestimated the strength of his nerves and was a nervous sufferer (zenuwlijder) from those years onwards. Ten years later I became one as well and, like him, I would never quite get rid of this ailment. Like Alex, I had to take a cure several times. Fortunately our children remained free of it.[77]

In 1915 Heldring declined an offer of the mayoralty of Amsterdam by the Dutch government. As he wrote in his reminiscences, he felt unable to cope with the job because: 'My nerves, already weak for some years, had been further undermined by the demands the war had made on me...'.[78] It appears that Heldring had been suffering from nervous complaints since 1912. He himself ascribed his complaints to 'all too ardent work and concerns about the health of my eldest child'.[79] He had already twice been forced to take a leave of several months, in winter 1913 at Pontresina and Meran in 1914 again at Pontresina. In December 1915 he had to take leave again, but this time, as it would turn out, during more than a year. He first took a cure in Laag-Soeren after which he stayed for a short while in De Bilt. Then, in April 1916, he travelled to Switzerland,

> where my ailment first developed into a distinct neurasthenia, but a seemingly complete recovery after one year, thank God, has been achieved, mainly thanks to the advice of the eminent psychologist

and sympathic human Dr. Bazzola in Celerina near St. Moritz. If only I had discovered him sooner.[80]

However, it would soon after become clear that Heldring's expectation, that he had been cured from his nervous complaints and his unremitting insomnia, would not come true. Thus he wrote in his diary on 27 April 1919: 'I sleep extremely badly and I am very frequently and very soon tired in the head.'[81] And on 25 November 1924, he miserably wrote: 'I give myself with so much difficulty and I radiate so little warmth. Having lost my mother too early myself, said Bazzola, my admired counsellor in Celerina (Engadin) in my neurasthenical period.'[82] Much later, in 1941, he wrote that he had suffered time and again from his nervous problems, and that he was just with great difficulty recovering from a severe disorder that had manifested itself in June 1940.[83]

So here we have a hard-working and involved businessman, frequently advising the Dutch government on international affairs, who calls himself a nervous sufferer (*zenuwlijder*), and reserves the qualification of neurasthenia for nervous complaints that are worse than just insomnia and fatigue in the head. Yet, the fact that he did use the term neurasthenia as late as 1916 would seem to indicate that neurasthenia's decline amongst the higher circles was by no means completed, if indeed it had already started. Heldring's therapeutical career until 1917 – in later years he does not dwell on the subject – shows that, although he did take some cures in Dutch sanatoria, Swiss mountain resorts were favourites with him. Whereas Van Deyssel had been quite content with a stay at five hundred metres altitude, Heldring preferred to go much higher up, to some 1800 metres. Especially the combination of skiing or walking in the mountains, a quiet life away from business and family concerns, and the presence of an understanding doctor turned out to be an attractive one. As it appeared, Dr. Bazzola had not been able to cure Heldring once and for all, for the insomnia and the fatigue in his head would return. However, the even worse condition of neurasthenia, as understood by Heldring, would belong to the past.

More neurasthenic patients: miscellanea from Atjeh to Amsterdam

Except for Van Renterghem and Van Eeden a few other Dutch physicians reported on their neurasthenic patients. Thus J.K. Jacobs, an army medical officer, reported in the early-1890s on four Dutch army officers in Atjeh suffering from 'cerebral neurasthenia'.[84] The most fully discussed patient, an officer of forty-two years with suicide plans, had, at the request of Jacobs, written down an outline of his life. It appears that several of his relatives had had mental problems, and that he himself, although nervous and impressionable since childhood, had been fairly healthy until his first stay in Atjeh in 1878-79 where he had suffered from fever and insomnia, as well as a tapeworm. During a particularly severe attack of fever he had thought that he was on fire and that he was in hell. He had regained consciousness for a short moment, long enough to grab a table knife and wound himself fairly dangerously. After he had been nursed for two months his fears had diminished, but he was still frightened at the sight of a bright light or an intensely red colour.

Three months later he had departed for the Netherlands. Aboard the ship he had continuously felt anxious, suffering from insomnia and melancholia. He had consulted professor Kooijker in Groningen who had diagnosed anaemia and a slight enlargement of the spleen, as well as anaemia of the brain. Kooijker had prescribed steel preparations and a particular regimen, and he had reassured his patient that he would recover completely. Three months later this had indeed been the case. As Jacobs observed, it was in all likelihood suggestion, besides the medication, that had restored the patient's health. The professor had moreover advised the patient to marry before returning to the Dutch Indies, 'if possible with a calm, sensible woman'.[85] The patient had fully succeeded in doing so and had returned to the Indies in 1882, feeling quite normal and healthy. Leading a happy family life he had, except for the odd setback, remained healthy until his second stay in Atjeh in 1891. There he had got fever, diarrhoea, insomnia and shortly after the earlier feeling of fear. Fearing that his earlier brain cramp, as he called it, would return, he was determined to commit suicide in case this should happen. Jacobs had tried to reassure the patient and had prescribed large doses of '*brometum kalicum*'.[86] Eventually the patient had been evacuated to Padang, from where he had been sent to the cool highlands for further recovery.

A few years later, in 1896, the medical superintendent of the Amsterdam Burgerziekenhuis, B.H. Stephan, reported on his results with Weir Mitchell's fattening cure.[87] He had treated 31 patients with nervous complaints, 28 of who were women. Only two male patients were diagnosed as neurasthenics, but at least three women had neurasthenic symptoms. Most patients had for many years been suffering from nervous complaints, they had tried nearly every possible medication, and all thinkable cures. One of them had even reported that the doctor who had referred (probably) her to Stephan, had said that 'if this cure would not help, he would have seen it all and would know of no other solution.'[88] According to Stephan the Mitchell cure was not suitable for people suffering from cerebral neurasthenia. He had, however, booked good results with nervous dyspepsia complaints.

These are usually cases of a chronical nature, which have obstinately defied both rational and irrational cures and drugs, and which become so complicated because of numerous accessory symptoms, that they finally get such a chameleon like appearance, that one can no longer tell whether they should be counted as belonging to hysteria, neurasthenia, primary gastroenteritis, anaemia, or something else...[89]

Stephan moreover emphasised that:

there exists, especially in our present time which is extremely demanding on the nervous system, another type of nervous patients, especially women, but also men, who drive the physician to true despair, I mean that large group of people that gets labelled as suffering from weakness of the nerves, spinal irritation, nervous debility etc., and is called hysterical or neurasthenic.[90]

According to Stephan a Mitchell cure could be extremely wholesome for such patients. Unfortunately it did not have this effect on one of Stephan's male neurasthenic patients, a forty-two-year-old, married stockbroker. For years he had been suffering from neurasthenic complaints: a feeling of pressure in his head, dizziness, congestion, perspiration, not being able to face things, irritability, insomnia, and fear to go out alone. However, nothing was wrong with his nutritional condition, or, for example, his pulse, heart, or urine. After seven weeks and an increase in weight of ten pounds he had been discharged without any improvement.[91] Others, especially a number of female patients, were luckier, for they not only put on weight but were also cured.

Finally one more voice of a neurasthenic himself. In 1901 a neurasthenic man wrote to the Dutch homoeopathic monthly journal that he had been suffering from his nervous complaints for nine years. Homoeopathic treatment had made his suffering relatively bearable. When he had tried the new treatment, as he called it, of hot baths and thereafter electricity, he had suffered a serious setback. He was quite certain 'that the allopathic treatment during two and a half months had caused more harm than homoeopathy during over nine years [sic].' He added the warning that no neurasthenic should ever let himself be treated by 'allopathy'. 'Suffering from nerves is a long-lasting companion throughout one's life; quiet resignation and not becoming impatient is an important prerequisite, but remain homoeopath.'[92]

Of course, only a small sample of Dutch neurasthenic patients has been presented here. Even so, their complaints, symptoms and therapeutical careers proved to be both diverse and similar. Diverse because of the variety of their exact complaints and symptoms, and their supposed origin: hereditary susceptibility (mainly a medical concern), whether or not in combination with for example business problems, the strain of exams, family problems or self-imposed standards of superior creativity. Also diverse were the cures that eventually brought relief: hypnotic suggestion, a cure in the hills or the mountains, the Weir Mitchell cure, homoeopathy or some other cure. Their complaints and therapeutical careers also showed resemblance to each other. Their suffering tended to be protracted, and their therapeutical careers correspondingly long-lasting and pluralist: they tried one doctor or cure after another until the right one was finally found. This may well have been the privilege of the relatively well-to-do. Neurasthenics of modest means would not have been able to afford shopping that widely, if at all, on the medical market. Certainly not the maid servants and labourers, mentioned by the homoeopathic physician Voorhoeve in the early-twentieth century.[93]

Conclusion: Dutch neurasthenics and the *fin-de-siècle*

Neurasthenia was a doctor's invention, the sufferer's complaints were not. Just like their colleagues abroad, Dutch physicians, psychiatrists, neurologists, or whatever they wished to call themselves, were highly instrumental in constructing neurasthenia and, for that reason, in creating neurasthenic patients. Of course this precludes by no means that the actual diagnosis of neurasthenia was subject to negotiation between the patient and the doctor. Unfortunately, it is hard to make out, at least for the Netherlands, to what extent the diagnosis was indeed affected by the ideas, wishes and expectations of the sufferers themselves.

On the whole, the Dutch medical profession appears to have been fairly slow in adopting the neurasthenia diagnosis. Once adopted, it would not nearly become as popular as in neighbouring Germany.[94] The diagnosis of neurasthenia tended to remain reserved for the educated and relatively well-off male members of society. Women from these circles and especially working-class people, whether male or female, were seldom diagnosed as neurasthenic, although they may well have been suffering from complaints that would have justified this diagnosis.[95] These findings are especially in contrast to those found for both Germany and England where women and working class people were much better represented amongst the neurasthenics.[96]

If neurasthenia kept a fairly low profile in the Netherlands, then the question is why. A general answer to this question would be that the Dutch experience of the *fin-de-siècle* was a relatively mild one. By the end of the nineteenth century it was optimism rather than pessimism that reigned, as has already been related by Vijselaar, in the wake of historians like Te Velde and De Rooy.[97] This picture may, however, be too rosy. Jelgersma, for example, judged differently when he wrote in 1897 about 'that pessimistic world view, that is increasingly taking root.'[98] And there were many pessimistically coloured voices to be heard in general magazines of the time. Modern times with their rapid pace and technical innovations such as the vacuum cleaner were considered to be one of the main causes of nervous diseases.[99]

However this may be, more specific answers seem to be called for, and, for that matter, more specific questions. To begin with, the slow adoption of neurasthenia may well have been a function of the relatively late development of Dutch academic psychiatry. Before the late 1890s Dutch psychiatrists were hardly in the position to help making neurasthenia fashionable. After all, pioneering physicians like Van Renterghem and Van Eeden were fairly atypical with their hypnotic suggestion therapy. But of course there was more to it. Well-to-do sufferers from nervous complaints in the Netherlands were quite used to taking cures abroad. They did not need Dutch physicians or psychiatrists to tell them that they were suffering from neurasthenia or whatever. They were primarily interested in being cured, preferably in attractive surroundings. They were not, so it seems, particularly keen on acquiring the label of neurasthenia, or it must have been that they (or their family) wanted to avoid the stigma of insanity. So it seems that it was the weak position of Dutch psychiatry rather than a lack of Dutch sufferers that was responsible for the slow adoption of neurasthenia.

After neurasthenia had indeed become integrated in the Dutch medical discourse, it still failed to become a truly widespread disease, nor was the sexual connotation particularly strong, as it was in Germany. Neurasthenia remained mainly associated with active, perhaps hyperactive, upper and middle class men. The diagnosis of neurasthenia did not fit women nearly as well, particularly if they were well-off, inactive, and therefore bored out of their mind. Although the emancipation of women had become an important issue by around 1900, its effects were still fairly modest. Concepts of masculinity and femininity were slow to change. Moreover, there was no Dutch Playfair for women with gynaecological problems. Dutch gynaecologists were not inclined to appropriate the diagnosis of neurasthenia, although some of them, like the feminist gynaecologist Catharine van Tussenbroek, were very much aware of the symptoms.[100] That neurasthenia failed to spread to the working-classes may be partly attributed to its relatively late take-off in the Netherlands, and partly to the lack of relevant legislation, like the accident insurance acts in Germany, which would have stimulated working class demand.[101]

There is another matter that still needs attention: religion. The Dutch were well on their way to form a pillarised society along mainly denominational lines. While some Calvinist sanatoria for neurasthenics and other mental patients were established from the 1890s onwards, it seems that Roman Catholics lagged behind in this respect. One wonders if this was due to a somewhat later organisation of the Roman Catholic pillar, a more wary attitude towards neurasthenia, in particular the sexual variant, or a greater trust in pastoral care. It would surely be one bridge too far to suggest that the Roman Catholic Church might have housed relatively few people with neurasthenic or other nervous complaints. Actually, very little is known about the religion of the neurasthenic patients we have come across so far, and the impact religion may have had on their mental well-being.

Generally speaking it has proved to be very difficult to get close to the sufferers themselves. Their emotions and experiences are seldom revealed to us. Sometimes we catch a glimpse of their despair when a cure failed, sometimes a sign of relief if at long last a cure had been successful. In this respect the Dutch sufferers were no exception.

Acknowledgements

My thanks to Leonie de Goei, Harry Oosterhuis, Jessica Slijkhuis, Cecile aan de Stegge and Joost Vijselaar for their help and comments.

Notes

1. People suffering form similar complaints as medically diagnosed or professed neurasthenics were suffering from, but who were not labelled as such, have not been included in this research. This is in a

way a pity, because including them would have clarified the
mechanism of labelling and diagnosing, especially at the level of
patient-doctor relationships. I have also left out people who were
diagnosed as suffering from insania neurasthenica. Again, it would
be interesting to find out how the boundary was actually drawn
between insania neurasthenica and neurasthenia. See for insania
neurasthenica in the patient's records of the asylum Meerenberg:
Pieter Eckhardt, *Neurasthenie-patiënten in Nederland, 1890-1900*,
unpublished essay Department of History, University of Amsterdam,
June 2000.

2. G. Jelgersma, *Leerboek der functioneele neurosen* (Amsterdam:
    Scheltema & Holkema, 1897), 4. From 1894 to 1899 Jelgersma was
    medical superintendent of a sanatorium for nervous disorders in
    Arnhem. He was also an unsalaried university lecturer in forensic
    psychiatry and criminal anthropology at the University of
    Amsterdam. See also Jessica Slijkhuis' contribution.
3. G.M. Beard, *Die Nervenschwäche (Neurasthenia). Ihre Symptome,
    Natur, Folgezustände und Behandlung*. Transl. from the English
    (Leipzig: F.C.W. Fogel, 1881).
4. Jelgersma, *op. cit.* (note 2), 5.
5. *Ibid.*
6. *Ibid.*, 18–22.
7. *Ibid.*, 23.
8. P.J. Moebius, *De zenuwachtigheid.* Adapted (from the German) by
    C.P. ter Kuile (Groningen: Noordhoff & Smit, 1884). S. Brosius,
    'Weir Mitchell's systeem bij de behandeling van neurosen',
    Psychiatrische bladen, 4 (1886), 215-22 and 5 (1887), 97–106. The
    subject was also treated by J. Hanlo, 'Bespreking van "De Weir-
    Mitchell-Playfairsche behandelingsmethode der neurasthenie"',
    Nederlandsch tijdschrift voor geneeskunde, 30, I (1886), 595–6.
    G.D.L. Huet, 'Over functioneele neurosen', *Nederlandsch tijdschrift
    voor geneeskunde*, 30, II (1886), 53–70. Paul Mantegazza, *Onze
    nerveuze eeuw*. Adapted by N.B. Donkersloot ('s-Gravenhage: W.P.
    van Stockum & Zoon, 1888).
9. Th. Swart Abrahamsz, 'Eduard Douwes Dekker (Multatuli). Eene
    ziektegeschiedenis', *De Gids* (1888) III, 1–75. Th. Swart Abrahamsz,
    'Neurasthenie en psychose', *De Tijdspiegel*, 3 (1889), 35–48. See
    also: Henk te Velde, '"In onzen verslapten tijd met weeke hoofden".
    Neurasthenie, fin-de-siècle en liberaal Nederland', *De Gids*, 151
    (1989), 14–24. Remieg Aarts, *De letterheren. Liberale cultuur in de
    negentiende eeuw: het tijdschrift De Gids* (Amsterdam: Meulenhoff,
    1997), 379.

10. E. Schneckenberg, *De zenuwachtigheid of zenuwzwakte en hare behandeling zonder geneesmiddelen*, adapted from the second German edition (Amsterdam: Seyffardt's Boekhandel, 1890).

11. H. van Ziemssen, *Die Neurasthenie und ihre Behandlung* (Leipzig: F.C.W. Vogel , 1887).

12. Huet, *op. cit.* (note 8), 69.

13. A.O.H. Tellegen, 'Eenige beschouwingen over krankzinnigheid, hare oorzaken en hare behandeling', *Psychiatrische bladen*, 2 (1884), 5–46: 35.

14. *Ibid.*, 44.

15. See Joost Vijselaar's contribution.

16. A.W. van Renterghem, *Autobiographie van Albert Willem van Renterghem CHs AlbT's zoon*, 2 volumes (s.l.: privately published, 1924 en 1927). Towards the end of his autobiography (II: 764) Van Renterghem mentions that Dr. J.M. Rombouts, second physician of 'Endegeest', the psychiatric hospital at Oegstgeest, will become his new partner on 15 December 1926. Van Renterghem was then 81 years old.

17. A.W. van Renterghem and F. van Eeden, *Clinique de psycho-thérapie suggestive. Compte rendu des résultats obtenus pendant la première période bisannuelle 1887-1889* (Bruxelles: A. Manceaux, 1889).

18. *Ibid.*, 80–81.

19. A.W. van Renterghem and F. van Eeden, *Psycho-thérapie. Communications statistiques, observations cliniques nouvelles. Compte-rendu des résultats obtenus dans la Clinique de Psycho-thérapie suggestive d'Amsterdam, pendant la deuxième période 1889-1893* (Paris: Société d'Éditions Scientifiques, 1894).

20. They for example distinguished neurasthenia with various fears, mental depression or asomnia, chronical neurasthenia, sexual neurasthenia, and cerebral neurasthenia with or without hypochondria, dyspepsia, traumatic experiences or agoraphobia.

21. Van Renterghem and Van Eeden, *op. cit.* (note 19), 31–40.

22. A.W. van Renterghem, 'Bericht omtrent de resultaten, verkregen in de Amsterdamsche Kliniek voor Psychotherapie gedurende het tijdvak 1893-1897', *Psychiatrische en neurologische bladen*, 2 (1898), 529–37.

23. Their names are for the first time on the 1889 list of members, published yearly in the *Psychiatrische bladen*.

24. See Vijselaar's contribution. And also: Annemarie Kerkhoven and Joost Vijselaar, 'De zorg voor zenuwlijders rond 1900', in Giel Hutschemaekers and Christoph Hrackovec (eds), *Heer en heelmeesters. Negentig jaar zorg voor zenuwlijders in het christelijk*

sanatorium te Zeist (Nijmegen: SUN, 1993), 27–58.

25. P.F. Spaink, 'De eerste honderd gevallen der neurologische kliniek te Apeldoorn', *Psychiatrische bladen*, 14 (1896), 203–10.

26. *Ibid.*, 207.

27. B.H. Stephan, *De behandeling van sommige vormen van zenuwlijders met mestkuren* (Amsterdam: W. Versluys, 1896).

28. J.K. Jacobs, 'Bijdrage tot onze kennis van de Neurasthenia Cerebralis', *Geneeskundig tijdschrift voor Nederlandsch-Indië*, 32 (1893), 693–725. J. van Deventer, 'Bijdrage tot de kennis der "neurasthenische verwardheid"', *Psychiatrische bladen*, 12 (1894), 32–40. *Idem*, 'Een geval van sexueele neurasthenie', *Psychiatrische bladen*, 12 (1894), 91-105. *Idem*, 'Bijdrage tot de leer van den waanzin op neurasthenischen bodem', in *Feestbundel uitgegeven door de Nederlandsche Vereeniging voor Psychiatrie ter eere van haar 25-jarig bestaan* ('s-Hertogenbosch: C.N. Teulings, 1896), 173–86. *Idem*, 'Bijdrage tot het begrip der insania neurasthenica', *Psychiatrische en neurologische bladen*, 3 (1899), 487–92.

29. See W. Koster, 'Het ziekelijke in den aanleg van genieën', *De Tijdspiegel*, 1 (1893), 265–89. And also: Te Velde, '"In onzen verslapten tijd met weeke Hoofden"'.

30. See for example: Jacqueline Bel, *Nederlandse literatuur in het fin de siècle* (Amsterdam: Amsterdam University Press, 1993). M.G. Kemperink, 'Medische theorieën in de Nederlandse naturalistische roman', *De negentiende eeuw*, 17 (1993), 115–71. Juke Fluitsma, *Zenuwziekte van Zola tot Maeterlinck. Neurasthenie in de naturalistische, de mystieke en de tendensroman in het fin de siècle van de negentiende eeuw*, unpublished essay Department of History, University of Amsterdam, May 2000.

31. A systematic search for neurasthenics in Dutch novels is not available.

32. See also on this subject: Te Velde, ' "In onzen verslapten tijd met weeke hoofden", *Idem*, 'Fin-de-siècle in de Nederlandse politiek', *Leidschrift*, 14 (1998), 45–55.

33. W.H. Cox, 'Eenige gevallen van sexueele neuro-psychose', *Geneeskundige bladen uit kliniek en laboratorium voor de praktijk*, 9 (1902), 27–55. M.J. van Erp Taalman Kip, 'De diagnose der neurasthenie', *Psychiatrische en neurologische bladen*, 8 (1904), 43–52. H. Breukink, 'Over vermoeieniscurven bij gezonden en bij lijders aan neurosen en psychosen', *Psychiatrische en neurologische bladen*, 9 (1905), 7–29. W.A. Betz, 'De classificatie der functioneele neurosen en psychosen volgens een natuurlijk stelsel', *Psychiatrische en neurologische bladen*,15 (1911), 57–94. A. Rijpperda Wiersma,

Moeilijkheden bij het beoordeelen van nerveuse toestanden (Baarn: Hollandia-Drukkerij, 1913). R. Bromberg, 'Sexueele neurasthenie', *Medisch weekblad,* 24, no. 32 (1917), 513–20.

34. From Dutch origin were for example: H. Bosma, *Zenuwachtige kinderen. Medische, paedagogische en algemeene opmerkingen* (Almelo: W. Hilarius Wzn., 1903). M. Juda Jr., *Hoe moeten wij zenuwziekten en zenuwachtigheid voorkomen? Wat is er tegen te doen?* (Amsterdam: H. Meulenhoff, 1905). J. Voorhoeve, *Zenuwzwakte, hare voorkoming en behandeling* (Zwolle: La Rivière & Voorhoeve, 1905). F.J. Soesman, *Hygiène van den geest. Tucht als middel tegen Zenuwzwakte* (Den Haag, 2nd revised edition: W.P. van Stockum & Zoon, 1908). J.P.F.A. Noorduyn, *De nerveusiteit van het kind* (Baarn: Hollandia-Drukkerij, 1912). P. van Utinga, *Het zenuwslopende van de onderwijzersarbeid* (Baarn: Hollandia-Drukkerij, 1919). Translated into Dutch were amongst many others: Otto Dornblüth, *Hoe verkrijgt men gezonde zenuwen?* (Utrecht: W. Honig, 1903). R. v. Krafft-Ebing, *Gezonde en zieke zenuwen* (Amsterdam: C. Bredée, 1903). Richard J. Ebbard, *Zelf-suggestie als radicaal geneesmiddel voor alle soort zenuwziekten. Moderne psycho-therapie* (Rotterdam: Meindert Boogaerdt Jun., 1905). H. Zbinden, *Raadgevingen aan zenuwlijders.* With a foreword by A.W. van Renterghem (Amsterdam: F. van Rossen, 1907).

35. See also Nelleke Bakker, *Kind en karakter. Nederlandse pedagogen over opvoeding in het gezin 1845-1925* (Amsterdam: Het Spinhuis, 1995).

36. J.V. [J. Voorhoeve], 'Neurasthenie', *Homoeopathisch Maandblad,* 12, 10 (1901), 267–70. Z., 'Neurasthenie', *Homoeopathisch Maandblad,* 12, 1 (1901), 199. Z., 'Neurasthenie', *Homoeopathisch Maandblad,* 12, 3 (1901), 215. Voorhoeve, *op. cit.* (note 34).

37. Voorhoeve, *op. cit.* (note 36), 269.

38. See Vijselaar's contribution, and also Kerkhoven and Vijselaar, 'De zorg voor zenuwlijders'. A guide of the mid-1930s mentions many more sanatoria and rest homes. See: B. Huddleston Slater, *Nederlandsche sanatoria en herstellingsoorden. Gids* (Den Haag: Ten Hagen, 1935).

39. The following has been derived from: H.G.M. Rooijmans, *99 jaar tussen wal en schip, Geschiedenis van de Leidse universitaire psychiatrie (1899-1998)* (Houten & Diegem: Bohn Stafleu Van Loghum, 1998), 19–29.

40. The following is mainly derived from: Giel Hutschemaekers, 'Variaties in C-groot. De identiteit van het Sanatorium becijferd', in *idem,* and Hutschemaekers and Hrackovec (eds), *op. cit.* (note 24) 81–98. See also Giel Hutschemaekers, *Neurosen in Nederland.*

Vijfentachtig jaar psychisch en maatschappelijk onbehagen (Nijmegen: SUN, 1990).

41. See Hutschemaekers, *ibid.*, 169.
42. *Ibid.*, 201–2, 210–14.
43. H. van der Hoeven, 'Neurasthenie', *Nederlandsch maandschrift voor geneeskunde*, 10 (new series 2) (1921), 35–46: 43–4.
44. *Ibid.*, 46.
45. The patients' records from Rhijngeest have only been kept from 1918 onwards. Most of the patient's records of the Christelijk Sanatorium in Zeist have been or will soon be destroyed; the remaining records are badly accessible. The patients' records of the Valerius kliniek at Amsterdam from 1911 onwards may still be analysed. Attempts to trace the archives of the smaller sanatoria and rest homes have so far been unsuccessful.
46. Van Renterghem and Van Eeden, *op. cit.* (note 17), 80–1.
47. Van Renterghem and Van Eeden, *op. cit.* (note 19), 165–6.
48. *Ibid.*, 166–8.
49. *Ibid.*, 168–70.
50. *Ibid.*, 168.
51. *Ibid.*, 171.
52. A.W. van Renterghem, *op. cit.* (note 16), 68.
53. *Ibid.*.
54. *Ibid.*, 110 and 146.
55. See the Frederik van Eeden Archive, University Library, University of Amsterdam, inv. numbers 235–237. Fontijn does not mention Van Eeden's medical practice in Bussum, after he stopped his cooperation with Van Renterghem. See Jan Fontijn, *Tweespalt. Het leven van Frederik van Eeden tot 1901* (Amsterdam: Querido, 1990), 243.
56. Frederik van Eeden Archive, inv.no. 236, no. 4.
57. Frederik van Eeden Archive, inv.no. 235.
58. See for information on their friendship and its ending in: Jan Fontijn, *op. cit.* (note 55), and *idem, Trots verbrijzeld. Het leven van Frederik van Eeden vanaf 1901* (Amsterdam: Querido, 1996).
59. *De briefwisseling tussen Lodewijk van Deyssel en Arnold Ising Jr. 1883-1904* I, edited by Harry G.M. Prick. ('s-Gravenhage: Nederlands Letterkundig Museum en Documentatiecentrum, 1968), 29: letter by Van Deyssel to Ising d.d. 1 March 1886. Van Deyssel used the Dutch words *zenuwzwak en -ziek.* See also Harry G.M. Prick, *In de zekerheid van eigen heerlijkheid. Het leven van Lodewijk van Deyssel tot 1890* (Amsterdam: Athenaeum-Polak & Van Gennep, 1997), 562–3. Prick somewhat relativises Van Deyssel's self-diagnosis, but he adds that in his most personal writings Van Deyssel used to

present himself as a nervous sufferer (*zenuwlijder*).

60. Prick, *ibid.*, 816.
61. *Ibid.*, 813.
62. *De briefwisseling tussen Frederik van Eeden en Lodewijk van Deyssel*, edited H. W. Van and Harry G.M. Prick ('s-Gravenhage: Martinus Nijhoff, 1981).
63. See the unpublished parts of Van Eeden's letters to Van Deyssel d.d. 1.11.1887, 17.12.1888, 2.4.1890, 7.8.1890. Van Eeden Archive, University Library, University of Amsterdam. I have not read the unpublished parts of Van Deyssel's letters because his letters are kept in Heerlen. Van Eeden was unwilling to assist with abortion. See also Fontijn, *op. cit.* (note 55), 220.
64. Diary 20.10.1889. Mentioned in: *De briefwisseling, op. cit.* (note 62), 50–1.
65. *Ibid.*, 66: letter by Van Deyssel to Van Eeden d.d. 6.4.1890.
66. *Ibid.*, 112–113: letter by Van Deyssel to Van Eeden d.d. 7.6.1891.
67. *Ibid.*, 89: letter by Van Deyssel to Van Eeden d.d. 31.7.1891. See *De briefwisseling, op. cit.* (note 62), 151: letter by Van Deyssel to Ising d.d. 17.7.1891 in which Van Deyssel mentions that, starting on 23 June, he had got into 'such a severe exaltation-crisis as I have probably never, but certainly not since spring 1886 experienced.'
68. *Ibid.*, 123: letter by Van Eeden to Van Deyssel d.d. 7.8.1891.
69. *Ibid.*, 123: letter by Van Deyssel to Van Eeden d.d. August 1891 (the first part and therefore the date of the letter has been lost).
70. *Ibid.*, 150: letter by Van Deyssel to Van Eeden d.d. 22.9.1891.
71. Van Deyssel also reported on his stay in Cleve in *Gedenkschriften* I, edited by Harry G.M. Prick (Zwolle: Tjeenk Willink, 1962), 389–97. See also Van Deyssel's fictional account of this episode: *Badplaats-schetsen* (Baarn: Uitgeverij De Prom, 1990).
72. *De briefwisseling, op. cit.* (note 62), 119: letter by Van Deyssel to Van Eeden d.d. 14.6.1892.
73. *Ibid.*, 163: letter by Van Eeden to Van Deyssel d.d. 16.6.1892.
74. *Ibid.*, 183: letter by Van Deyssel to Van Eeden d.d. 25 October 1892.
75. *De briefwisseling tussen Lodewijk van Deyssel en Arnold Ising Jr.*, *op. cit.* (note 59), 143: letter by Van Deyssel to Ising d.d. 16.6.1893.
76. The correspondence between Van Eeden and Van Deyssel after 1893 contains no further information on the subject. The correspondence between Van Deyssel and Ising reveals that Van Deyssel continued to suffer from nervous complaints. See: *De briefwisseling, op. cit.* (note 62), 267, 289–290, 298, 300, 315: letters by Van Deyssel to Ising d.d. 19.12.1897, 4.3.1899, 28.9.1899, 14.4.1900, 16.9.1901. Ising

died in 1904.

77. *Herinneringen en dagboek van Ernst Heldring (1871-1954)*, edited by Joh. de Vries (Groningen: Wolters-Noordhoff, 1970), 33.

78. *Ibid.*, 180.

79. *Ibid.*, 203.

80. *Ibid.* Bazzola treated psycho-analytically and apparently attributed Heldring's problems to the early death of his mother in 1876, when Heldring was (nearly) five years old. See also Heldring's diary of 25 November 1924, 592.

81. *Ibid.*, 331.

82. *Ibid.*, 592.

83. *Ibid.*, 204.

84. Jacobs, *op. cit.* (note 28).

85. *Ibid.*, 699.

86. *Ibid.*, 701.

87. Stephan, *op. cit.* (note 27).

88. *Ibid.*, 97–8.

89. *Ibid.*, 99.

90. *Ibid.*, 110.

91. *Ibid.*, 68–70.

92. Z., 'Neurasthenie', *Homoeopathisch maandblad*, 12, 3 (1901), 215.

93. Voorhoeve, *op. cit.* (note 36), 269.

94. See the contributions by Doris Kaufmann, Volker Roelcke, Joachim Radkau and Heinz-Peter Schmiedebach. See also: Joachim Radkau, *Das Zeitalter der Nervosität. Deutschland zwischen Bismarck und Hitler* (Munich and Vienna: Carl Hanser Verlag, 1998).

95 The Meerenberg patient's records contain between 1890 and 1900 forty cases of insania neurasthenica. This group shows a much less one-sided class and gender distribution than I have found for neurasthenia. See Eckhardt, *op. cit.* (note 1).

96. See the contributions by Roy Porter, Mathew Thomson, Chandak Sengoopta, Hilary Marland and Michael Neve. See also: Janet Oppenheim, *'Shattered Nerves'. Doctors, Patients, and Depression in Victorian England* (New York and Oxford: Oxford University Press, 1991).

97. Henk te Velde, *Gemeenschapszin en plichtsbesef. Liberalisme en Nationalisme in Nederland, 1870-1918* ('s-Gravenhage: Sdu Uitgeverij, 1992). Idem, '"In onzen verslapten tijd met weeke hoofden"'. Piet de Rooy, 'De groote puzzles van onze maatschappij', in: Frits Boterman and Piet de Rooy, *Op de grens van twee culturen. Nederland en Duitsland in het Fin-de-Siècle* (Amsterdam: Balans, 1999), 17–38.

98. Jelgersma, *op. cit.* (note 2), 5.

99. Annejet Kluin and Anne-Marie van Meel, *Een zenuwslopende moderne tijd. Een onderzoek naar zenuwziekten in tijdschriften van 1873 tot WOI*, unpublished essay Department of History, University of Amsterdam, June 2000.

100. See Lidy Schoon, *De gynaecologie als belichaming van vrouwen. Verloskunde en gynaecologie 1840-1920* (Zutphen: Walburg Pers, 1995), 179–90. Van Tussenbroek advocated that the best remedy for nervous, idle middle class women was work. Schoon suggests a connection with chlorosis rather than neurasthenia, a diagnosis she does not mention at all.

101. See Heinz-Peter Schmiedebach, 'Post-Traumatic Neurosis in Nineteenth-Century Germany: A Disease in Political, Juridical and Professional Context', *History of Psychiatry*, 10 (1999), 27–57. And also Radkau, *op. cit.* (note 94), 215–232.

14

A Harmless Disease:
Children and Neurasthenia in the Netherlands

Nelleke Bakker

Introduction

In 1949 a Dutch mother sent a letter to the Neo-Calvinist women's monthly magazine *Moeder* (Mother) asking for advice on her troublesome eight-year-old daughter, whom she herself labelled as 'a neurasthenic child'. Unlike her older brothers and sisters, who all did 'very well at school', the little girl was constantly causing teachers' complaints of unruliness and lack of attention in the classroom. This mother's interpretation of the girl's symptoms as well as her diagnosis corresponded very well with the ones presented by the editor himself to the many desperate mothers seeking his advice on their 'nervous' children. Nevertheless, the editor reproached her for not giving enough information to allow proper counselling. According to him, she had better realise that, although 'neurasthenic children give trouble, not all difficult children are therefore neurasthenic'. For a correct diagnosis, which of course was the expert's prerogative, he ought to be informed as to whether or not the little girl bit her nails, wet her bed, was suffering from temper tantrums or fits of weeping. As long as he was not informed about these topics, which he considered valuable indications to diagnose the disease, he could not give sensible advice. The diagnosis, he explained, should determine the treatment of the child: 'If she is not a neurasthenic, but simply a demanding and naughty child, she ought to be treated with authority and firmness. If, however, she is really suffering from neurasthenia, she has to be treated in a totally different way.'[1]

This example of public use of expert terminology shows that children's nervous disorders and their labelling as neurasthenia were well known and widespread in the popular educational discourse in the Netherlands as late as the middle of the twentieth century. Whereas the diagnosis began to disappear from adult neurology and psychiatry from about 1920, as the other Dutch contributions to this

309

volume show, neurasthenia seems to have been granted a second life in child-rearing advice. It is tempting to suggest that this is simply another proof of children's fate to have to do with second-hand theory and expertise, as is often claimed by defendants of children's rights. Rather, one could try to explain this long-lasting popularity of a worn-out adults' disease in terms of its use for those involved as compared to alternative interpretations of a child's awkward behaviour. For different groups of child-rearing experts as well as for their audiences, especially parents struggling to raise their children in conformity with the prevailing standards of good family upbringing, neurasthenia may have been attractive as a label for a problem child for different reasons. If adult psychiatry and its shifting agenda of interest in particular mental illnesses is not developing in a social and cultural vacuum, this is certainly true of the changing concerns of child-rearing experts and their clients: teachers, parents and children.

This chapter traces the use of the psychiatric concept of neurasthenia and its more popular equivalents 'nervousness' and 'weak nerves' in relation to children and their upbringing in the Netherlands during the first half of the twentieth century. The focus is directed at the attractiveness of these concepts for the respective users at different times and at different levels of professionalism. Therefore, however real the symptoms may have been, the illness is neither conceived of as an intrinsic children's reaction to unsatisfying educational relationships, nor as a typical early-twentieth-century paediatricians' answer to trends in adult psychiatry. Children's neurasthenia is considered a cultural construct in its own right.

Pedagogical prophylactics and treatment

Neurasthenia as a functional disease of the nervous system first appeared on the Dutch stage of child-rearing expertise immediately after 1900. The ground had been prepared by an evolving specialisation, educational pathology, which claimed authority for educationalists next to physicians in the field of diagnosing, categorising, and treating mentally handicapped children. This specialisation developed in close relation to special education, another rapidly growing phenomenon at the time[2] and one of the many turn-of-the-century expressions of an increased interest in children's condition and treatment. At the time Germany was the model country for Dutch educationalists. In his *Pädagogische Pathologie* (Educational Pathology, 1890) the founding father of late-nineteenth-century educational pathology, the philosopher Ludwig Strümpell, proposed collaboration between physicians and educationalists. According to him, after a collective diagnosis, the former would take charge of children with physical or organic faults, whereas the latter would take authority over all other faults, particularly their prevention and treatment.[3]

His Dutch follower, the deputy director of a youth penitentiary Jan Klootsema, a former teacher in special education, claimed an even larger piece of the pie for pedagogues. In his influential study on children's disorders, *Misdeelde kinderen* (Deprived Children, 1904), he discredited Strümpell's emphasis on the aetiology of children's problems as too theoretical. As he saw it, aetiology stood in the way of proper diagnosis and therapy. Educational pathology, in his interpretation, simply related to all 'those disorders of the object of education (mind, nerves, and senses) which show during a child's development and which interfere with the process of upbringing'. Nevertheless, he suggested collaboration between pedagogues and psychiatrists. Neurasthenia, for example, which Klootsema defined as instability of the child's consciousness, was to be diagnosed by medical pathology. If a child's nervous predisposition was recognised at an early age, it could be treated successfully by prophylactic pedagogy. Although Klootsema did not systematically discriminate between disorders that were or were not determined by heredity, in case of neurasthenia it is clear that its seriousness made it an illness more likely caused by degeneration than by deprivation.[4]

Educational pathologists like Strümpell and Klootsema published handbooks of children's disorders, ranging from physical, mental, moral, and emotional handicaps to the effects of parental faults, neglect or a bad environment. Whatever their, according to modern standards often curious, organising principle, they had one thing in common. These books violated neurologists' authority as to the treatment of diseases of the child's mind, senses and particularly the nervous system. The answer of these high-status academic medical specialists to this professional claim of the low-status and non-academic educationalists was emphasising the neurological character of children's mental disorders and making the diagnoses fit children's condition.

In Germany around the turn of the century two versions of the concept of neurasthenia were circulating among medical practitioners, one emphasising hereditary determinism and one stressing the possibilities of prevention and cure by creating a positive environment. As eugenics had only a limited influence in the Netherlands[5] and particularly in the Dutch educational discourse,[6] the latter naturally prevailed. The social-democratic teacher

311

H. Bosma represents the less popular pessimistic 'eugenic' version. He stressed heredity (which included drunkenness of one of the parents at the time of conception and strong emotions of the mother during pregnancy) as the main cause of children's 'nervousness'. Next, he mentioned illnesses from which a child had not recovered properly and frightening experiences such as accidents as additional sources of weak nerves. But he did not deny that wrong treatment at an early age or overburdening at school could turn a child with only a minor disposition into a serious case of neurasthenia. As symptoms of the disease he listed: weariness, irritability, and lack of classroom attention. Order and regularity, calmness and a positive approach of the educators, as well as a whole range of nineteenth-century hygienist panaceas such as fresh air and physical exercise would certainly help. Bosma agreed with the German eugenicists, that it was parents' foremost obligation to scrutinise their own hereditary predisposition and to prevent nervous children from being born.[7]

The more popular optimistic version, stressing the possibilities of sensible upbringing and a healthy environment to prevent nervousness among children, is represented for example by the homeopathic practitioner J. Voorhoeve. His *Zenuwzwakte: hare voorkoming en behandeling* (Weak Nerves: their Prevention and Treatment, 1905), which ran through five editions until 1939, called neurasthenia the disease of a lack of hygiene *par excellence*. As causes of weak nerves he mentioned first the misuse of stimulants like alcohol, tea, coffee or tobacco. Next he pointed at social conditions such as the speed of modern life, monotonous labour, lack of fresh air and rest at the workplace, or exacting school curricula. Heredity he mentioned only as the third cause of the 'rapidly spreading disease'. Children, he claimed, might be spared the suffering of a nervous constitution by a healthy diet and, particularly in case of a hereditary predisposition, good upbringing, which implied early habituation to obedience and self-control.[8]

Likewise, the neurologist F.J. Soesman stressed the importance of discipline in child rearing as a means to promote what he called 'rational mental hygiene'. As he saw it, discipline was the most effective prophylactic against weak nerves. He blamed the high incidence of the disease on 'modern society'. Like tuberculosis 'neurasthenia is not just an individual illness but a social phenomenon', he insisted. The economic growth in the Netherlands during previous years had, according to him, created a series of undesired effects: a quest for luxury, complacency, the denial of authority, and 'with each footstep a lack of self-control and a lack of discipline'. Each of these might be a possible source of nervous complaints. School children, especially adolescents, were particularly vulnerable in this respect, as they were lacking self-confidence and the mental force necessary to resist the temptations of luxury. Too much intellectual effort as against a weak moral development could easily unbalance their nervous system, the neurologist explained. Proper moral upbringing both in the family and at school was the most powerful means to prevent the epidemic from further growth, he insisted.[9]

In the early-twentieth-century discourse on nervousness and children in educational journals, however, neither heredity nor the failures of modern society figured frequently.[10] Pedagogues preferred the concept of neurasthenia as a physical illness that could be treated successfully in education. This approach fitted smoothly in the prevailing concept of child rearing, which showed an almost unlimited belief in the possibilities of educating and improving the individual.[11] It was a German neurologist, who had published extensively on adult neurological diseases, Adolf von Strümpell, who successfully introduced a corresponding view on children's neurasthenia. In 1905 he lectured on 'Nervousness and education' at the Faculty of Medicine of the University of Amsterdam. He described nervousness as a mental illness showing an enlarged irritability, caused by an unbalanced, namely 'abnormal lively', imagination which in turn inspired uneasy feelings such as fears. For children, whose emotional sensitivity resembled the emotional habits of the 'uncivilised people of nature', this was nothing but natural. However, the child definitely needed a hereditary predisposition for the disease to become manifest, he claimed. Nervous parents, on the other hand, were not doomed to have nervous children. In spite of heredity, he explained, they could counterbalance the child's lively imagination as much as possible with healthy, rest-inspiring impressions. A quiet, harmonious environment offered the best chances for a nervous-born child to avoid the symptoms and develop a steady character, notwithstanding the inborn inclination to the contrary, he concluded optimistically.[12]

Von Strümpell's lecture was published in 1905/06 in an educational journal, co-edited by paediatricians and educationalists. His interpretation of neurasthenia immediately became authoritative among Dutch educational professionals. Apparently, they wanted to believe that it was in the power of child-rearing to spare a child with a neurasthenic predisposition the suffering of the symptoms. Moreover, this concept of neurasthenia still had the aura of a real, medically defined illness. Until the First World War educational journals published articles on nervous children on a fairly regular basis. Educational optimism is their most conspicuous characteristic. As in adult psychiatry neurasthenia was presented as a not too serious and curable failure of the nervous system of an otherwise normal child. Although a hereditary predisposition determined the risk of becoming nervous, education was considered a powerful remedy if not a cure. This approach clearly pleased the readership of teachers and parents. They were told that if they acted in a sensible way a child with a nervous constitution would be all right and could perhaps even function as a normal child. Medical professionals in particular explained to the public that it was extremely important to prevent excessive stimulation of the nerves, to provide for regular activities and relaxation, radiate calmness, and prevent any suggestion of danger. In every classroom and in every family there would be potentially nervous children, the treatment of whom would decide their future, these experts claimed.[13]

Thanks to neurasthenia, adult upper-class victims of mental illness could be spared the stigma of insanity, as several contributions to this volume show. Likewise, for bourgeois parents of trouble-making children the diagnosis may have had a similar attractiveness. Neurasthenia prevented their difficult child from any association with child protection, the newly created network of institutional measures to counteract deprivation or indeed the incapacity of the lower classes to raise their children according to the standards of 'civilised' society. If a problem-child was diagnosed as victim of a 'nervous predisposition', parents could never be pointed at as the sole cause of the trouble. In spite of statements of the contrary[14] deprived children were clearly associated with the conditions of lower-class life, such as inadequate housing and food, frequent parental absence, drinking, and family violence. Because children's neurasthenia was on the other hand frequently mentioned as an effect of luxury and the exacting school curricula of higher secondary schooling, the disease seems indeed to have had the same upper-class bias as its adult counterpart. For teachers in special education, particularly those at the recently introduced schools for 'backward and nervous' children,[15] this medically-defined concept of a disease inflicting part of their pupils may have promised a positive effect on their still relatively low professional status.

Nevertheless, at the time neurasthenia did not become a major concern of Dutch pedagogues. In the educational journals nervousness was mentioned in relation with children's insubordination, irritability, fear, eating or sleeping problems, bed-wetting, or nail biting.[16] Apart from the first one, none of these problems figured in the nucleus of their attention. Moreover, they were discussed more often without any reference to weak nerves. At the time in the Netherlands child-rearing was conceived of primarily in terms of character formation. In the process of raising a child, parental authority was to create morally good individuals. Accordingly, children's behavioural problems were considered almost exclusively in moral terms. Educational professionals even discarded references to children's faults in terms of illness as attempts to deny the reality of sin.[17] Because of this predominantly religious interpretation of child-rearing, they considered children's moral failures like lying or resistance to parental authority by far the most important issues to discuss. This one-sided experts' orientation at children's morality explains not only early-twentieth-century Dutch educationalists' lack of interest in neurasthenia in general, but also the refusal of some contributors to the debate to accept the diagnosis of a nervous constitution. In their opinion, these children were not ill in the real sense but suffered from a lack of self-control or will power, perhaps from parental suggestion, or they might simply be the victims of too indulging parents. In those cases, the experts recommended firmness as the key to the solution of the problem.[18] However, on a modest scale the concept of neurasthenia as a disease made its way among pedagogues, precisely at the time when it began to disappear from the psychiatric discourse and practice.

School mental hygiene during the interbellum period

In spite of its fairly limited circulation and acceptance, neurasthenia as a concept survived into the inter-war educational discourse. Two reasons seem to be important in this respect. Both relate to the growing interest in school mental hygiene.

First, the paediatric discourse continued to use neurasthenia as a concept referring to a serious illness. For example, the most authoritative textbook on children's health and development by the first female Dutch paediatrician, Cornelia de Lange, *De geestelijke en lichamelijke opvoeding van het kind* (Rearing the Child's Mind and Body, 1907), modelled after a German example, discussed neurasthenia as one of the so-called 'school diseases'. The textbook had gone through eight editions by 1927. The content of the heading 'nervous and neurasthenic children' – put in between more serious school diseases like tuberculosis, scoliosis etc. – was never changed. This means that several generations of teachers were trained to recognise the symptoms of the illness, which according to De Lange were to be interpreted as the effects of either too much blood in the brains or of mental overburdening. A nervous schoolchild could suffer from headache, bellyache, heart palpitation, dizziness, weariness, lethargy, lack of interest, fits of weeping, in short from almost every symptom of the disease mentioned for adults. Students learned that the little victims were often pale in their faces, had a bad sleep, or were tormented by frightening dreams. De Lange explicitly discriminated between neurasthenia on the one hand and 'psychopathic inferiority' on the other hand. The latter she called a halfway stage between normality and insanity. Both were hereditary diseases, but the symptoms of neurasthenia were much easier to prevent. Good school furniture, enough fresh air, regular physical exercise, and a sensible timetable were effective prophylactics, we learn from the textbook. Most important, however, was a child's right to play and to move freely. From the perspective of mental hygiene, particularly homework and additional private lessons at home were scorned at.[19]

This hygienist concern for the child's physical and mental welfare at school is closely linked to the second reason why neurasthenia survived as a diagnosis. Since the turn of the century nervousness was recognised as one of the foremost risks of the so-called mental overburdening of school children. Particularly the pupils of secondary schools were considered likely victims of the disease.[20] The concern for pupils' mental health was most prominent during the early decades of the century. From its very beginning it was mixed up with another pedagogical hot issue: the one-sided intellectual orientation of higher secondary schooling. Again, the medical profession provided the arguments.

In 1907, at the opening of an international psychiatric conference in Amsterdam, the famous Dutch psychiatrist Gerbrandus Jelgersma had lectured on 'Civilisation as the cause of neurasthenia'. The editor of the important educational journal, *Het Kind* (the child), immediately seized the opportunity to make this distinguished professor an ally in his own battle against 'one-sided intellectualism' at school. Since 1898 he had agitated for educational reform, particularly for a delay of serious study until after the initial puberty crisis, that is not before fourteen or fifteen years of age. Thanks to Jelgersma's 1907 reference to the occurrence of neurasthenia among children he now could include a medical argument against too much emphasis on intellectual labour in general. The editor himself, J.H. Gunning Wzn., added a totally new aspect to the psychiatrist's analysis of what was wrong with Dutch culture. According to him, religion and good old training in self-control were the best prophylactic means.[21] 'Nerves' and the risk of weakening them by too many hours of school and homework and too little opportunity to play or to move freely featured in the New Education Movement's rhetoric until World War II.[22]

These complaints about schools producing nervousness because of their one-sided intellectualism related primarily to secondary education and consequently at the time to the children of the upper and middle-classes. That is why there is often reference to parents sending their children, especially boys, to schools that did not fit their talents. For those victims of adults' pride school could become a burden, particularly during early adolescence when young people's mental vulnerability and morbidity reached the highest level, experts explained.[23] As to girls, it is interesting to note that neurasthenia came in as an argument only after they had entered secondary education in large enough numbers not to run the risk of being excluded on the pretext of 'feminine' mental deficiencies. They were simply doing too well at school.[24] Therefore, the debate on secondary schooling as a source of mental illness hardly related to issues of gender. The only restriction we ought to make in this respect is the frequent qualification of girls as more diligent than boys are.[25] Together with the less gifted and the more ambitious ones, diligent pupils were often mentioned as likely victims of mental illness or indeed neurasthenia.[26]

From neurasthenia to nervousness

This increased awareness of environmental risks for a child's mental health coincided with a process of psychologisation of the liberal educational discourse. From the 1920s, Dutch educational experts showed much more interest in children's emotional troubles like bed-wetting, eating disorders, anger, and especially fear. At the same time these problems began to be interpreted in a different way. Fear for example was not only discussed more frequently, but its meaning also changed. From an expression of a child's lack of self-control it turned into a normal aspect of a young child's inner feelings, which deserved understanding and help instead of hardening.[27] Moreover, traditional concerns like violations of the educators' rule began to be approached from a different angle as well. Henceforth, lying or self-willed children were not just naughty but victims of either emotional neglect or discouragement.[28] Experts began to recognise behaviour problems as disorders that could not easily be redressed by teaching the difficult child self-control. In the more serious cases a child might need therapy or clinical treatment. This implies a gradual shift from a moral or religious interpretation of children's faults to a psycho-medical interpretation of children's disorders as deviations from healthy emotional development. In other words, difficult children were no longer vice-ridden but suffered a more-or-less serious illness.

This process of medicalisation of child-rearing implied that children stopped being held responsible for their own 'bad' behaviour. The message for parents, however, was less clear. It was indeed a double-edged one. On the one hand they were less easy to blame for bad upbringing, as a child's mental illness could result from either nature or an exacting school curriculum. On the other hand parents moved front and centre as the prime cause of children's emotional trouble, because the new dynamic psychology focused on the family as the foremost developing ground of the personality. Psychoanalysis in particular considered parent–child interaction during early childhood the most important source of neurosis. The German analyst Wilhelm Stekel introduced 'nervousness' as children's expression of a neurotic or indeed oedipal conflict.[29]

In the Netherlands, however, it was not so much orthodox psychoanalysis but the oldest heterodoxy, Alfred Adler's Individual psychology, which acted as the main theoretical force in leaving behind the idea of a problem child as sinner. During the 1930s and 1940s Individual psychology was the dominant theoretical influence on child-rearing literature. Orthodox Freudianism had a much more limited impact, because the majority of Dutch educationalists showed a clear-cut dislike of its 'pansexualism'. Adler denied the sexual origins of mental illness and considered physical experiences during early childhood, especially diseases and infirmities, the prime cause of neurosis. In his early work, physical distress explained the development of 'feelings of inferiority'. Later he attributed these feelings to every child. Throughout his work the focus is directed at parent–child interaction, conceived of as a power-relationship. In a young child's mind, he claimed, a battle is fought between two opposite drives: one to defend the self and one to belong to the community. Frustration of either of the two would trigger off a compensatory 'pursuit of power'. Parents could easily 'discourage' a child by failing to appreciate her/his true individuality. Both spoiling and emotional neglect might be the cause. In either case parents were to blame. However, it was not Adler's own work but his follower Fritz Künkel's which gained most popularity in the Netherlands, particularly among liberals. By calling the infantile drives 'egotism'

318

and 'realism' he turned Adler's unconscious drives into normative categories of behaviour. This preference is easy to understand because of the consistency of the revived concept of the good–bad child with the former moral approach of child-rearing.[30]

In the meantime, in the liberal educational discourse children's behaviour problems were more often interpreted as expressions of a nervous constitution. Sometimes the concept of 'nervousness' was used as a collective but unspecific label for all difficult or otherwise abnormal children. They were described as oversensitive and therefore easily aroused and quickly exhausted by schoolwork. They suffered tics, temper tantrums, nail biting, bad sleep and lack of classroom attention.[31] For an explanation some experts pointed at 'modern' ways of child rearing: too little discipline surely caused too little self-discipline.[32] Others pointed precisely into the opposite direction: traditional authoritarianism made children fear their educators, frustrated their self-confidence, and stimulated feelings of inferiority.[33] Certainly, children with a hereditary predisposition and the unfortunate ones who grew up in unstable families, were the most likely victims. Consequently, nervousness was no longer conceived of as the illness itself, but as a set of symptoms with a deeper cause, to be found in parents' attitude. The experts agreed that a hereditary predisposition alone was not enough to bring about the symptoms. Parents' faults on the other hand, no matter if it was spoiling or neglect, always played a role.[34]

Some contributors to the educational debate did know for sure that the number of nervous children was rising. Others were of the opinion that experts had just become fond of using the label. They might even use it too easily, for example in cases of psychopathy, which happened to be a more serious disease, as the psychiatrist H. van der Hoeven explained.[35] He indeed stressed the normality of nervous children, who were 'normal or, if heredity counts, born with normally developed useful capacities, but raised in the wrong way'.[36] Anyway, among the public the concept seems to have gained popularity too. Experts complained that parents liked the diagnosis because it could hide bad parenting. This is for example true of one of the earliest individual-psychological studies of problem children, which happened to be also one of the earliest translations from across the Atlantic. The author, the American psychiatrist Frank H. Richardson deliberately chose 'nervousness' to indicate all difficult children, no matter if they were insubordinate or fearful, precisely because parents preferred the concept. According to him 'nervous' children were simply the victims of parents who were incapable to really understand their children's needs. There was nothing wrong with the child's nervous system and there was no reason to blame heredity, he claimed.[37]

Gradually, during the inter-war era 'neurasthenia' was replaced with 'nervousness' to describe mentally unbalanced children. At the same time there was a shift of emphasis in the use of 'nervousness' from a neurological to a psychiatric interpretation, pointing at family relations as pathogenic conditions. Psychoanalysis and its heterodoxies paved the way in this respect. But even those medical practitioners who continued to believe in a physiological basis of the disease agreed upon the decisive influence of child-rearing.[38] Therefore, we may conclude that 'nervousness' became both more important, because it was referred to more often, and less specific, as it lost the status of an explanatory category. In the liberal educational discourse of the time, which drew heavily upon broad psychoanalytical categories like 'the unconscious', a nervous child became synonymous with a difficult child. This child suffered from a set of symptoms that were more often attributed to feelings of inferiority than to proper neurosis.

No neurosis

Thanks to the development and success of their own 'pillarised' organisations during the inter-war era denominational groups, particularly orthodox Calvinists and Roman Catholics, became very powerful in politics and culture. They were, of course, more reluctant than liberals to interpret children's behaviour problems as illnesses instead of sins. Nevertheless, they too made the transition to a psycho-medical discourse on child rearing. As a consequence of pillarisation they now started their own educational journals, in which they presented their blueprints of an ideal family and school upbringing. Though later, not before the mid-1930s, and accompanied by much more resistance, particularly of clerics, these magazines show the same developments in the discourse.[39] In these cases, however, psychologisation and medicalisation were closely linked with the end of a traditional authoritarian approach. Nervousness seems to have been functional in this respect. One could even say that it helped to trigger off the modernisation of child-rearing.

This is particularly true of Roman Catholics. Contributors to the Catholic journal for parents and other educators first introduced 'nervousness' to explain readers the dangers of the medical view. This approach, conservative Roman Catholics insisted, did not only deny the reality of sin but propagated understanding instead of disciplining a child's unacceptable behaviour.[40] Soon, however, more progressive Catholic educationalists began to refer to 'weak nerves' in an attempt to convince Catholic parents of the risks of too much authoritarianism in child-rearing. Lack of mutual trust between parents and children, too much strictness in discipline and particularly spanking were totally inadequate means as regards 'nervous children', they explained. These problem kids, Catholic parents had better understand, were not sinners but sufferers of a hereditary illness of the nervous system, for which they could not be held responsible. Anger and fear could be symptoms of the disease rather than reasons to discipline a child, they pointed out. Calmness instead of strictness had to instill what these children lacked most of all: self-confidence.[41]

From the late 1930s a young Catholic woman educationalist, Sis Heyster, successfully took the next step in the process of medicalisation and modernisation of child-rearing advice. She introduced Individual psychology into the Catholic discourse. Her books became very popular among parents, especially mothers. She propagated a gentle style of upbringing, in which confidence and understanding had replaced parents' authority as the central means.[42] The concept of 'nervousness' may have prepared the ground for this approach. Attached to nervousness was the aura of medical science. Moreover, belief in a nervous constitution as cause of a whole range of children's behaviour problems was easy to combine with individual-psychological concepts like the 'unconscious' and 'feelings of inferiority', as Heyster's work shows.[43] Most important perhaps, like Individual psychology, nervousness provided a perfect opportunity to avoid the introduction of sexuality and related psychoanalytical concepts like neurosis into the educational discourse. For Roman Catholics, until the 1960s, this would have been two bridges too far.

Among orthodox Calvinists the editor of the mothers' journal this chapter opened with, the Free University professor of Education and Psychology Jan Waterink, embodies the two transitions in the Calvinist discourse on child-rearing in one person: medicalisation and the promotion of a less authoritarian style of upbringing. To him, neurasthenia as well as hereditary dispositions in general, were very important. In his textbooks he dismissed not only Freud's psychoanalysis (because of its pansexualism, materialism, and lack of respect for morality and religion), but Individual psychology as well (it left out heredity and it was too positive about the lower human instincts). Nevertheless, he valued Individual psychology as a heuristic means.[44] Later on, however, he added an extensive discussion of Künkel's work. According to this Calvinist professor it offered a key to the understanding of lots of everyday problems in child rearing. Unlike psychoanalysis, he pointed out, this theory pressed the individual to accept full responsibility for her/his own behaviour. Nonetheless, there were drawbacks, he explained. Religion was for instance ignored and a number of 'serious disorders like for example neurasthenia' could not be reduced to a lack of 'realism'.[45]

However, in Waterink's popular mother's monthly *Moeder*, edited between 1934 and 1961, and particularly in his answers to letter-writing mothers, not only neurasthenia but indeed also Adlerian concepts like 'feelings of inferiority' or 'frustrated assertiveness' were important explanatory categories. Neurasthenia was even the most frequently used diagnosis. It was given as an answer to a whole range of mothers' complaints. From bed wetting to stammering, from night-time fright to masturbation, from insomnia to eating disorders, almost every problem a Dutch Calvinist mother could possibly come up with in a letter, could be attributed to a neurasthenic predisposition. If a letter-writing mother mentioned the right symptoms and certainly if she mentioned being nervous herself, the diagnosis was easily given. But neurasthenia was not only popular at the level of diagnosis. Nervousness was also the most frequently mentioned problem in the letters women sent to the editor. These worried women asked for expert confirmation of their own lay intuition. In a sense, they begged for the diagnosis. It was a safe and therefore attractive one; children's disorders were not ascribed to parents' faults but to hereditary predisposition. And, as many letters show, these women used the professor's diagnosis to promote a gentle approach of children among their husbands, whom they often blamed of a more conservative attitude. As dedicated readers of the journal they were convinced that nervous children deserved understanding, if not right away than at least on medical grounds.[46]

In the post-war period, Calvinist mothers did not stand out among the general public in calling their problem children 'nervous'. Between 1928, when the Amsterdam Child Guidance Clinic was established, and 1970 nervousness continued to be one of the most important reasons for parents to apply for treatment of their child.[47] However, the liberal middle-class parents who did so would not be given the blessings of absolution. As orthodox psychoanalysis dominated the clinic's work,[48] their children were certainly diagnosed as the victims of neurotic family relationships, for which parents were held fully responsible. Therefore, it is no wonder that a popular series on child rearing issued a most reassuring volume on nervous children as late as 1960. The authors, two psychiatrists, advised old-fashioned quiet and regularity in the treatment of these victims. And, perhaps even more important, they pointed at an inborn predisposition as the cause of most cases of 'real nervousness'.[49]

Conclusion

Neurasthenia seems to have been functional as a diagnosis for experts, teachers, parents and children in a variety of ways. Thanks to the disease educationalists could approach with a few more steps the almost unattainable status of medical practitioners. At the beginning of the twentieth century the very belief in pedagogical prophylactics turned the quality of education and consequently the work of teachers into a decisive aspect of public hygiene. Educational reformers' arguments also seem to have gained importance from medical language and particularly from the idea that school hygiene could prevent serious illnesses like nervousness or weak nerves. During the inter-war era in the liberal educational discourse neurasthenia was replaced with the less specific concept of 'nervousness'. This coincided with a shift from a neurological to a psychiatric interpretation. At the same time the disease lost the status of an explanatory category and turned into a set of symptoms. However, neurasthenia as an illness caused by hereditary predisposition was granted a second life in the educational discourses of orthodox Calvinists and Roman Catholics, particularly among those experts who wanted to modernise the traditional authoritarian mode of child-rearing. Thanks to this medical concept they could promote their ends without running the risk of being blamed of denying religious dogma as to the God-ordained authority of parents. As compared to Freudian neurosis neurasthenia provided parents with freedom of guilt of a child's fate. If a child suffered it was not their fault. Moreover, bourgeois parents were spared the association of their difficult child with child protection intervention. If a child failed at school, neurasthenia could also conceal a lack of intelligence or bad teaching. The child, finally, gained a position in which she/he was not held responsible for her/his behaviour. The boy or girl was not just difficult but ill and in need of help instead of punishment. If not rewarding, neurasthenia was at least a harmless disease.

•

Nelleke Bakker

Notes

1. J. Waterink, 'Vragen van moeders', *Moeder* (1949), no. 4, 152.
2. J.J.H. Dekker, 'An Educational Regime: Medical Doctors, Schoolmasters, Jurists, and the Education of Retarded and Deprived Children in the Netherlands around 1900', *History of Education*, 25 (1996), 255–68.
3. Ludwig Strümpell, *Die pädagogische Pathologie oder die Lehre von den Fehlern der Kinder. Versuch einer Grundlegung für gebildete Eltern, Studierende der Pädagogik, Lehrer, sowie für Schulbehörden und Kinderärzte* (Leipzig: Ungleich, 1899, 3rd).
4. J. Klootsema, *Misdeelde kinderen. Inleiding tot de paedagogische pathologie en therapie* (Groningen: Wolters, 1904), 184,189.
5. Jan Noordman, *Om de kwaliteit van het nageslacht. Eugenetica in Nederland 1900-1950* (Nijmegen: SUN, 1989).
6. Ernst Mulder, 'Patterns, Principles, and Profession: The Early Decades of Educational Science in the Netherlands', *Paedagogica Historica*, Supplementary Series, III (1998), 231–46; Nelleke Bakker, *Kind en karakter. Nederlandse pedagogen over opvoeding in het gezin 1845-1925* (Amsterdam: Het Spinhuis, 1995).
7. H. Bosma, *Zenuwachtige kinderen. Medische, paedagogische en algemeene opmerkingen* (Almelo: Hilarius, [1903]).
8. J. Voorhoeve, *Zenuwzwakte: voorkoming en behandeling* (Zwolle: La Rivière & Voorhoeve, 1936, 4th). The first prints appeared with 'hare' in the title.
9. F.J. Soesman, *Hygiène van den geest. Tucht als middel tegen zenuwziekte* ('s-Gravenhage: Van Stockum, 1908), 15, 30, 39.
10. An important exception is the psychiatrist Noorduyn, who used both arguments in a plea for educational reform: J.P.F.A. Noorduyn, *De nerveusiteit van het kind. Uit zenuw- en zieleleven*, II no. 6 (Baarn: Hollandia, 1912).
11. Bakker, *op. cit.* (note 6).
12. A. von Strümpell, 'Zenuwachtigheid en opvoeding', *Tijdschrift voor Kinderverzorging*, 3 (1905/6), 73-5, 82-5, 91-2, 99-100, 108-9, 118.
13. E.g. dr. Wiardi Beckman , 'Achterlijke en nerveuse kinderen', *Tijdschrift voor Kinderverzorging*, 1 (1903/4), 55–7, 64–7, 74–5; N. Knapper, 'Het zenuwachtige, lastige kind', *Het Kind*, 15 (1914), 129–31, 149–52, 156–8, 165–6; T.A. Williams, 'Zenuwachtigheid en opvoeding', *De Vrouw*, 18 (1910/1), 75–6.
14. For example Klootsema explained that deprivation was not the prerogative of the lower classes and that it could be found both in huts and in palaces: Klootsema, *op. cit.* (note 4), 79.

15. The organisation of professionals in special education was for example called Association of Teachers and Medical Practitioners Working at Schools for Backward and Nervous Children. See: Dorien Graas, *Zorgenkinderen op school. Geschiedenis van het speciaal onderwijs in Nederland, 1900-1950* (Leuven/Apeldoorn: Garant, 1996).

16. Bakker, *op. cit.* (note 6), 164-7, 248.

17. Most explicitly formulated by: F.W. Foerster, *Karaktervorming. Een boek voor ouders, onderwijzers en geestelijken* (Zwolle: Ploegsma, 1913), 421; *Idem, Opvoeding en zelfopvoeding. Voornaamste gezichtspunten voor ouders en onderwijzers, opvoeders en verzorgers der jeugd* (Zwolle: Ploegsma, 1926), 31-7.

18. F. van Raalte, *De ziel van het kind. Opstellen van ...* (Nijmegen: Robijns, 1916), 159-69; L. de Jager, *Onthouding in de opvoeding* (Leeuwarden: Meijer & Schaafsma, 1911), 22.

19. Cornelia de Lange, *De geestelijke en lichamelijke opvoeding van het kind. In vrije navolging van prof. Biedert 'Das Kind'* (Amsterdam: Meulenhoff, 1908, 2nd), 407-33.

20. G. Oosterbaan, 'Praeadvies: Medisch toezicht op de scholen', *Tijdschrift voor Sociale Hygiëne,* 7 (1905), 270-82; T.H. de Beer, *Steenen voor brood. Het doel van het onderwijs en dat van de nieuwe onderwijswetten* (Baarn: Hollandia, 1904); J. Kleefstra, *Wat maken wij van onze jongeren?* (Haarlem: Bohn, 1905).

21. J.H. Gunning Wzn, ' Op het psychiatrisch congres', *Het Kind,* 8 (1907), 153-5; *Idem, Zenuwachtigheid en opvoeding* (s.l. [1929]).

22. For example: C.P. Gunning, 'Geestelijke gezondheid', *Het Kind,* 27 (1926), 107-12; C. Wilkeshuis, ''t Zenuwachtige kind', *School en Huis,* 6 (1926/7), 517-9, 533-5; J. van Mourik, 'Overlading op de L.S.', *Onze Kinderen en hun Toekomst,* 15 (1936), 11-5, 215-20.

23. A. Cramer, *Puberteit en school* (Groningen: Noordhoff, 1912); Voorhoeve, *op. cit.* (note 8). See also: Nelleke Bakker, 'The Lamp in the Living Room. Dutch Family Educationalists on Adolescence, 1915-1950', *Paedagogica Historica,* 29 (1993), 241-55.

24. Nelleke Bakker & Mineke van Essen, 'No Matter of Principle—The Unproblematic Character of Coeducation in Girls' Secondary Schooling in the Netherlands, ca. 1870-1930', *History of Education Quarterly,* 39 (1999), 454-75.

25. Nelleke Bakker, 'A Curious Inconsistency: Coeducation in Secondary Education in the Netherlands, 1900-1960', *Paedagogica Historica. ,* IV (1998), 273-92.

26. J.P.F.A. Noorduyn, *op. cit.* (note 10); Cramer, *op. cit.* (note 23).

27. Nelleke Bakker, 'The Meaning of Fear. Emotional Standards for Children in the Netherlands, 1850-1950: Was there a Western

Transformation?', *Journal of Social History,* 34 (2000), 369–91.

28. Nelleke Bakker, 'Van kindergebreken naar opvoedingsfouten: Een historisch onderzoek naar de bespreking van gedragsproblemen in opvoedingsvoorlichting aan Nederlandse ouders, 1890-1940', in J.R.M. Gerris & J. van Acker (eds), *Gezinsrelaties onderzocht* (Amsterdam/Lisse: Swets & Zeitlinger, 1988),161–72.

29. Wilhelm Stekel, *De oorzaken der zenuwachtigheid. Een psychanalytische beschouwing* (Leiden: Leidsche Uitgeversmaatschappij, [1924]). See also: L.F. Groenendijk, 'Masturbation and Neurasthenia: Freud and Stekel in Debate on the Harmfull Effects of Autoerotism', *Journal of Psychology and Human Sexuality,* 9 (1997), 71–94.

30. Nelleke Bakker, 'Child-rearing Literature and the Reception of Individual Psychology in the Netherlands 1930-1950: The Case of a Calvinist Pedagogue', *Paedagogica Historica. op. cit. (note 6),* 585–602.

31. A.M.E. Beernink-Trip, 'Zenuwachtige kinderen', *Het Kind,* 26 (1925), 4–7; M. Dekker-Benjamins, 'De zenuwachtige kleuter', *Zuigeling en Kleuter,* 5 (1935), no. 9, 1–3; M.J. Langeveld, 'Tics', *Zuigeling en Kleuter,* 5 (1935), no. 2, 3–4.

32. I.C. van Houte & G.J. Vos, *Moeilijke kinderen. Een boek voor ouders en opvoeders* (Utrecht 1929, Keming & Zn.), 38.

33. H.G. Hamaker, 'Geneeskundige voorlichting', *School en Huis,* 1 (1921/2), 709–12, 739–43, 772–5, 805–8 and 2 (1922/3), 8–12, 39–42, 71–4.

34. C. Wilkeshuis, 'Over opvoeding: 't zenuwachtige kind', *School en Huis,* 6 (1926/7), 517–9, 533–5; G.J.E. Ruysch, 'Het nerveuse kind', *Het Kind,* 27 (1926), 92–3.

35. H. van der Hoeven jr., 'Psychopathische kinderen', *Tijdschrift voor Ervaringsopvoedkunde,* 2 (1923), 1–8.

36. H. van der Hoeven jr., 'Nerveusiteit en opvoeding', *Tijdschrift voor Ervaringsopvoedkunde,* 10 (1931), 76–9, especially 79.

37. Frank H. Richardson, *Het nerveuse kind en zijn ouders* (Amsterdam: Van Holkema & Warendorf, 1929). This was an adapted translation of the original American edition: *Parenthood and the Newer Psychology: Being the Application of Old Principles in a New Guise to the Problems of Parents with their Children* (New York: Putnam, 1926).

38. For example: Dekker-Benjamins, *op. cit.* (note 31); A.M.E. Beernink-Trip, 'Zenuwachtige moeders—lastige kinderen', *Zuigeling en Kleuter,* 2 (1932), 3–4; P. Tilma, 'Prophylaxis en therapie van de neuropathie bij het kind', *Het Kind,* 34 (1933), 371–7; J.C. van Andel & O. van Andel-Ripke, *Gezonde kinderen, evenwichtige*

mensen (Utrecht: Bijleveld, 1939), 159; N.I. Heijbroek, C.J. Heijbroek-d'Ancona, & C.G. Querido-Nagtegaal, *Onze kinderen. De lichamelijke verzorging en geestelijke ontwikkeling, van geboorte tot puberteit* (Amsterdam: Meulenhof, 1949), 193–6.

39. Bakker, *op. cit.* (note 30).
40. H. Woltring, 'Over zenuwen en opvoeding', *Tijdschrift voor R.K. Ouders en Opvoeders*, 1 (1919), 61–3, 69–71, 85–8, 93–6; dr. E., 'Zenuwachtige kinderen', *Tijdschrift voor R.K. Ouders en Opvoeders*, 4 (1922), 255–9, 265–8 and 5 (1923), 95–6, 110–2.
41. A. Hulsmans, 'Buskruit', *Tijdschrift voor R.K. Ouders en Opvoeders*, 3 (1921), 134–5; L., 'Opvoeding van zenuwachtige kinderen', *Tijdschrift voor R.K. Ouders en Kinderen*, 8 (1926), 273–6, 289–91, 309–12.
42. Bakker, *op. cit.* (note 30), 590.
43. Nervousness figured only in her later work: Sis Heyster, *Levende opvoedkunde ten dienste van kleinere en grotere kinderen* (Leiden: Nederlandsche Uitgeversmaatschappij, [1947]), 176-82. Individual psychology was already adapted in the 1930s: Sis Heyster, *Opvoeden in de practijk. Het boek voor iederen opvoeder* (Den Haag/Gent: Populair Wetenschappelijke Bibliotheek, 1935); Sis Heyster, *Opvoedingsmoeilijkheden van iederen dag* (Amsterdam: Kosmos, 1938).
44. J. Waterink, *Hoofdlijnen der zielkunde* (Wageningen: Zoomer & Keuning, 1934), 211.
45. J. Waterink, *Ons zieleleven* (Wageningen: Zoomer & Keuning, 1946, 5th), 176–202.
46. Bakker, *op. cit.* (note 30), 596–7.
47. A. van der Wurff, '"Niet zoo maar een mening, doch een welbewust gegeven psychiatrisch advies". Aspecten uit de MOB-geschiedenis 1928–ca.1975', in Joost Vijselaar (ed.), *Ambulant in zicht. Geschiedenis van de ambulante geestelijke gezondheidszorg in Nederland* (Utrecht: NCGV, 1987), 83–101.
48. A. van der Wurff, 'Aspecten van medicalisering en normalisering bij de opkomst van het medisch-opvoedkundig werk in Nederland in het begin van de twintigste eeuw', *Pedagogisch Tijdschrift*, 15 (1990), 102–10.
49. C. Rümke & Th. Hart de Ruijter, *Het nerveuze kind. Het ABC der opvoeding*, no. 4 (Nijkerk: Callenbach, [1960]).

15

Neurasthenia and Manhood in *fin-de-siècle* France[1]

Christopher E. Forth

Let's not forget that the vigour of humanity is composed of the
vigour of men.

Dr. F. Aumont, L'Estomac des gens du monde[2]

Nervous weakness, the protean heart of neurasthenia, sits
uncomfortably alongside modern representations of manhood. This
is partly the case because, thanks to the association of nervousness
with hysteria, it has historically been viewed as a quality more
properly found among women. Due largely to the etymology of the
term and the traditionally female constituency of those who were
diagnosed with the malady, it is undeniable that during the
nineteenth century hysteria carried definite connotations of
femininity, which is partly why the 'discovery' of male hysteria during
the 1870s caused such a furor in medical circles. Yet did being
diagnosed with neurasthenia truly represent a way for men to be
safely nervous without compromising their sense of manhood?
Edward Shorter has suggested that many *fin-de-siècle* men welcomed
the neurasthenia diagnosis as a more flattering alternative to the
overtly feminising implications of hysteria. After all, he reasonably
wonders, 'What forty-year-old businessman would want to see
himself as hysterical?'[3] It is also true that physicians emphasised the
indiscriminate nature of neurasthenia's reach and demonstrated how,
by being fuelled by all sorts of exhaustion and hyperstimulus, it
respected neither boundaries of sex nor of class. Despite his insistence
that male hysteria did not necessarily entail any loss of manly vigour,
however, in his diagnostic practice the famed neurologist Jean-
Martin Charcot seems to have reserved the neurasthenia label for
bourgeois male patients with hysteria-like symptoms while placing
working-class men into the category of male hysterics.[4] Charcot even
extended this division into his description of the varieties of
neurasthenia, indicating that traumatic 'hystero-neurasthenia' was

most often experienced by working-class men. This quarantining of proletarian neurasthenia from its bourgeois counterpart indeed suggests, as Sonu Shamdasani points out, a divergence between a formal medical desocialisation of neurasthenia and the lingering tendency to carve out in practice class distinctions that doubled as markers of gender difference.[5]

Historical accounts of neurasthenia often follow a medical and psychiatric trajectory, plotting a course from Beard's resurrection of the term through its falling out of favour during the 1920s, citing along the way key intellectual changes from a belief in the somatic foundations of mental disorders to more strictly psychological explanations epitomised by Freud and his followers. This chapter rather moves between the world of official medical discourses on the disorder and wider cultural understandings of what being a neurasthenic male meant in France at the *fin de siècle*. By situating itself within the very divergence that Shamdasani has observed, it is concerned less with the rise and fall of neurasthenia as a diagnostic category than with the shifting fortunes of male nervousness during a period when masculinity was said to be in a state of crisis. Beyond the question of the gender strategies of medical practice – that is, the subtle efforts of physicians to shield bourgeois men from too close an association with femininity – it inquires into the success of these strategies within a culture where the 'real' man was viewed as a vanishing breed. What did it mean for a man to be diagnosed with a disorder like neurasthenia during such a crisis period? How did fashionable affirmations of neurasthenia sit alongside competing claims that nervousness and emotivity in general were incompatible with manliness? In short, what cultural forces were at play to render the very notion of a 'neurasthenic man' somewhat oxymoronic?

There are no simple answers to such questions. If the pervasiveness of what Robert Nye has called an 'organicist discourse of national decline' highlights the difficulty of confining a discussion of neurasthenia and manhood to strictly medical parameters, it also illuminates how events that are often considered eminently 'political' were themselves cast in the language of such discourses.[6] This chapter thus argues that the shifting status of the neurasthenic male in France was as much a social and political phenomenon as it was a medical issue, and that any attempt to answer the questions posed above necessarily entails juggling a wide range of contemporary concerns. Similarly, it also means adopting a selective approach to a complex issue that has more dimensions than can be coherently broached within current space restrictions.

Neurasthenia and masculinity:
Work and the problem of fatigue

As a continuation and refinement of the myriad forms of nervousness that had plagued westerners since the eighteenth century, neurasthenia was a remarkably elastic category that could encompass a stunning array of symptoms and causes, thus rendering it virtually meaningless in the eyes of some critics. For most French physicians the aetiology of '*la maladie de Beard*' often came down to *surmenage*, an overtaxation of the nervous system that stemmed from any number of physical and moral sources. 'In a word, all surmenage, that is to say, all fatigue leading to the exhaustion of one or more functions of the nervous system, prepares the ground for and favours the development of neurasthenia'.[7] A hereditary predisposition to nervousness, usually cited as the common denominator of most cases of neurasthenia, could be activated by a variety of factors, particularly by the accelerated pace and sensual distractions of modern existence. 'Ours is the century of accelerated movement', explained one physician.' We are in a perpetual effervescence; our nervous systems remain in a state of tension which never relaxes.'[8] People dubbed 'true neurasthenics' by Gilles de la Tourette, however, were those who displayed the stock symptoms of nervous weakness without any hereditary taint, and represented an even more troubling category of sufferers. These were otherwise healthy people literally worn down by the overstimulating effects of modernity and who now risked passing their debilities on to their children, thus exacerbating and expanding the anxieties about hereditary degeneration that marked the *fin de siècle*.[9]

Yet while many women were diagnosed with the malady, neurasthenia was first and foremost considered a problem of men. 'Neurasthenia is more common among men than among women', observed Adrien Proust and Gilbert Ballet in their authoritative study, though they were quick to note that (unlike women) men shared no innate weakness that made them particularly prone to this unfortunate condition. Rather, hard work, worries, and excess were 'consequences of the more active and more militant role of the man in the struggle for existence'.[10] Whatever consolation could be found in such claims was also potentially diminished due to neurasthenia's effects on the person: the disorder robbed a man of the ability to continue fulfilling this 'more militant role', thus generating what Anson Rabinbach has rightly termed a 'negative work ethic'.[11] Modern men, whether bourgeois or proletarian, have generally found something validating in hard work, at once in the expressive potential of the labour itself, in its capacity (by the mid-nineteenth century) to separate men from women along a public/private divide, and even in the gratifying effects of fatigue that it sometimes wrought. A man's capacity for labour power thus represented a terrain upon which aspects of masculinity could be tested, defended, and critiqued. 'To dispute our ability to work', wondered health reformer Jules Payot, 'isn't that to reproach our weakness and our cowardice?'[12]

Although modern men often registered a common disdain for the principled idleness of the traditional aristocracy, they have remained considerably divided over the relative merits of mental as opposed to physical labour. The 'ideology of adventure' that had since the Middle Ages structured the expectations and emotional investments of western men lingered on in the social imagination, and represented a persistent source of anxiety among men involved in contemplative, non-manual activities. Having excluded themselves from a martial lifestyle that in the modern period was lived by only a select few, men of thought (whether clerics or bourgeois) nevertheless appropriated the physicalist language of warfare and craftsmanship as a means of masculine compensation.[13] Faced in the early-nineteenth century with forging a definition of manhood that did not rely primarily on demonstrations of physical strength and risk-taking (qualities that were crucial for working-class men as well as soldiers), many bourgeois males incorporated the rhetoric of combat and conquest into discussions of economic activity while implicitly valorising rationality as an inherently masculine trait.[14] Hence the 'more militant' quality that Proust and Ballet attributed to male labour.

By the end of the century, however, amid what historians have identified as a widespread rediscovery of the body in western culture, the heroic deeds of certain men were being viewed in overtly physical terms that were not so amenable to metaphorical appropriation. Across the western world bourgeois professionals found their manhood called into question in a debate that pitted the 'man of thought' against the 'man of action', a dispute that invoked the question of the male body in a manner that was potentially embarrassing for the bourgeois 'brain worker'. Some were thus left in a defensive posture that led them to insist upon the burden that cerebral labour wrought as a means of manly redemption. Aside from being potentially harmful in the long run, the physical and mental evidence of wear and tear was often offered as proof of the difficulty (and therefore superior masculinity) of the professions. Arguably, such evidence functioned at once as a health warning to bourgeois professionals and as a mild form of flattery that invoked the conventional bourgeois acceptance of nervousness as a sign of an elevated sensibility. Physicians may have maintained that neurasthenia struck men of every profession and social class, but such claims flew in the face of prevailing popular associations of nervous fatigue with the bourgeoisie.

This ambivalence about fatigue was to a significant degree generated by physicians, perhaps explaining why some men may have considered it acceptable to be neurasthenic. In a regular medical column in the highbrow *Annales politiques et littéraires,* Dr. Henri de Parville assured his readers that mental labour was just as burdensome, if not more so, than manual exertion. 'It's always the same prejudice', he lamented. 'For the worker, intellectual labour does not count'. Little did the manual labourer know what hardships were endured by the white collar professional, for whereas the former might work outdoors and remains free in his toil, the intellectual worker is 'a prisoner to his chair'. As the effects of such labour had a cumulative effect, the difference between the two men at age forty would be quite striking: 'The worker is solid, healthy; *l'homme de plume* is deformed; he digests badly, and is already gouty or rheumatic'. In terms of fatigue and the expenditure of energy there could be no comparison between these two forms of work, for 'mental labour uses up its man more quickly than does muscular labour'. A worker who swapped places with a bourgeois professional for just one year would not be able to hack it, Parville averred, and would quickly discover that the 'building site and the workshop are preferable to the office'.[15]

At once destructive and validating, nervous fatigue was an ambiguous phenomenon. Yet there are other reasons that men may have embraced neurasthenia during this time. For instance, concern with one's health was quite fashionable among the bourgeoisie, and functioned as a preoccupation that at once affirmed the older image of the superior but delicate sensibility of that class and provided an easy rationale for a three-week sojourn at a health spa or seaside resort. Admitting the discomfort of fatigue was, in a word, to anticipate the potential pleasure of a cure. Although space does not permit an elaboration of this latter development, its importance for the social image of neurasthenia must be noted. Douglas Mackaman has recently shown that after 1850 many people who flocked to French sanatoria failed to register as curists, thus slowly giving rise to the bourgeois holiday as a mode of leisure that did not require a strictly medical justification. Yet the *fin de siècle* was a transitional phase of this process during which complaints about fatigue, nervousness, and other pitfalls of modern urban life still lent an air of respectability to *les vacances* that the simple desire for leisure failed to confer. This interaction of modernity, medicine, and tourism may have helped to render neurasthenia fashionable among both men and women, thus mitigating for a time its destructive implications for masculinity.[16]

Emotional control and failed boundaries

Despite the anticipated pleasure of rest and relaxation, fatigue's potential as a bulwark of masculine identity was fatally limited by its capacity to leave a man so weakened as to be incapable of labour. Viewed from a social as well as a medical perspective, neurasthenia represented not only physical and moral weakness, but a certain *vulnerability* that undermined what had come to be viewed as normative conceptions of the bounded and autonomous male self. Of course neurasthenics manifested a variety of symptoms, including headaches, insomnia, loss of appetite, indigestion and constipation, that did not in themselves pose immediate threats to their sense of manhood. Yet from the viewpoint of *fin-de-siècle* understandings of masculinity, two sets of related symptoms proved most vexing about the neurasthenic man. There was on the one hand his extreme susceptibility to external physical stimuli, manifested in an inability to withstand loud noises, crowds, movement, and even changes in the weather. On the other hand, neurasthenics suffered from more internal weaknesses, especially psychic disorders like memory lapses, anxiety, short attention spans, and a slavish submission to their own inner passions, all symptoms of a troubling inability to exercise willpower and a collapse of personal boundaries. Spatial and martial metaphors abounded in the medical discourses on mental illness at the *fin de siècle*, and often referred to 'floods', 'waves' and 'invasions' of excitations from the outside as well as crumbling inner resistance to such dangerous stimuli. Compromised boundaries and weakened inner forces were intimately related, and illuminate a spatial dimension to masculine identity that is rarely observed in the existing historiography.

In keeping with the materialist terms of the nineteenth century human sciences, the spatiality of male identity was to a great extent constructed through the interarticulated domains of medicine and morality. First, the ideal male was one who in medical terms was seen as capable of maximising his vitality and resisting illness. According to Anne C. Vila, during the late-eighteenth century the normative

334

male body was defined in part by its natural ability to 'resist or overcome unwelcome irritants and obstacles, whereas women cede involuntarily to the multiple stimuli to which they are subject because they have no more power to resist than do children'.[17] This association of proper physiological manhood with optimal health and vitality persisted throughout the nineteenth century, and posed a stark contrast to artistic and literary depictions of invalid and consumptive women whose physical ailments only seemed to confirm the inherent frailty of femininity.[18] In an 1874 entry in his *Journal intime*, Henri-Frédéric Amiel also equated manliness with physical robustness in terms of the capacity for resistance that was lacking in more refined social circles: 'The stronger one is, the less sensitive he is to all that torments, agitates, worries and upsets worldly people. Robustness is a suit of armour and consequently a source of freedom. Vulnerability is a hard servitude. *Vae debilibus!* Woe to the weaklings!'[19]

This medical view of an ideal male who was insulated from pathogens was inextricably bound up with a parallel discourse about the maintenance of strong ego boundaries, a psychic investment in one's bodily peripheries that effected a gradual closing (and, one might say, a closing off) of the male body, at once from the outer world of dangerous stimuli and from the inner world of threatening passions. Without a doubt, as Norbert Elias has shown, in the western world both men and women experienced a shift in their sense of personal boundaries during the early modern era where, amid changing social circumstances, rising thresholds of repugnance and shame were manifested among the upper-classes as a growing aversion to their own bodily functions and to the bodies of others. The changes wrought by new developments in table manners and etiquette were extended by the introduction of hygienic practices in the eighteenth and nineteenth centuries that endeavoured to maximise the order and cleanliness of the social body while further compartmentalising the bourgeois self as a discrete bodily unit.[20] As the schoolbooks of the Third Republic suggest, children were taught to view health and subjectivity as the results of constant vigilance and self-surveillance, and illness as evidence of a moral flaw. 'The microbe can invade us despite everything', cautioned one text. 'It is necessary to resist... Be strong and disease will not vanquish us. But if we are not strong, it is our own fault. We deliver ourselves to our vices and they kill us.'[21]

This process of boundary formation reached its apotheosis by the end of the nineteenth century, when across the western world male

335

displays of emotion, particularly grief and fear, were increasingly being viewed with derision. In the early-nineteenth century, for example, Evangelical Christianity in Britain had seen no contradiction between manliness and displays of tears, and often congratulated the father who was moved to emotion. Not so by the end of the century, where British men were increasingly expected to maintain strict control over such emotions.[22] In France too representations of the weeping man underwent significant changes. The emotional release whereby in earlier decades a man may have easily melted or dissolved into tears was by the 1880s replaced with metaphors of explosion, catharsis, and violent eruption. Anne Vincent-Buffault has vividly captured this shift in her history of tears:

> Explosion, tearing, trembling, shaking, suffocation, smothering, the body was overcome with crises, with convulsions, with nervous spasms.... A man wept when he could not act. The metaphors which illustrated male sobs revealed an image of the sealed body which began to explode.[23]

Whether a question of pent-up emotions or resistance to external influences, changes in male identity, often directly linked to perceived crises of manhood, were here manifested in the formation of a new sensibility, a new way of managing emotions and of maintaining boundaries around the self that could nevertheless be breached under circumstances of extreme pressure or constitutional weakness. This phenomenon was short-circuited through the emotional disorders that were frequently generated by neurasthenia. As Vincent-Buffault astutely observes: 'In the excess of his nervous despair, the man who sobbed found himself relegated to femininity and childhood.'[24]

Each of these two discourses, the medical and the moral, were grafted onto and articulated the other, often in a manner that confounded causality. This is why neurasthenia itself could be described alternately as the cause or the effect of will pathologies and moral contagion. From the perspective of an embattled masculine identity, then, the emotivity, fear, and loss of control wrought by neurasthenia counted among the more problematic aspects of the disorder. Sketching a tense dynamic between inner and outer realms, Borel spoke of how neurasthenics suffered from 'great moral susceptibility: a trifle, the smallest obstacle, the slightest reproach, the lightest emotion agitates *le malade*, who is ready to burst out in anger or pity.'[25] The neurasthenic was also no longer capable of enduring the accelerated pace of urban life, where 'the crowd, movement, a noise, a gesture, [or] a trifle are unbearable.'[26] The movement described in such accounts is one of collapse: emotions that should be contained flow outward while the sensorial stimuli from the outside world rush inside unchecked. A neurasthenic suffering from morbid fear displayed even more pronounced symptoms: 'he pales, his pulse and respiration accelerate, his head reels, a cold sweat breaks out on his face and extremities, his legs tremble and waver.'[27] Symptoms such as these were incompatible with conventional ideals of the self-sufficient and courageous male.

An inability to control one's emotions was paralleled in the inability to control oneself sexually, and genital disorders ranked high on the list of neurasthenic complaints. Sexual or genital neurasthenia was isolated as a special disorder, one where the fatigue experienced was due primarily to childhood masturbation or homosexuality, both of which were believed to produce dangerously high expenditures of nervous energy. 'Pederasty', especially among active partners, was reputed to play an especially significant role in the etiology of genital neurasthenia.[28] Many men experienced 'a progressive diminution of sexual appetite and virile power' that could result in complete impotence.[29] Even when able to perform sexually many neurasthenic men found intercourse to be a challenge and often suffered from premature ejaculation and post-coital fatigue, if not depression. Spermatorrhea, the uncontrollable loss of semen while urinating, was also a common genital symptom that represented perhaps the most vivid example of failed boundaries. As great emphasis was placed on the invigorating power of semen retention, uncontrolled outpourings of the valuable substance was the *ne plus ultra* of manly decline.[30] Such genital crises represented both 'a cause of fatigue for the organism and despair for the sufferer.'[31]

Neurasthenia left the male in a state of profound vulnerability, rendering him at once incapable of withstanding the sensory overload of the urban environment and of quelling the passions that they inevitably stirred up. Although in many quarters nervousness continued to be prized as a sign of a refined artistic sensibility, it also produced, according to the brothers Edmond and Jules Goncourt, 'a kind of skinned and chafed moral and sensitive being, wounded by the minutest impressions, defenseless, without a casing, all bloody and raw'.[32] However fashionable it may have been in certain circles to suffer from *la maladie du siècle*, there is little doubt that around 1900 emerging styles of masculine identity vigorously protested against such weakness. By the *fin de siècle* critics began to wonder what had happened to the 'real' man of the past, and bemoaned the loss of autonomy and willpower that afflicted so many in the modern world. 'Most men are governed by what's outside of them', lamented Jules Payot in his popular self-help manual *L'Éducation de la volonté*: 'they are "marionettes"' moved primarily by 'involuntary desires and external suggestions'.[33] Those who hid behind the convenient excuse of innate temperament committed themselves needlessly to physical decline by neglecting basic hygienic calls to exercise, to take clean air and sun, and to display moderation at the table. Such men were, according to another reformer, 'victims of engulfment' [*l'enlizement*]. 'We are all perpetually drowning, or navigators on the open sea in a cockleshell: if we cannot grasp, just in time to recover our breath, a providential twig on the bank, or if we do not succeed in emptying our bark of every wave that fills it, all of which is up to us, we perish.'[34]

The nervous nineties

Although neurasthenia invoked the symptoms associated with a more general sense of *nervosité* and in many respects furthered eighteenth century treatments of the condition, one may also view it in terms of the specific circumstances of France under the Third Republic, where in the wake of a national catastrophe a new class of men rose to social prominence. During the closing decades of the nineteenth century there were many reasons for people to question the state of French manhood. Not only had Prussia brought the nation to its knees in 1870, but the French birth rate seemed to lag dangerously behind that of other countries, particularly the newly-formed German empire. The gender anxieties of the *fin de siècle* were to a significant degree structured by these martial and reproductive anxieties, and all of these worries were imbricated in medical discourses about degeneracy and national decline. It is true that academic medical texts rarely condemned neurasthenia among men as a form of effeminacy; yet whether he suffered from muscular weakness, morbid fear, or sexual impotence, in the wider culture the neurasthenic man was increasingly seen as a living testimony to French weakness, a weakling who was ill-equipped for action should the nation require it.[35]

1. Republican manhood

With neurasthenia evidently on the rise among the bourgeois elite during the Third Republic, it became impossible simply to relegate neurasthenics to the margins of social life. The specifics of the French experience resonated with developments across the western world where, in addition to the preoccupation with homosexuals, criminals, and the insane, physicians began to focus more closely on those men who had been long considered normal. As George Mosse observes, during this time attention was increasingly drawn to 'otherwise respectable middle-class men who could not live up to the manly ideal because in some manner they were considered sick or unmanly. They seemed to narrow the gap between true masculinity and its foil in a dangerous way.'[36]

Despite the cultural demand that men defend their honour through duelling, the men who rose to positions of power and prestige in the new republican system were somewhat removed from any military ideal of masculinity, primarily because their livelihood was based on mental rather than physical labour. By the 1880s, and partly in response to the growing awareness of neurasthenia, the schools that produced the nation's elite came under scrutiny for promoting a dangerously excessive cerebralism. Attempts had been made in previous decades – particularly after 1870 – to incorporate physical education into the *lycées*, but most schools either lacked the facilities or the will to do so.[37] Among many specialists neurasthenia represented a logical progression of the mental fatigue incurred during one's school days. With mental strain and sedentarity came physical debility, and the thoracic capacities of schoolboys were found to be alarmingly limited, thereby potentially exempting them from military service. All of this served to 'annihilate individual initiative, force of will, moral energy, [and] firmness of character.'[38] It was no wonder that boys were growing up to be neurasthenic, noted Borel: 'Look at the soft, enervating, effeminate education to which we submit the child whose faculties are just beginning to develop.'[39] The result of this *surmenage intellectuel* was a steady deterioration of the French elite, leading one physician to note with irony that, when it comes to neurasthenic men, 'the classes that are called *dirigeantes* furnish the strongest contingent.'[40]

Yet most physicians were quick to point out that intellectual exhaustion alone was not enough to cause neurasthenia, and usually argued that moral exhaustion, brought on either by overindulgence in pleasures like the theatre, novels, café-concerts, and cabarets, or by depressive states like worry and jealousy, was even more damaging. Indeed, concerns about *surmenage intellectuel* among adolescents were generally conceived alongside the moral turpitude that seemed so rampant in boarding schools, and consequently recommendations for preventing neurasthenia often went hand-in-hand with desires to ensure the reproduction of the heterosexual norm. For Bouveret it was the 'frightful contagion' of certain 'bad habits' that, while normally curtailed by the healthy at an appropriate age, proved especially dangerous for children with 'hereditary defects' and represented 'a very powerful cause of nervous exhaustion'.[41] Proust and Ballet also indicted the moral environment of *lycées* by citing experiments where male animals that had been placed in situations of 'restrictive domesticity', being deprived access to females, experienced a 'great excitation of reproductive instincts followed by a dreadful perversion of those instincts'. Admitting that the 'evil' of boarding students was a necessary one, the authors nevertheless recommended that children issuing from nervous backgrounds should be prevented from rooming with other students. Such boys should be educated as 'external' students, where 'some honourable family' would offer them room and board in exchange for a modest compensation.[42] Those predisposed to nervous disorders would thus be shielded from the unhealthy conditions of school life, while their more vigorous comrades would likewise be spared excessive contact with noxious elements. Indeed, for all of their Lamarckian insistence on the formative role of the environment in the aetiology of nervous disorders, French physicians underscored the importance of heredity in the generation of neurasthenia while nevertheless agreeing that hereditary predisposition needed to be triggered through environmental factors. Some physicians even invoked conceptions of individual temperaments (nervous, sanguine, bilious, and lymphatic) as a way of thinking about nervous heredity, while others went so far as to suggest separate schools altogether for congenitally nervous students.[43]

2. Jewish nerves

Although medical texts said little about different types of nervous adolescents, Jewish people figured prominently among those considered congenitally prone to neurasthenia. Indeed, under the Third Republic neurasthenia was a racial as well as a gender issue, and during the late 1880s anxieties about national decline and the fitness of the bourgeoisie were often concentrated in representations of the Jewish man, a stock cultural figure whose close association with intellectuality, nervousness and physical frailty contributed to impressions of his effeminacy. Such stereotypes received considerable medical support, and physicians often followed Charcot's authoritative lead by asserting that Jews were particularly susceptible to nervous exhaustion, diabetes, gout, and arthritis.[44] In addition, the observations of one of Charcot's students, Henri Meige, about the nervous disposition of the proverbial 'wandering Jew' were frequently echoed in works on neurasthenia.[45] Such images were readily invoked by physicians like Henry Labonne, who deplored the exhaustion that came with the competition and 'struggle for money' in overly refined cultures. Labonne echoed a common medical assumption when he declared that 'half of all Jews are neurasthenics', though he believed that this was amply supported by his claim that 'in no other race is suicide so common'.[46] Finally, by citing both scholarly opinion and cultural stereotypes in his immensely popular anti-semitic diatribe, *La France juive*, Édouard Drumont cemented for many the dangerous connections between Jews, mental labour, and nervousness.[47]

Insofar as he seemed to epitomise the dire consequences of modernity, the neurasthenic Jew crystallised the anxieties that haunted many bourgeois men: the very labour that bolstered their sense of manhood could also undermine it. In an age when the boundary between the normal and the pathological was becoming increasingly uncertain, 'Jewishness' was perceived less as the absolute 'other' of bourgeois manhood than as a metaphor for a set of negative qualities that awaited less vigilant modern men.[48] Indeed, in his well-known attack on antisemitic dogma, Anatole Leroy-Beaulieu reinforced a number of old stereotypes about male Jewish effeminacy. In a move common among champions of Jewish assimilation, ancient beliefs were qualified rather than dismissed: the Jew's 'narrow chest' was due less to heredity than to the 'sedentary habits' encouraged by city life, and this physical deterioration was only compounded over several generations. Thus did Leroy-Beaulieu explain the 'unmanly appearance' of many Jewish men, why they were so unattractive to women and why they seemed so 'puny, weak, and frail'. In the Jewish man muscular weakness accorded his nervous system a certain prominence: 'he is all nerve. . . . The Jew is the most nervous of men, perhaps because he is the most "cerebral", because he has lived most by his brain'. The neurasthenic Jew was one of the most telling symptoms of modern urban life and seemed to foreshadow the fate of all modern men: 'The Jew is the most nervous and, insofar, the most modern of men... it will not take the Christians long to catch up to the Jews in this respect'.[49]

There is perhaps more than a trace of melancholy in Leroy-Beaulieu's assessment, for by the *fin de siècle* modernity was viewed both as the embodiment of western cultural progress and as a major source of contemporary decay. Hygiene reformers like Jules Payot, for instance, lamented how the contemporary *lycéen* had become a 'New

Wandering Jew' who, in his scholarly trek through subject after subject, was slowly being reduced to a 'scattered personality' [*un éparpillé*].[50] While in general agreement with Leroy-Beaulieu, sociologist Émile Durkheim tried to put a more positive spin on the connection between nervousness and modernity that necessarily implicated Jews. Although for Durkheim the neurasthenic's muscular weakness and extreme sensitivity admittedly 'disqualify him for action', he admitted that such a man nevertheless possesses 'an ambiguous power' that is crucial for the advancement of society:

> precisely because he rebels against tradition and the yoke of custom, he is a highly fertile source of innovation.... Although the degenerate multiply in periods of decadence, it is also through them that States are established; from among them are recruited all the great innovators.[51]

'Ambiguity' has proven to be problematic in most cultural systems under the best of conditions, and during the gender crises of the *fin de siècle* few French Jews were willing to wear such a label. Max Nordau, who had inveighed unequivocally against degenerates in his 1892 study *Degeneration*, insisted that Jewish men abandon their largely cerebral and sedentary lifestyles for the conscientious development of their bodies, thus giving birth to a new 'muscle Jew' who would recapture the heroism of their Hebrew heritage. Nervousness was for Nordau a trait that was incompatible with manhood, one that only lent credence to anti-semitic accusations of Jewish effeminacy and cowardice.[52] Yet Nordau's appeal for a muscle Jew was hardly an unprecedented notion at the *fin de siècle*, and had been a de facto aspect of acculturated Jewish male identity throughout the nineteenth century – historically, Jewish assimilation has always meant an incorporation of the martial styles of manhood privileged in the west.[53] The widespread Jewish reaction against Nordau thus had less to do with the specifics of his plan than with his scandalous assumption that modern Jewry was in a state of effeminacy. Few Jews had illusions about what they risked as men by being too closely associated with nervousness, and their discomfort at being saddled with such a label illuminates how feminising neurasthenia could be, both personally and publicly. While agreeing that Jews were especially nervous, sensitive, and impressionable, the journalist Louis Lévy maintained that 'it was not necessary to exaggerate this sensitivity and make of the Jew one of these pansies [*femmelettes*] who are made to swoon by a loud noise or a slightly disagreeable odour'.[54] Other Jewish commentators seemed to echo Zionist appeals for physical rejuvenation:

[Jews] have lost the habit of physical exercise.... Indeed, we have observed among them a progressive diminution of bodily health, a disturbing augmentation of nervous illnesses. In the future it will be necessary [for them] to fortify their muscles and nerves.[55]

3. The Dreyfus Affair

Medical and popular discourses thus evince a great deal of tension between, on the one hand, a desire to stress the ecumenical scope of neurasthenia and, on the other, the stigmatising reductions of the disorder to specific and potentially blameworthy individuals and groups. Repeated medical insistence that men and women from all walks of life were susceptible to neurasthenia seems to have been partly designed to counter the lingering popular belief (or fantasy) that the opposite might be true. They also suggest ambivalence about the proper social view of neurasthenia. From a strict medical perspective no single style of masculinity could be seen as being entirely beyond reproach, for all professions – even a military one – potentially created the conditions for some form of emotional or physical weakness that threatened to undermine one's sense of mastery.[56] Nevertheless there was an obvious assumption, even within the medical community, that certain types of men were more prone than others to nervousness. This tension furthered confusion about what precisely constituted true manhood, and only generated disagreement about which social group most embodied this quality.

Many of these issues were brought to the forefront of national discussions about masculinity during the Dreyfus Affair, the most divisive political and social crisis of the *fin de siècle*. Although medically the Affair added nothing new to the neurasthenia problem, it upped the ante considerably by underscoring the shifting relationships among manhood, nervousness, profession and race, on the one hand, and the prognosis for an apparently ailing body politic on the other. Following Carole Pateman and other feminist thinkers, it is now fairly commonplace to describe participation in the public sphere as having traditionally been considered a male prerogative that was in the eighteenth century founded on the exclusion of women, proletarians, and other 'feminised' populations.[57] By calling into question the masculinity of those who would have hitherto been considered eminently fit to fulfil such a role, however, the gender crisis of the late-nineteenth century effected a wholesale reconsideration of the manly credentials of 'the normal', and in so doing posed a challenge to those public men who dominated the political sphere. The Dreyfus Affair provided an opportunity to canvas such issues on a national scale, for within the more prominent question of whether or not Captain Alfred Dreyfus was guilty of treason lurked a deeper uncertainty about the gender credentials of those whose opinions on this issue purported to represent the good of the nation during this crisis period.

As long as the Dreyfus case was perceived as an unproblematic case of treason, as it generally was in 1894-5, such anxieties were safely contained within the parameters of the Jewish question. The alleged treason of Dreyfus was often described as a form of cowardice that, coming on the heels of anti-semitic claims that Jews were congenitally unfit to serve in the military, reflected badly on the masculine identity of male Jews. While it is true that many assimilated French Jews opted to remain detached from the Affair in order to allow the republican process to correct the judicial error (and thereby exempting themselves from 'action') it is also revealing that Jewish journalists, as they had often done during periods of anti-semitic agitation, recounted the martial glory of the Hebrew past as a means of affirming at once the virility of male Jews and their steadfast loyalty to France.[58] Not content to reminisce about glory days, Nordau chastised French Jews for remaining 'flabby spectators' on the sidelines while other, more manly men took up their cause.[59]

Increasingly vocal calls for a revision of the Dreyfus case widened the scope of the crisis beyond the Jewish community, and in turn implicated a broader range of men. Insofar as it was closely associated with the very outspoken contingent of 'intellectuals', the public reputation of the pro-Dreyfus camp suffered from the nervous connotations of mental labour. The negative implications of shattered nerves for masculinity were eagerly invoked by anti-Dreyfusard Maurice Barrès in his characterisation of opponents. When at the height of the Affair nationalist hero Paul Déroulède rudely interrupted a pro-Dreyfus rally, Barrès reported how 'some "intellectuals", weak masters of their nerves, displayed on their faces the convulsions of satyrs and, under the scorching light, in this terrible atmosphere of the masses, delivered themselves to the rut of hatred'.[60] Representations such as these abounded in anti-Dreyfusard imagery, and often contrasted the physically hardy officer with what would have been recognised as a neurasthenic intellectual, figured as exceptionally thin, physically weak, and repulsive to women (Fig. 15.1).[61] Here was an extension of the conflict between men of thought and men of action on a national scale, and anti-Dreyfusards were quick to emphasise how nervous and 'pale intellectuals' failed to

Fig. 15.1

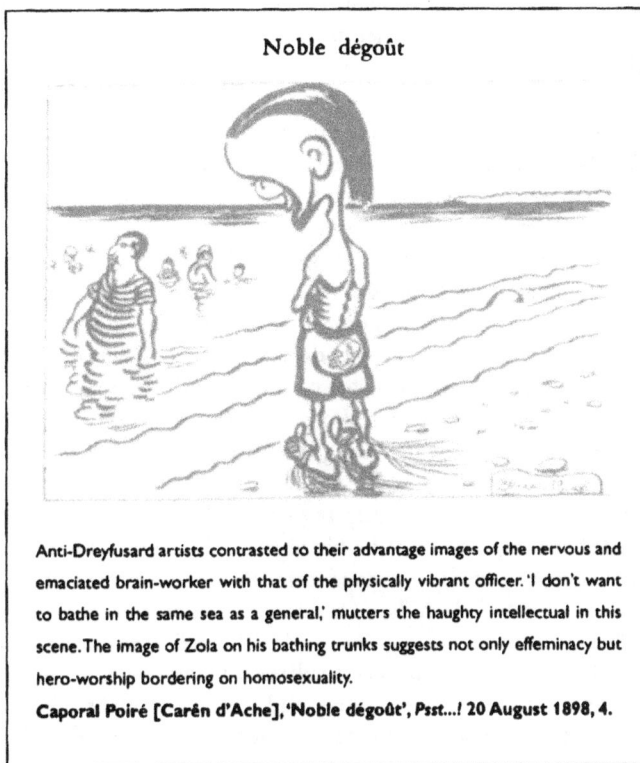

Noble dégoût

Anti-Dreyfusard artists contrasted to their advantage images of the nervous and emaciated brain-worker with that of the physically vibrant officer. 'I don't want to bathe in the same sea as a general,' mutters the haughty intellectual in this scene. The image of Zola on his bathing trunks suggests not only effeminacy but hero-worship bordering on homosexuality.

Caporal Poiré [Carên d'Ache], 'Noble dégoût', *Psst...!* **20 August 1898, 4.**

measure up to the more physically robust style of manhood embodied in the unjustly condemned military. One even facetiously declared his opposition to the pro-Dreyfus camp as the president of a 'group of neurasthenics', while another saw his intervention as a way to help 'reawaken traditional French virility'.[62]

In light of the gathering criticism of mental labour in French culture one should not narrowly interpret this tension as being germane only to students, professors, and artists in their immediate confrontation with the military and religious establishments. While the so-called 'Manifesto of the Intellectuals' of early 1898 brought together men (and sometimes women) from literary and academic circles, it also included many from the bourgeois professions who, while rarely engaging directly in the judicial or journalistic sparring of the Affair, were beneficiaries of the educational system that promised ascension within the new meritocratic order. Of course many poets and academics were careful to distance themselves from the bourgeoisie in the interests of asserting their own autonomy, yet from a medical perspective men in such groups represented extreme (and thus easily caricatured) instances of a more or less widespread shift toward mental labour among the republican elite. In this sense they may be viewed as grotesque distortions of a more general type.

Unable to measure up to the robust manhood of soldiers, the typical response of Dreyfusards was to assert their capacity for moral as opposed to strictly physical courage, which they identified with the apparent passive automatism required for the military lifestyle. For them pathological nervousness was clearly situated in the opposing camp—not only was the real traitor, Major Walsin-Esterhazy, marked by all sorts of moral and mental defects, but the violence of anti-semitic crowds demonstrated what could happen when mass hysteria manifested itself.[63] Yet there is also evidence of a shift in the public image of male neurasthenia during the Affair, for even self-professed 'intellectuals' acknowledged an incommensurability between nervousness and manhood. Despite their emphasis on ideas they too conceded the importance of bodily vigour. This rethinking of male nervousness was vividly conveyed through representations of arch-Dreyfusard Émile Zola. When Dr Édouard Toulouse examined Zola in 1896 as part of an ongoing study of creative men, his work revealed the novelist's constant vacillation between heroic creative effort and periods of nervousness and morbid thoughts. Having always been frank about his nervous tendencies, Zola found no shame in being exposed as having suffered from a nervousness that compromised his bodily strength, for it only attested to his ability to struggle victoriously against considerable odds. Yet it is also worth noting that by the time of the Affair, Zola was a changed man. Having scrupulously adhered since the late 1880s to a dietary and exercise regimen that resulted in considerable weight loss, Zola appeared to his champions as a new man whose apparent vigour represented a manly triumph over his old nervous self. The writer Octave Mirbeau directly linked this physical and mental change to the novelist's intervention in the Affair: 'since these events, Zola is less nervous, less febrile than usual, he is more in possession of himself – body, mind, and soul.'[64] Overcoming nervousness was for Mirbeau clearly a positive development, and served to enhance the public image of Zola's manly sacrifice for humanity.

•

Recapturing manhood

'It is to you *fin-de-siècle* young men that I address myself, a
generation of playboys [*noceurs*] and pleasure-seekers [*viveurs*],
anaemic and neurasthenic, bereft of both will and courage; to you,
the impotent and the tubercular, who lie about in your scrawny
carcasses in café-concerts and fashionable brasseries.'[65] Thus did the
hygiene reformer and professor of law Louis Bally introduce in 1901
the first major book by Edmond Desbonnet, the undisputed guru of
physical culture in France. The tone of Bally's remarks suggest that
Janet Oppenheim's observation about male neurasthenia in Britain
holds true for France as well:

> The man with shattered nerves was not merely pitiable, but also
> somehow blameworthy, and by the Edwardian period male
> neurasthenics were becoming almost as suspect as male hysterics.
> Whereas in the past, medical authorities had interpreted a paralysed
> will as the result of nervous exhaustion, they now began to suspect
> that it belonged at the origins of the disaster.[66]

Although during the 1890s one can find scattered voices expressing
such opinions, by the first decade of the twentieth century they had
become a veritable chorus as the bourgeois fashion for neurasthenia
underwent serious criticism.

In the wake of the Dreyfus Affair the line between complacent
and embarrassed neurasthenics was sketched most sharply, and here
too social and political developments lent a certain urgency to
demands that men conquer nervousness. The Dreyfusards had for
the moment emerged victorious when in 1899 they secured a
revision of the Dreyfus case and enjoyed an important electoral
victory through a coalition of republicans and socialists. Yet the
mounting critique of the government by both leftist and rightist
political extremes after 1905 – and the belief that Dreyfusards were
in the service of the Jews – coloured French political life in the years
leading up to World War I, and often amounted to a reassertion of
rivalries that had solidified during the Affair. A reinstallation of
boundaries and the reconstruction of self-mastery were central to
these assertions of masculinity, and the spectre of neurasthenia
allowed many anti-republican critics to condemn the weakened
condition of the bourgeoisie and the need for a new, virile political
culture. The identification of a new generation of young men who
grounded their identities on being distinct from their elders provided
yet another powerful critique of the status quo.[67] Dreyfusard

'intellectuals' may have won the immediate political battle, but they were losing the more protracted war between competing styles of manhood.

Yet the rhetoric of energy and new-found virility reverberated throughout French culture during the *Belle Epoque*, and one did not have to be an outright enemy of the Third Republic to condemn the current state of the bourgeoisie or the health problems wrought by intellectualism. The tensions described above were coupled with a new and widespread interest in sports and exercise that represented a more personal side to what many have seen as a revival of nationalism during the pre-war years. Drawing inspiration in part from Pierre de Coubertin's campaign for fitness during the 1890s, this functioned, according to Robert Nye, as a 'profoundly compensatory movement. It took the place of an unrealisable military revenge on Germany, while helping to convince the French that they had not fallen into an irremediable moral and physical decadence.'[68] Sports was often promoted explicitly as a means of overcoming nervousness, and while they often condemned the effeminacy wrought by modern life and spoke of the need to fortify the race, physical culturists and hygiene reformers framed male weakness as a reversible condition and welcomed neurasthenic men to the challenge of 'educating the will' for the good of the nation. With the aim of sculpting male bodies that were as beautiful as they were powerful, Edmond Desbonnet's chain of physical culture centres specifically targeted emaciated neurasthenics and the obese, men who suffered from either the pressures or the abundance of modern life.[69] Above all, such a return to the body would prepare young men for combat if the need arose, and whereas mental work produced nervous men physical exercise would forge men with nerves of steel. 'Nervous force and enervation are not the same thing', explained J. de Lerne in *Comment devenir fort*. 'Unhealthy, uncertain and ephemeral enervation is the lot of weaklings, of the enfeebled. Nervous force, healthy and salutary, is the great resource of the strong, of the fortified.'[70]

Lack of attention to hygienic issues was cited as a central cause of the decline of French vigour, leading one physician to note that 'if our children are less and less fit and virile, the cause is there – at least indirectly – and there is no need to look elsewhere'.[71] After 1900 or so popular health manuals adopted a moralising tone that condemned the blithe acceptance of neurasthenia among the upper-classes. Placing much more emphasis on muscular strength or 'force' than manuals from earlier decades, they exploited the popular demand for rejuvenation in such 'how-to' titles as: *Comment devenir énergique?* (1901), *Comment devenir fort* (1902), *Comment on devient beau et fort* (1905), and *Comment on devient robuste* (1909). Underscored quite frequently were the martial weaknesses of neurasthenic men so easily vanquished in the everyday struggle for existence. Viewing the disorder as 'a well-armed adversary' prone to ruses and other manoeuvres, Dr Aumont found that the neurasthenic was 'a sad fighter' in his daily conflicts. 'Taken unawares in battle, he receives blows that he cannot return. Life, mother to the strong, is a harsh stepmother to weaklings. The neurasthenic is a weakling and succumbs.'[72] Unlike those men with 'more hardened bodies and solid nerves', the underdeveloped musculature of such weaklings rendered them incapable of enduring physical pains and shocks.[73] A manual entitled *Comment on se défend dans la rue* (1909) even taught nervous men how to bravely face adversaries on the street and, when necessary, to return blows. Even physical violence could be edifying, suggested this author, and cultivating such abilities promised to build him up physically and to 'make nervousness disappear.'[74]

Shifts in literary tastes at once reflected this trend and provided it with some of its most vivid imagery. It was during this period that in France the colonial adventure novel came into its own, transporting readers to exotic locales where physical courage was essential for conquest, if not survival.[75] Not only had the radical right launched an all-out attack on the 'decadence' of contemporary literature, but even the literary avant-garde, long considered a hotbed of nervousness and degeneracy, dispensed with many of its decadent 'romantic' themes to embrace new forms of classicism. Indeed, left-leaning writers like Saint-Georges de Bouhélier and his fellow 'naturists' praised the 'everyday heroism' of peasants and sailors, thus celebrating more robust forms of manhood that bore little resemblance to the 'morbid heroism' of the decadent era.[76] Significantly, changes such as these were not confined to rarified discussions of style, but were meant to be embodied in the everyday lives of the writers themselves. Paul Léautaud, a young secretary at the *Mercure de France*, reflected this mood when describing his older colleague Jacques Morland, an erstwhile symbolist who had withered into:

> the type of sick, worn-out, dejected, even unhealthy man, *l'homme à régime*, who is disturbed... by trifles, who grasps furniture in order to walk, who does not say a word without becoming exhausted, [a man] without will, personality, or character.[77]

Yet physical culture was not for everyone, and for men like Morland who did not commit to an arduous exercise regimen, the world of patent medicines and nostrums promised an easy path back to full manhood.[78] *Le Vin Désiles* was a popular 'regenerating tonic' that seemed perfect for all ailments, and while it promised some benefits for women (as did most products), men clearly formed its target group. An intriguing blend of quinine, coca, kola, cocoa, lime phosphate, iodo-tannic solution and an unnamed but 'special' ingredient, this product promised to restore to men the 'force, vigour, and health' that had been sapped away due to the 'muscular or nervous weakness caused by fatigue, long nights, [and] study'.[79] The list of such questionable remedies and devices for combatting neurasthenia is extensive, and worthy of a study in its own right. 'Do you lack vigour?' asked one especially provocative advertisement in 1902: 'Do you feel the need for renewed force? Have the abuses of youth or the excesses of adulthood left an imprint on you, such as: spermatorrhea, kidney problems, seminal losses, nervousness, impotence, varicoceles, atrophy of the organs?' If so, then 'Dr. Sanden's "Herculex" electric belt' would be ideal, allowing the wearer to be rejuvenated overnight while 'a real current of life and force [penetrates] the weakened organs, curing them while you sleep.' In promoting this veritable 'fountain of youth for men', the Herculex ad skilfully invoked French anxieties about depopulation and physical decline through its explicit emphasis on muscular and sexual potency – in the image accompanying the text, a rejuvenated nude man lifts a baby boy (presumably the fruit of his invigorated loins) while electric sparks fly from his Herculex-clad waist (Fig. 15.2).[80]

Other remedies operated in a less spectacular manner, and took advantage of the period's obsession with nutrition and autointoxication. 'Digestion,' observes Joachim Radkau, 'is perhaps the most neglected major theme of psychohistory', and this is so even in studies of neurasthenia.[81] This oversight is surprising considering that intestinal complaints were considered a virtually universal feature of nervous exhaustion, so common in fact that physicians like Frantz Glénard and Charles Bouchard were convinced that neurasthenia was itself an effect of more fundamental gastro-intestinal disorders.[82] The fact that most authors mentioned Glénard and Bouchard only to dismiss their theories did not prevent the makers of patent medicines from capitalising on the widespread belief that constipation, indigestion, and suralimentation were at the heart of most modern ailments. Anxieties about the dangers of autointoxication would persist in the popular imagination despite the drift away from such theories by physicians in the twentieth century. For many members of the bourgeoisie purgatives had

Fig. 15.2

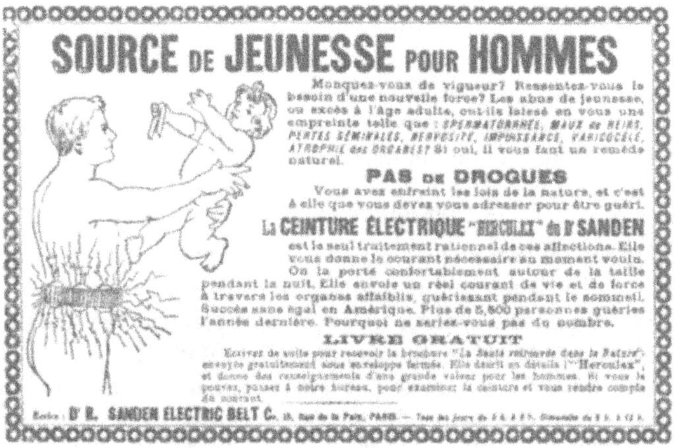

'A fountain of youth for men,' the Herculex electric belt situated neurasthenia and other disorders in the context of contemporary anxieties about national depopulation and the diminished muscular force of bourgeois men.
Advertisement, *Le Petit Journal*, 24 September 1897, 29.

become a quasi-ritualistic aspect of personal hygiene, a practice even extended to infants and carried out as often as five times a day. Taking it as given that 'the habitual laziness of the intestine is the source of the most dangerous diseases', from neurasthenia and gout to diabetes, obesity, typhoid, and even appendicitis, the makers of 'Grains de Vals' could confidently offer the public a gentle laxative that had allegedly earned 'the favour of the medical body across the world'.[83]

While physical exercise was often recommended for reversing the effects of overwork and sedentarity, physicians also recommended electrotherapy, hydrotherapy, psychotherapy, and holidays at the seaside or a health resort. Yet whether administered at home or on holiday, the treatment of men suffering from genital neurasthenia sometimes called for special measures. Sexual impotence was an especially delicate issue that cut to the heart of male anxieties about neurasthenia, and Proust and Ballet were sensitive to the need for tact when it came to this disorder. In cases of total impotence Proust and Ballet felt it was prudent to 'prove' to patients that 'they are still capable of strong erections' through electrical means, thus enlisting

351

electrotherapy in the service of psychotherapy. With one pole inserted into the rectum and the other attached to the urethra, erections could be artificially provoked in order to demonstrate the psychical (rather than somatic) source of the dysfunction. Bolstering a sense of manhood in this manner was not to be frowned upon, for it is sometimes 'an imperious necessity to give the patient confidence in his own powers, since the despair into which this functional incapacity plunges him can lead to suicide'.[84]

Conclusion: the new man

Like most western nations, by the time of the Great War France believed that it was well on the way to creating a new man whose physical vigour and superior willpower would weather any crisis and vindicate decades of lassitude and decadence. With the cultural stock of brain workers clearly in decline, men of action emerged victorious, at least in terms of styles of manhood considered worth cultivating. In 1912 Hugues Le Roux revelled in how completely *la culture de la force* seemed to have penetrated a generation of young men who refused to develop their minds at the expense of their muscles. Their republican professors, he charged, had acted in a manner similar to the *clercs* of the time of Charlemagne: they too had struggled against men of arms who preferred to make history rather than merely write about it: 'They invented, unfortunately, the word "intellectual" to oppose it to "man of action".' In this respect they had manifested along with traditional Catholics a 'disdain for the body' that no longer commanded the allegiance of young men, whose wholehearted embrace of physical force had produced a superior nervous system. An American track and field coach had assured him of this in a manner that was most flattering to French pride:

> These Germans... have neither the muscles of our young Anglo-Saxons nor the nervous systems of you Frenchmen.... What magnificent powers of energy have accumulated in your race! ... Thanks to the nervous system you have inherited from your elders, the day will come when you . . . will be unbeatable.[85]

Le Roux's remarks suggest a sharp division between the 1890s and his own time, and while they conform to the generationalist rhetoric that abounded in the pre-war years, they also capture a mood that affected both young and old in France. To some extent this mood can be chalked up to a sensitivity to the latest cultural trends, and one observer even recognised that 'Fashion has implanted in our time the need to preach energy and to glorify action.'[86] At the same time, however, there is evidence that educated men raised during the 1890s also regretted their own upbringing – even as committed an intellectual as Julien Benda would later lament that he grew up at a time when the promotion of 'energy' had not yet penetrated bourgeois circles.[87] Thus, while it is appropriate to consider this a transitional period where a new emphasis on muscular manhood proceeded by way of uneven development, in this era of mounting international tension, national self-consciousness about physical decline, and obsessive assertions of willpower and courage, the critique of the neurasthenic male was an essential part of a counter-model of masculinity that called into question the viability of the hitherto accepted gender norm. The doctors had always admitted that neurasthenia could befall any man, but with manhood increasingly described less as a fixed entity than as the result of endless struggle, the very fact of succumbing to nervousness signified that one had indeed lost the battle. In the pre-war years it was often agreed that such men would be useless in the battles to come.

Notes

1. I am grateful for the comments and suggestions offered by Marijke Gijswijt-Hofstra, Stephanie Liau, Robert Nye, and Sonu Shamdasani on earlier versions of this chapter. Thanks also to my research assistant Francine Morgan for tracking down many of sources cited herein.

2. Dr F. Aumont, *L'Estomac des gens du monde: Neurasthénie digestive* (Paris, n.p., 1908), 28.

3. Edward Shorter, *From Paralysis to Fatigue: A History of Psychosomatic Illness in the Modern Era* (New York: The Free Press, 1992), 220.

4. Mark S. Micale, 'Charcot and the Idea of Hysteria in the Male: Gender, Mental Science, and Medical Diagnosis in Late Nineteenth-Century France', *Medical History*, 34 (1990), 363–411: 379.

5. See Sonu Shamdasani's contribution in this volume. Traumatic hystero-neurasthenia was diagnosed when the typical symptoms of neurasthenia were accompanied by the 'anguished paroxysms' so often confused with hysteria, most of which were sparked by external shocks like fires, railway accidents, and physical assaults. Following Charcot, Gilles de la Tourette too observed that on the whole men were more likely to suffer from hystero-neurasthenia, but claimed that while members of the liberal professions figured prominently among true neurasthenics, those suffering from hystero-neurasthenia tended to be working class, thus reflecting the findings of Charcot on the high incidence of male hysteria among proletarians. Gilles de

la Tourette, *Les états neurasthéniques* (Paris: Baillière, 1898), 68.
Among men the line between hysteria and neurasthenia was often
superimposed over pre-existing class divisions, a practice that
continued through the Great War, where men suffering from shell-
shock could be diagnosed with either neurasthenia or hysteria
depending upon whether they were officers or privates. Joanna
Bourke, *Dismembering the Male: Men's Bodies, Britain, and the Great
War* (London: Reaktion, 1996), 112. See also Robert A. Nye,
Masculinity and Male Codes of Honor in Modern France (New York:
Oxford University Press, 1993), 226–7.

6. Robert A. Nye, *Crime, Madness, and Politics in Modern France: The
Medical Concept of National Decline* (Princeton: Princeton University
Press, 1984).

7. Ferdinand Levillain, *La neurasthénie: Maladie de Beard* (Paris: A.
Maloine, 1891), 28.

8. A. Cullère, *Nervosisme et névroses: Hygiène des énervés et des
névropathes* (Paris: Baillière, 1887), 12.

9. Robert A. Nye, *op. cit.* (note 6); Daniel Pick, *Faces of Degeneration: A
European Disorder, c. 1948-c. 1918* (Cambridge: Cambridge
University Press, 1989).

10. Adrien Proust and Gilbert Ballet, *L'Hygiène du neurasthénique* (Paris:
Masson et cie., 1897), 11–2.

11. Anson Rabinbach, *The Human Motor: Energy, Fatigue, and the
Origins of Modernity* (Berkeley: University of California Press, 1993).

12. Jules Payot, *L'Éducation de la volonté*, 37th edition (Paris: Alcan,
1912 [1893]), 17.

13. Michael Nerlich, *Ideology of Adventure: Studies in Modern
Consciousness, 1100-1750,* Wlad Godzich, trans. (Minneapolis:
University of Minnesota Press, 1987), 2 vols. Among intellectual
communities in the west, verbal sparring was often cast in strictly
martial terms. See Walter Ong, *Fighting for Life: Contest, Sexuality,
and Consciousness* (Amherst: University of Massachusetts Press,
1989), 119–48, and Dena Goodman, *The Republic of Letters: A
Cultural History of the French Enlightenment* (Ithaca: Cornell
University Press, 1994).

14. Peter N. Stearns, *Be a Man! Males in Modern Society*, 2nd edition
(New York, London: Holmes and Meier, 1990), 112.

15. Henri de Parville, 'Psychologie: Travail de tête et travail manuel',
Annales politiques et littéraires, (September 1896), 189–90. See also
Aimé Riant, *Hygiène du cabinet de travail* (Paris: Baillière, 1882), 60.
Such consolations did not prevent some scholars from feeling self-
conscious about their physical state, and Julien Benda admitted such

insecurities in his memoirs: 'Si j'eusse été d'un grand aspect physique avec les dilatations temporelles que tout jeune on en ressent, eussé-je tout de même un clerc? J'avoue ne me poser la question que par honnêteté.' Benda's encounter with a true 'man of action' like Georges Clemenceau is also telling: 'Un mot sur l'attitude de Clemenceau à mon égard. Bien que je n'eusse que vingt-deux ans, j'incarnais pour cet homme d'action l'intellectuel pur: je ne prenais part à aucune discussion politique, ne lisais pas un journal, passais toute la journée dans ma chambre à lire des ouvrages théoriques ou à jouer du piano. J'ai l'impression qu'il éprouvait devant cette race d'hommes de la pitié en même temps que de la gêne et une certain estime.' Julien Benda, *La jeunesse d'un clerc* (Paris: Gallimard, 1965 [1937]), 71, 96.

16. Douglas Peter Mackaman, *Leisure Settings: Bourgeois Culture, Medicine, and the Spa in Modern France* (Chicago: University of Chicago Press, 1998), and Eugen Weber, *France, Fin-de-Siècle* (Cambridge: Belknap Press, 1986), 177–9. The pleasures of seeking a cure were also one aspect of a 'new narcissism' that during the nineteenth century encouraged members of the bourgeoisie to pay close attention to their bodily states, thus helping to concretise a sense of subjectivity centred around a kinesthetic grasp of one's embodied self. On this topic see Alain Corbin, *The Lure of the Sea: The discovery of the seaside, 1750-1840*, Jocelyn Phelps, trans. (London: Penguin, 1994), 57–96.

17. Anne C. Vila, *Enlightenment and Pathology: Sensibility in the Literature and Medicine of Eighteenth-Century France* (Baltimore: Johns Hopkins University Press, 1998), 248.

18. See the discussion of the 'cult of invalidism', in Bram Dijkstra, *Idols of Perversity: Fantasies of Feminine Evil in fin-de-siècle Culture* (Oxford: Oxford University Press, 1986), 25–63.

19. Henri-Frédéric Amiel, *Journal intime*, (Clausinne: Editions l'Age d'Homme, 1989) vol. IX, 10 June 1874, 1236.

20. Norbert Elias, *The Civilising Process* (Oxford: Blackwell, 1997 [1939]); Georges Vigarello, *Concepts of Cleanliness: Changing Attitudes in France since the Middle Ages*, Jean Birrell (trans.) (Cambridge: Cambridge University Press, 1988); Alain Corbin, *The Foul and the Fragrant: Odor and the French Social Imagination* (Cambridge: Harvard University Press, 1986); Klaus Theweleit, *Male Fantasies*, vol. I (Minneapolis: University of Minnesota Press, 1987).

21. Rolland, *Lectures encyclopédiques*, cited in Dominique Maingueneau, *Les livres d'école de la république, 1870-1914* (Paris: Le Sycomore,

1979), 329.

22. Janet Oppenheim, '*Shattered Nerves*': *Doctors, Patients, and Depression in Victorian England* (New York: Oxford University Press, 1991), 146–51. For an analysis of similar developments in the United States, see Peter N. Stearns, *American Cool: Constructing a Twentieth-Century Emotional Style* (New York: NYU Press, 1994).

23. Anne Vincent-Buffault, T*he History of Tears: Sensibility and Sentimentality in France* (London: Macmillan, 1991), 183, 186.

24. *Ibid.*, 246.

25. V. Borel, *Nervosisme ou neurasthénie: La maladie du siècle et les divers moyens de la combattre* (Lausanne: F. Payot, 1894), 51–2.

26. Dr Foveau de Courmelles, *Comment on se défend contre la neurasthénie: La lutte contre le surmenage mentale* (Paris: L'édition médicale française, 1900), 14.

27. Léon Bouveret, *La neurasthénie, épuisement nerveux* (Paris: Baillière, 1891), 88.

28. Levillain, *op. cit.* (note 7), 45.

29. Bouveret, *op. cit.* (note 27), 144.

30. Tourette, *op. cit.* (note 5), 23–4.

31. Émile Laurent, *La neurasthénie et son traitement* (Paris: Maloine, 1897), 20. On male sexual complaints see Joachim Radkau, in this volume.

32. Edmond and Jules Goncourt, quoted in Deborah L. Silverman, *Art Nouveau in fin-de-siècle France: Politics, Psychology, and Style* (Berkeley: University of California Press, 1989), 37–8.

33. Payot, *op. cit.* (note 12), 24–5.

34. E. Detois, *La santé virile par l'hygiène* (Aurillac: Roux, 1901), 16, 23.

35. For a succinct description of these concerns, see Edward Berenson, *The Trial of Madame Caillaux* (Berkeley: University of California Press, 1993), 113–7, 189–93.

36. George Mosse, *The Image of Man: The Creation of Modern Masculinity* (New York: Oxford University Press, 1996), 83.

37. Eugen Weber, 'Gymnastics and sports in fin-de-siècle France: Opium of the Classes?' *American Historical Review*, 76 (1971), 70–98.

38. Jadwiga Szejko, *Influence de l'éducation sur le développement de la neurasthénie* (Lyon: A Rey et cie., 1902), 59.

39. Borel, *op. cit.* (note 5), 44.

40. Foveau de Courmelles, *op. cit.* (note 26), 24.

41. Bouveret, *op. cit.* (note 27), 40.

42. Proust and Ballet, *op. cit.* (note 10), 134–5.

43. Borel, *op. cit.* (note 5), 31.

44. Jan Goldstein, 'The Wandering Jew and the Problem of Psychiatric

Anti-Semitism in fin-de-siècle France', *Journal of Contemporary History*, 20 (1985), 521–52.

45. See Charles Féré, *La famille névropathique* (Paris: Alcan, 1898), 82; Laurent, *op. cit.* (note 31), 7; and Bouveret, *op. cit.* (note 27), 19.

46. Henry Labonne, *Comment on se défend des maladies nerveuses: La lutte contre la neurasthénie et les névroses* (Paris: Société d'éditions scientifiques, n.d.), 33. Assertions such as these were usually supported by little or no data, and it is telling that, when armed with statistical data on the percentages of suicide in various religious groups, Durkheim found that, regardless of their professions or propensity to nervousness, Jews were less prone to suicide than Protestants, largely due to the close social ties engendered by Judaism itself.

47. Édouard Drumont, *La France juive: Essai d'histoire contemporaine* (Paris: Marpon and Flammarion, 1886), I, 105–9.

48. This metaphorical expansion of Jewishness beyond its original seat in ethnic bodies was an early form of what the twentieth century would call 'Jewification'.

49. Anatole Leroy-Beaulieu, *Israel Among the Nations: A Study of the Jews and Anti-semitism*, translated by Frances Hellman (New York: G.P. Putnam's Sons, 1904), 163–4, 165, 168, 169. On Jews and nervousness see Edward Shorter, *From the Mind into the Body: The Cultural Origins of Psychosomatic Symptoms* (New York: The Free Press, 1994), 95–108, and Sander Gilman, *The Jew's Body* (New York: Routledge, 1991).

50. Payot, *op. cit.* (note 12), 12–13. For the problems with attention that attended such disorders, see Jonathan Crary, 'Attention and Modernity in the Nineteenth Century', in Caroline A. Jones and Peter Galison (eds), *Picturing Science, Producing Art* (London: Routledge, 1998), 475–99.

51. Émile Durkheim, *Suicide: A Study in Sociology*, translated by John A. Spaulding and George Simpson (New York: The Free Press, 1951 [1897]), 76–7.

52. Max Nordau, 'Discours prononcé par M. le Dr. Max Nordau', in Théodore Herzl and Max Nordau, *Discours prononcés au IIe congrès sioniste de Bâle*. Translated by Jacques Bahar. (Paris: Aux bureaux du Flambeau, 1899), 24–8.

53. Daniel Boyarin, *Unheroic Conduct: The Rise of Heterosexuality and the Invention of the Jewish Man* (Berkeley: University of California Press, 1997).

54. Louis Lévy, 'M. Max Nordau et le Sionisme (deuxième article)', *L'Univers israélite*, (March 1899), 42–3. This term, *la femmelette*, also

had definite homosexual connotations which Lévy would have also
disavowed. See Vernon A. Rosario, *The Erotic Imagination: French
Histories of Perversity* (New York: Oxford University Press, 1997), 87.

55. Mathieu Wolff, 'Soyez forts!' *L'Univers israélite* (December 1899),
398–400.

56. 'No craft', noted Jules Payot, 'no career, no matter how elevated, ever
suffices to safeguard personality, vigour, and energy'. Payot, *op. cit.*
(note 12), 5. One means of refuting antisemitic critiques was for
Jews to reaffirm their patriotism and martial prowess while
distancing themselves from associations with nervousness and
cerebrality. Yet even soldiers, long depicted as the epitome of virile
manliness, were by the end of the century being depicted as prone to
nervousness. Indeed, many of Charcot's students produced theses
that identified the military profession as also playing a predisposing
role in the cause of male hysteria. Such analyses obviously threatened
to undermine the purported virility of the military life, and in a
1904 article on neurasthenia and hysteria in the army, a military
physician tried to discourage the chuckling that would inevitably
greet the association of such apparently incongruent terms. This
medical attention to the minds and bodies of soldiers was
complemented by increasing critiques of the severity and even
immorality of the military life that at best cultivated mindless
automata, at worst promiscuous men ill-equipped to function in
society. Alain Flambart, 'L'Hystérie masculine en France à travers la
littérature médicale', Doctoral Dissertation, Faculté de Médecine,
Université de Caen, 1981, 59; Dr. Émile Lux, 'Névropathie et
neurasthénie: Les neurasthéniques dans l'armée', *La Revue de
l'hypnotisme* 19 (1904), 179–91.

57. Carole Pateman, *The Sexual Contract* (Stanford: Stanford University
Press, 1988).

58. Michael R. Marrus, *The Politics of Assimilation: A Study of the French
Jewish Community at the Time of the Dreyfus Affair* (Oxford:
Clarendon Press, 1971), 205. On Jewish defensiveness about their
honour, see Louis Lévy, 'Les vertus militaires de juifs', *L'Univers
israélite*, (February 1897), 632–4; Louis Lévy, 'Le soldat juif',
L'Univers israélite, (May 1897), 204–6; and R.T., 'Le duel et les
juifs', *L'Univers israélite*, (November 1897), 293–6.

59. Nordau, *op. cit.* (note 62). Non-Jewish Dreyfusards like Jean Ajalbert
shared Nordau's contempt for the apparent non-involvement of
'certain dirty Jews' in the Affair, an abstention that was often read as
a typical sign of Jewish cowardice. Despite having the right and even
the duty to defend themselves against anti-semitic outrages, Ajalbert

explained, French Jews have done nothing on their own behalf. 'We have seen little of them; they have marched off—as they tend to do—under a variety of pretexts, to such an extent that for their cowardice they deserve the panegyrics of La Libre parole'. Jean Ajalbert, *Sous le sabre* (Paris: Éditions de La Revue blanche, 1898), 221.

60. Maurice Barrès, *Scènes et doctrines du nationalisme* (Paris: Émile-Paul, 1926 [1902]), 226.

61. Ironically these caricatures contained a germ of medical truth, for it was commonly accepted that excessive intellectual labour augmented the volume of the brain while diminishing musculature throughout the body. With a bit of imagination one could easily arrive at such grotesque imagery. See Szejko, *op. cit.* (note 38), 64–7.

62. Pierre Quillard (ed.), *Le Monument Henry* (Paris: Stock, 1899), 405–6. This slippage from bona fide intellectuals to educated men of the liberal professions is evident in the growing concern that academic over-production contributed to what some critics called an 'intellectual proletariat' which, when it did not leave men unemployed and rebellious, produced sedentarity and nervous weakness. See Christopher E. Forth, 'Intellectual Anarchy and Imaginary Otherness: Gender, Class, and Pathology in French Intellectual Discourse, 1890-1900', *The Sociological Quarterly*, 37 (1996), 645–71: 656–8, and Venita Datta, *Birth of a National Icon: The Literary Avant-Garde and the Origins of the Intellectual in France* (Albany: SUNY Press, 1999), 121–4.

63. For more on these themes see my 'Intellectuals, Crowds, and the Body Politics of the Dreyfus Affair', *Historical Reflections/Réflexions Historiques*, 24 (1998), 63–91, and 'The Novelisation of the Dreyfus Affair: Women and Sensation in *fin-de-siècle* France', in Andrew Maunder and Grace Moore (eds): *Crime, Madness, and Sensation, 1800-1900* (Associated University Press, forthcoming).

64. Octave Mirbeau, 'Un matin, chez Émile Zola', in *Livre d'hommage des lettres françaises à Émile Zola* (Paris: Société libre d'Édition des Gens de Lettres, 1898), 73.

65. Louis Bally, Preface to Edmond Desbonnet, *La force physique: Culture rationnelle* (Paris: Berger-Levrault et Cie., 1901), ix–x.

66. Oppenheim, *op. cit.* (note 22), 151.

67. Robert Wohl, *The Generation of 1914* (London: Weidenfeld and Nicolson, 1980), 5–41.

68. Nye, *op. cit.* (note 6), 328–9. See also Nye, 'Degeneration, Neurasthenia and the Culture of Sport in Belle Epoque France', *Journal of Contemporary History*, 17 (1982), 51–68.

69. Of course Desbonnet was merely cashing in on what many physicians had since the eighteenth century recommended as a cure for modern nervousness. For Proust and Ballet an effective prophylaxis against neurasthenia was an education that would 'assure the development of force and what is called physical health. That is the highest priority, since physical health is the essential condition or, if you like, the foundation of mental health'. Moral health would stand upon this overtly somatic foundation. Proust and Ballet, *op. cit.* (note 10), 128.

70. J. de Lerne, *Comment devenir fort* (Paris: Baillière, 1902), 131.

71. E. Detois, *op. cit.* (note 34), 8.

72. Aumont, *op. cit.* (note 2), 8, 35.

73. *Ibid.*, 42.

74. Edmond Vary, *Comment on se défend dans la rue et chez soi: Manières multiples de se mettre partout en garde contre les agressions* (Paris: La Nouvelle populaire, 1909), 6.

75. Pierre Jourda, *L'Exoticisme dans la littérature française depuis Chateaubriand: Tome II: Du romanticisme à 1939* (Geneva: Slatkine Reprints, 1970), 217–42.

76. Louis Estève, *De Nietzsche à Bouhélier: Essai de philosophie naturiste* (Paris: Figuière, 1912), 4, 7.

77. Paul Léautaud, 24 June 1908, *Journal littéraire* (Paris: Mercure de France, 1955), II: 234.

78. On advertisements for neurasthenia cures see the chapters by Heinz-Peter Schmiedebach and Michael Neve in this volume.

79. Advertisement, *Le Rire*, 182 (1898), 11.

80. Advertisement, *Le petit journal*, (November 1902), 375. As was the case with many cures for male weakness discretion remained paramount, and the makers of the Herculex assured interested men that a free brochure would be sent to them 'in a sealed envelope'.

81. See Radkau in this volume.

82. Dr. Frantz Glénard, *A propos d'un cas de neurasthénie gastrique: Entéronéphroptose traumatique* (Paris: Masson, 1887).

83. Advertisement, *Je sais tout*, 1 (1905), Supplement, xxii; James C. Whorton, *Inner Hygiene: Constipation and the Pursuit of Health in Modern Society* (New York: Oxford University Press, 2000). Note also that health reformers sometimes drew parallels between proper digestion and manly vigour, and that physical culturists often suggested that well-developed abdominal muscles were evidence of well-tuned inner processes. See Tamar Garb, *Bodies of Modernity: Figure and Flesh in fin-de-siècle France* (London: Thames and Hudson, 1998), 68.

84. Proust and Ballet, *op. cit.* (note 10).

85. Hugues Le Roux, 'La culture de la force et la jeunesse d'aujourd'hui', *La Revue hebdomadaire*, 26 (1912), 607–8.

86. A. Cartault, *L'Intellectuel: Étude psychologique et morale* (Paris: Alcan, 1914), 276.

87. Benda, *op. cit.* (note 15), 56–8.

16

Claire, Lise, Jean, Nadia, and Gisèle: Preliminary Notes towards a Characterisation of Pierre Janet's Psychasthenia

Sonu Shamdasani

Do you suffer from obsessions, impulsions, mental manias, the madness of doubt, tics, agitations, hypochondria, phobias, deliriums of contact, anguish, feelings of estrangement or depersonalisations? Do you dream of sacrilegious acts, of exposing your body to random passers by? Do you daydream and ruminate (perhaps you are doing so now)? Then you, as Pierre Janet would have it, may well suffer from psychasthenia.

For historians suffering from 'hysteria studies fatigue syndrome' – HSFS, to give it an acronym – the study of psychasthenia has much to recommend it. For it is a field as yet unpopulated by literary critics, post-colonial theorists, feminists, art critics, post-structuralists, and last but by no means least, psychoanalysts of all persuasions. And it is likely to long remain so.[1]

Having just completed a work, which as William James put it, has clung too long to my fingers, the symptoms of psychasthenia – exhaustion and the quest for excitement and stimulation – are not foreign to this contributor.[2] Thus this essay, as opposed to simply being a study of psychasthenia, is likely to bear its stigmata. So if there be a psychasthenic style, somewhat akin to the neurasthenic discourse identified by Tom Lutz,[3] this chapter is proffered as an exhibit.

The advent of psychotherapy

In the medical world at the end of the nineteenth century, a new configuration came into being. A plethora of self-styled psychotherapies emerged, replete with clusters of practitioners, diseases and patients. This was achieved through complex negotiations between medicine, psychiatry, neurology and psychology. As Charles Rosenberg notes, until the middle of the nineteenth century, 'all medicine was necessarily and ubiquitously 'psychosomatic' and 'every clinician had to be something of a psychiatrist and family therapist.'[4] It was in the last third of the century that 'emotional ills, altered mood states, and even patterns of behavioural deviance were for the first time widely advanced, if not universally accepted, as legitimate diseases in and of themselves.'[5] Concepts of functional nervous disorders and psychoneuroses arose, which gave rise to new ways of framing distress and of being distressed, together with new forms of self-identity, that are still with us today.

According to the still persistent Freudian legend, the birth of modern psychotherapy is solely ascribed to the sign of Freud. This has obscured the breadth and multifaceted nature of these developments, leading to the mystification not only of the development of psychotherapy, but also of psychoanalysis itself. As John Burnham perceptively noted decades ago:

> In the United States Freud became the agent not so much of psychoanalysis as of other ideas current at the time. Psychoanalysis was understood as environmentalism, as sexology, as a theory of psychogenic etiology of the neuroses. Likewise when Freud's teachings gained attention and even adherents, his followers often believed not so much in his work as in evolution, in psychotherapy, and in the modern world.[6]

Misunderstanding the nature of these substitutions has led to the vastly over-inflated view of the significance of psychoanalysis in twentieth century culture. In 1929 the Bostonian psychopathologist Morton Prince noted: 'Freudian psychology had flooded the field like a full rising tide, and the rest of us were left submerged like clams buried in the sands at low water.'[7] One of these clams was Pierre Janet (1857-1947). Speaking of Freud and Breuer, he complained:

> They spoke of 'psychoanalysis' where I had spoken of 'psychological analysis'. They invented the name 'complex', whereas I had used the term 'psychological system'... They spoke of 'catharsis' where I had spoken of the 'dissociation of fixed ideas' or of 'moral disinfection'. The names differed, but the essential ideas I had put forward... were accepted without modification.[8]

After decades of vilification by psychoanalysts, Henri Ellenberger commenced the reappraisal of Janet's work and its historical study.[9] More recently clinicians have taken an interest in his early studies of trauma.[10]

Janet (1857-1947) initially trained in philosophy. From 1883 to 1889, he taught at Le Havre. Under the influence of Dr Gibert, he commenced studying hypnosis and suggestion.[11] His investigations of telepathic hypnotism attracted the interest of the English psychical researchers, Frederic Myers and Edmund Gurney, who travelled over to France to participate in them, as well as that of Jean-Martin Charcot. Janet's investigations resulted in a series of landmark articles, culminating in 1889 in *Psychological Automatism.*[12] Continuing his research under Charcot at the Salpêtrière hospital in Paris, he completed his medical studies in 1893 with a dissertation, *The Mental States of Hysterics.* That year, Charcot opened a psychological laboratory at the Salpêtrière, which he entrusted to Janet. Though prominent in his lifetime, Janet never formed a school or movement, and did not cultivate disciples.[13]

In 1902, he succeeded Théodule Ribot in his post at the Collège de France, thanks to the support of Henri Bergson. In 1903 – Lutz's neurasthenic year – he published a work entitled *Obsessions and Psychasthenia*, which launched a disease entity of psychasthenia, complete with a psychotherapy linked to a system of dynamic psychology. Before considering this, we need to consider the French importation of Beard's neurasthenia, and Janet's relation to Charcot in more detail.

Neurasthenia: the French connection

If Beard was the father of neurasthenia, it was Charcot who was its French godfather, wrote Fernand Levillain in 1891.[14] As Roy Porter has shown, late-nineteenth century neurasthenia followed a long train of nervous disorders from the eighteenth century.[15] José López Piñero also notes that neurasthenia first made its appearance in France in 1883, with Huchard's revised edition of Axenfeld's *Treatise on the Neuroses*, and the translation of Silas Weir Mitchell's *Lectures on the Diseases of the Nervous System, Especially in Women.*[16] It was Charcot and his students who took up neurasthenia, and this led to its rapid dissemination. The issue of neurasthenia appears in Charcot's lectures at the end of the 1880s, and works appeared by L. Bouveret in 1890, F. Levillain in 1891 and A. Mathieu in 1892.

For Levillain, the significance of Charcot's work on neurasthenia was that he did to it what he had done to hysteria.[17] Charcot approached neurasthenia in the same way as he did hysteria. He held that epilepsy, hysteria and kindred states (such as neurasthenia):

> come to us like so many Sphynx, which deny the most penetrating anatomical investigations. These symptomatic combinations deprived of anatomical substratum, do not present themselves to the

mind of the physician with that appearance of solidity, of objectivity, which belong to affections connected with an appreciable organic lesion.[18]

His assumption was that such conditions could be approached like any other disease, and that the symptomatology of the neuroses came close 'to that which belongs to maladies having organic lesions... Thus we are brought to recognise that the principles which govern pathology as a whole are applicable to neuroses.'[19]

This was one reason why he laid stress on the universality of hysteria. He claimed that one found the same lawlike regularity in hysteria 'in private or hospital practice, in all countries, all times, all races.'[20] For Charcot, Beard's merit was to have sorted out the chaos of the old 'nervosisme.' The description that he gave of neurasthenia, for the most part, was 'excellent,' corresponding to 'the reality of things.'[21] What was still required was a process of nosographical purification. Charcot held that neurasthenia was by no means an American disease. Beard had erred in his understanding of the demography of the disease, for neurasthenia was not the exclusive preserve of 'the man of privileged classes, softened by culture, weakened by the abuse of pleasures and the excess of intellectual work.'[22] On the contrary, it could be found among the proletariat, artisans and manual labourers.[23] Charcot was essentially desocialising the disease so as to give it a universal basis as a neuropathological condition. Thus the symptomatic complexity had a 'nosographical fixity' and the disease maintained its essence and identity in whatever circumstance it developed in.[24] Despite the fact that different etiological factors could result in neurasthenia, the 'morbid type' was everywhere the same.[25] Various authors, including Beard, had also erred in grouping under neurasthenia the symptoms of other disorders, such as agoraphobia, and the varied stigmata of hereditary degeneration. Such a mistake arose as these conditions were often found together. Charcot claimed that neurasthenia was sometimes found in combination with hysteria, and that it was 'one of the nervous affections which become developed most frequently in consequence of a shock, particularly in railway accidents.'[26] His desocialising of neurasthenia gave it a far wider social penetration. According to Levillain, nearly a quarter of the patients who presented themselves at the Salpêtrière were neurasthenics.[27] Thus Levillain dutifully claimed that Charcot's accomplishment lay in establishing the stigmata (ie. the necessary symptoms) of neurasthenia. In Beard's work, the symptoms of neurasthenia had been put forward in a jumbled manner, and Charcot had distinguished from these what were the most important and frequent symptoms.[28] Levillain set out the following stigmata of neurasthenia: neurasthenic headaches, insomnia, spinal hyperasthesia (what was previously called spinal irritation), muscular weakness, dyspeptic troubles, troubles of the 'genital apparatus' and a mental state characterised by intellectual and moral depression, which he called '*asthénie psychique.*'

Moral and hypnotic cures

The therapeutic application of hypnosis and suggestion spread thanks to Hippolyte Bernheim and the Nancy school. In 1886, Hack Tuke's *Illustrations of the Influence of the Mind Upon the Body* appeared in French translation. Tuke had proclaimed the advent of a new science of Psycho-Therapeutics, which consisted in the practical application of 'the Influence of the Mind on the Body to Medical Practice.'[29] That year, the second edition of Bernheim's work on suggestion appeared, utilising the term 'psycho-therapeutic' [*psychothérapeutique*] in Tuke's sense.[30] A few years later, he employed the word again, this time without a hyphen. Thus it may have been through the effect of translation that psycho-therapists became unhyphenated, as it was principally through Bernheim's work that the term and practice of psychotherapy – and critically, the notion that 'most neuroses are amenable to psychotherapy' became disseminated.[31]

Bernheim's work was not oriented towards nosological questions. He recognised the existence of neurasthenia, and more importantly, that it too was amenable to cure through hypnotic suggestion. He argued that it was important to differentiate between acquired or hereditary neurasthenia. The former could be cured or significantly improved through suggestion. The latter was usually incurable, though suggestion could provide some temporary relief.[32] The following capsule descriptions of Bernheim's cases may give some indication:

> Observation 44. (Catherine M.) Neurasthenia dating back eight months. Pains in the right iliac fossa (below the costal margin). Laryngeal constriction, dyspepsia, etc. Right hemianesthesia. Rapid restoration of sensitivity as a result of suggestion. Notable and lasting improvements obtained in 10 days.

> Observation 45: (Marie B.) Nervous problems dating back 15 months. Continuous pain in the head, back, and legs. Sensation of

a lump in the throat. Melancholia. Suppression of the symptoms for a month after 16 days of suggestion.

Observation 46: (Charles S.) Nervous difficulties. Epigastric pain. Melancholia for three and a half months. Vomiting. Immediate improvement, and cure in 12 days as a result of hypnotic suggestion.[33]

Other hypnotic practitioners argued that neurasthenia was less amenable to suggestion than hysteria. Joseph Grasset considered them to be harder to hypnotise, and as having less clear and localised symptoms.[34] In contrast to Bernheim, the Salpêtrière school were as reluctant to employ suggestion and hypnosis in the cure of neurasthenia as they were in hysteria. Thus they utilised a modified form of 'moral treatment', harking back to Pinel and Esquirol. Levillain argued that the use of hypnotism in cases of neurasthenia led to a new form of weakening, and hence could not play an efficacious role. Besides, hypnotism was itself a morbid state of neuropathology. Whilst suggestion in a hypnotised case of neurasthenia might have some results, it was not prudent.[35] Instead, he suggested the use of moral persuasion, hydrotherapy, and above all, Weir Mitchell's and Playfair's 'isolation method.' Charcot had recommended the same methods for the treatment of hysteria.

Léon Bouveret argued that 'the moral influence which the doctor can exercise over the patient plays the greatest role in the treatment of neurasthenia.'[36] The physician had to gain the confidence of the patient, and required an incontestable authority. This was because many neurasthenics needed to find moral guidance from their physician. To win the confidence of the patient, one had to listen to all his sufferings, and even appear to take a real interest in him. Bouveret recommended that one should also awaken the hope of a cure, and cite examples of cured patients.

In a similar vein, Adrien Proust (the father of Marcel) and Gilbert Ballet stressed the moral action of the physician on the neurasthenic, and the importance of listening to a patient's history and gaining their confidence. The physician should proceed in a genealogical manner:

When his special object is to counteract a fixed idea, a hypochondriacal obsession, he should contrive, by persuading the patient to confide in him, to trace up to the incident, the morbid derangement, that set the spark to it. He will then be in a position to show the invalid the emptiness of his fears, by making him understand that his attention is fixed on a disorder that is real but purely functional and without gravity, and that he has accustomed himself little by little to interpret it wrongly, to ascribe it a significance that it does not possess, a significance that is not the true one.... This proceeding, which consists in retracing to the patient in a correct and precise manner the stages of his hypochondriacal preoccupations, and in some sort the genesis of his obsessions, is well calculated to impress him.[37]

Exemplary errors

After Charcot's death, Janet wrote an article on his psychological work. In the course of this, he signalled out the significance for Charcot of the pathological or morbid type:

> To study a disease, Charcot *chose* amongst different subjects with this condition one particular individual who he presented and described in preference to all the others. Without doubt the other patients weren't entirely neglected, they were signalled in their turn, but on a second level, after the first subject who remained the model, the perfect type of the disease.[38]

He added that Charcot often chose the rare and exceptional cases to typify a disease, such as in his work on hysteria. What Charcot looked for was a case which presented the clearest, cleanest and most intelligible form of the disease:

> The type was an ensemble of symptoms, which clearly depended upon one another, and which were in a hierarchy, and could be classed in well defined groups, which above all by their nature and by their combination distinguished their characters from their neighbouring diseases.[39]

Thus the individual, and hence the type, was chosen thanks to the requirements of the classificatory system. Janet was critiquing Charcot's concept of exemplarity, and hence his manner of establishing the demarcation between diseases. In the case of his work on hypnosis, Janet noted the curious parallel between Charcot's conceptions of the three stages of lethargy, catalepsy and somnambulism with the work of the old magnetists, such as Despine. A number of years later, he argued that Charcot's cardinal error was that he never hypnotised his patients himself, and that they had often been 'trained' by local magnetisers.[40] Whilst critiquing Charcot's concept of exemplarity and method of procedure, Janet did not abandon Charcot's conception that the neuroses constituted fixed diseases, or his classificatory project. He saw the weakness of Charcot's work, and that of his rival Bernheim, as the lack of an adequate psychology, and it was this gap which he sought to fill.[41]

The birth of psychasthenia

Between 1892 and 1894, Janet put forward his concept of psychasthenia, arguing that the field of the neuroses was divided between hysteria on the one side and neurasthenia on the other. Psychasthenics constituted a category of patients, on the limits of insanity with varied symptoms, including deliriums of doubt, obsessions, impulsions and phobias. Psychasthenia was closely related to hysteria, and some patients suffered from both. In both neuroses, one met with a diminution of the mental synthesis and an emancipation of automatic phenomena.[42] Janet was essentially employing the model of mental functioning which he had developed in *Psychological Automatism*. The difference between the two neuroses was that in hysteria, the psychological phenomena were clearly separated or dissociated into independent groups, and at times, independent personalities. The subject did not know or express their fixed ideas. This was not the case with psychasthenia. Here, the deliriums did not remain subconscious, but formed the content of the patient's obsessions and ruminations.

In 1903, psychasthenia featured as the main subject of Janet's two volume study, *Psychasthenia and Obsessions*. The first volume was written by Janet, and the second volume, written in conjunction with Fulgence Raymond, consisted of clinical observations. Psychasthenia was a 'major psychoneurosis' on the model of hysteria and epilepsy.[43] It was 'very close' to neurasthenia.[44] Rather than Beard's neurasthenia, it was the neurasthenia of Charcot and his followers that Janet was reformulating. In other words, it was a neurasthenia which had already been desocialised and turned into a universal disease. Psychasthenia comprised of 'simple' neurasthenia, depression, phobias and obsessions. Janet based his study on 325 patients - 230 women and 95 men. Most patients were between twenty and forty. A number of these were recycled from his 1898 study, *Neuroses and Fixed Ideas*. In a similar manner to his procedure in *Psychological Automatism*, he focussed on five of them: Claire, Lise, Jean, Nadia, and Gisèle. This was to obviate the problems of employing Charcot's concept of the pathological type. What did psychasthenia encompass? Obsessions: religious, and, above all, sacrilegious. Phobias, hallucinations, forced agitations, ruminations, indecision, interminable deliberation, hypochondria, depersonalisation, estrangement, fatigue, indolence. After eighteen months, Claire, whose chastity, Janet informs us, cannot be doubted, confessed to him that she sees to the left a naked man in the act of soiling a consecrated host. Za..., a man of thirty-two, dreams of raping an old woman in front of a church. Leb, a woman of thirty-five, feels possessed by Satan to masturbate each time she prepares a confession.[45] It was not only members of the 'congregation' who were so afflicted. Janet reports the case of a priest who became obsessed with genitals after listening to an adulterer:

> He always has in his mind the thought and the same image of these two lovers in each others arms. After a year, the image simplified, only to become more bizarre and embarrassing. He only thought of and saw female genital organs, he could not see a woman, or speak to any woman, without becoming convinced that he could see her genital organs beneath her clothes. After many years, he noticed a new change in the form of the illness. 'To reason the thing, I began to think of my own sexual organs, and no longer of those of women. But this preoccupation led to another annoyance, it soon produced a physical irritation and led to a very disagreeable hypersensitivity of the penis and the scrotum.' The same patient ended up with a final form fifteen years after the beginning. He constantly thinks that his genital organs are attached to his body as to a foreign body and do not belong to him. He is no longer aware if it is he who is conscious of impressions made on them.[46]

Claire has a phobia of bottles. Lod... has a terror of spit on the pavement. Jean has a phobia of trams. If he mounts a tram, the proximity of women evokes his obsession with Charlotte, or he sees the face of the chamber maid, Élise, mocking him. Nadia looks in the mirror and asks herself if she is looking pale, and if she is as pale as the day before. Re... indefinitely asks if she loves her fiancé or not.[47] Loy..., a notary gives up his job because he can't sign a single act:

> each signature which he has to give awakens the idea of a dishonesty he is about to commit, he interrogates himself as to whether he can pay no heed and commit the dishonest act, if he should not get carried away, if he should consider the act to be insignificant, if he should consult before signing, etc.[48]

Janet's work is filled with a procession of patients like these, meticulously recorded. 'Nothing is more instructive and captivating,' wrote Théodore Flournoy in his review, 'than this gallery of tragicomic portraits where each reader can in some degree recognise himself and his neighbour.'⁴⁹ Implicit in Flournoy's point was the manner in which psychiatric and psychological texts, particularly concerning the 'psychoneuroses', were becoming sites that conferred new forms of identity, and that in no small measure, their power and persuasiveness resided in the manner in which they generated these identity-effects.

Beneath the plethora of symptoms, psychasthenia was characterised by three factors: the 'sense of incompleteness,' the loss of the 'function of the real' and the physiological symptoms of nervous exhaustion. To explain psychasthenia, Janet presented a new model of mental functioning. In his view, his earlier distinction between synthetic and automatic activity was only clearly applicable to hysteria, where the automatic activity was sharply distinguished from the voluntary mental synthesis. The hierarchy of mental phenomena required further differentiation. Psychasthenics

> continue to have the sensation and the perception of the external world, but they have lost the sentiment of reality which is ordinarily inseparable from these perceptions.⁵⁰

Their mental functions were not troubled concerning the imaginary, but only when it was a question of application to reality.⁵¹ Similarly, whilst they were fine in matters pertaining to the past and the future, they had difficulties with the present. These particularities justified the assumption that the relation to reality constituted a specific psychological function which was deficient in such individuals, the function of the real.⁵² He added that this corresponded to what Bergson in *Matter and Memory* had called attention to life.⁵³ The function of the real represented one of a hierarchy of mental functions. Each function was characterised by a level of psychological tension - the superior functions having the highest level. In a schema which recalls Hughlings Jackson's model of the dissolution of the nervous system, Janet claimed that the superior mental functions, such as the function of the real, were the most complicated and hardest to perform, and hence the first affected by psychological difficulties, which led to a reversion to inferior functions. The function of the real was itself sub-divided into several components: voluntary action on external objects, attention, self-consciousness and presentification, the ability 'to make present a state of mind and a group of phenomena.'⁵⁴ Ranged below this function were disinterested action, such as habits, which were marked by an indifference to reality; the function of images, which contained imagination and abstract reasoning; and below this, visceral emotional reactions and useless muscular actions.

The effects of physical illness, fatigue and certain emotions led to a lowering of the mental level, which, if sufficiently prolonged, led to the development of a psychasthenic state. When someone was unable to complete an act at a certain mental level, he reverted to a lower one, which gives rise to a sense of incompleteness.[55] The lowering of the mental level was also present in other neuroses and psychoses. To compensate for this, people sought to stimulate themselves. Hence alcoholism, drug addiction and fetishism represented failed attempts at self-cure.

The notion that disorders had a psychological origin was by no means new. The novel element which was emerging in works such as Janet's was that the psychological factor acted in a uniform, universal and lawlike manner. This came about through the transposition and extension of medical and neurological concepts of disease – in this instance, Janet's employment of a revised Charcotian concept of disease.

Janet claimed that the physical symptoms of psychasthenia corresponded to the symptoms of neurasthenia. He effectively reversed the order of causation: the physical symptoms were now the sequelae of a psychological state.[56] He dismissed the category of dementia praecox, claiming that the sense of the term had become over extended, and that it was wrong to turn a bad prognosis into the diagnostic of a disease.[57]

From moral treatment to a new cure of souls

We pass now to the treatment of psychasthenia. Janet considered isolation, the use of suggestion, moral direction, the re-education of emotion and the re-education of attention. He referred to all of these as 'moral treatment.' Isolation had some use, as it created a simple artificial milieu, which was less taxing to the patient. Whilst suggestion could be of some assistance, he considered obsessives as neither hypnotisable nor suggestible.[58]

Of more significance was moral direction. He made the observation that when patients found a friend or someone whom they could obey, their problems ceased. Priests had formerly fulfilled this function, and doctors could now do the same. Priests had done this in a haphazard manner, and no longer had the authority that they once had. Hence it was:

a characteristic of our time that this work of moral direction has sometimes returned to the doctor, who is now often charged with this role of moral direction when the patient does not find enough support around him."

It was easy for doctors to fulfil this function, besides which, they had certain powers that made it easier:

> he [the doctor] can menace him, he can speak to him of the known consequences of the disease, of the isolation it ends in or of the internment that the subject dreads, he can make him hope for a treatment, and medical prescription still has prestige.⁶⁰

The doctor had to indicate that he was interested in the patient, and had to behave in a commanding manner. Whilst taking charge of the patient in this way represented the utilisation of a symptom, it was an important palliative, as it was hard to directly attack the obsession. Fundamentally, treatment consisted of a re-education of the function of the real and a raising of the mental level. To re-educate the attention, military exercises, gardening, bicycling and gymnastics were useful. One of the ways in which the mental level was raised was through the clinical encounter:

> Already at the first visit to the doctor, the examination is done in a manner which astonishes the subject in showing him that his illness is well known, the demonstration that one has made to him that his state is an illness and that this illness is in general curable, all this has given rise to a happy emotion and has made the mental level rise.⁶¹

Thus the very act of being baptised with a diagnosis was of important therapeutic significance. A paradox enters here. From this perspective, the precise nosological schema is irrelevant. What was critical was that the psychological state was considered to be a real illness. Thus there was a tension between Janet's attempt to construct a complex hierarchical nosography of psychasthenia, and its therapeutics.

If part of the therapeutic efficacy in psychotherapy consisted in being diagnosed, and hence having a real illness conferred on one, patients were not long in requesting precisely this as a form of validation. This issue was highlighted by Jean-Paul Sartre:

> The psychasthenics whom Janet studied suffer from an obsession which they intentionally enter into and *wish* to be cured of. But, to be precise, their *will* to be cured has for its goal the confirmation of their obsessions as *sufferings* and consequently the realisation of them in all their strength. We know the result; the patient can not confess his obsessions; he lies sobbing on the floor, but he does not

determine himself to make the requisite confession. It would be useless to speak here of a struggle between the will and the disease; these processes unfold within the ecstatic unity of bad faith in a being who is what he is not and who is not what he is.[62]

For Sartre, the medical approach to existential suffering, such as represented by Janet's treatment of obsessions, was itself a mark of bad faith.

A number of further questions arise here. After the work of Ellenberger, Léon Chertok and Raymond de Saussure, psychoanalysis, psychotherapy and dynamic psychiatry have been seen as having arisen out of the practice of hypnosis and suggestion at the end of the nineteenth century, which in turn arose out of the practice of animal magnetism at the end of the eighteenth century.[63] In 1986, Marcel Gauchet and Gladys Swain in effect challenged this view, pointing to the significance of the role of moral treatment. They argue that an important part was played by a return to moral therapy in the first decade of the twentieth century, as a reaction against suggestion therapy. This represented an 'invention-reinvention of the therapy of the soul by the soul.'[64] The two main protagonists of this that they refer to were Paul Dubois and Jules Déjerine, who were friends (Déjerine wrote a preface to Dubois' work). Déjerine claimed that the problem with suggestion therapy was that it was directed to the symptom, as opposed to the causes, and hence only worked on the surface.[65] For Dubois, suggestion increased the state of servitude of patients. Psychoneurotics needed to be immunised from suggestion, so that they would accept 'nothing but the councils of reason.'[66] Patients needed to regain their self-mastery. In place of suggestion, Déjerine and Dubois spoke of moral persuasion. For Déjerine, hysterics and neurasthenics were only cured

> when they come to believe in you. In short, psychotherapy can only be effective, when the person on whom you are practising it has confessed his entire life, that is to say, when he has absolute confidence in you.[67]

In contrast to Dubois, Déjerine stressed the affective dimension. The doctor had to seek out the emotional cause of the disturbance, no matter how far back in time it lay. Gauchet and Swain point out that these forms of arguments participate in the myth of all powerful suggestion, and that ironically, this total confidence in the physician was the equivalent of the patient supposedly being placed completely at the physician's disposition through hypnotic induction.[68] The power over the subject gained through hypnosis was to be replaced by the power gained by possession of the narrative of his life. Whilst Janet sought to ground psychotherapy within a scientific psychology, Déjerine and Glaucker claimed that in psychotherapy no profound psychology was necessary, and that 'the psychology of every-day life, such as that which a good artisan or honest farmer would use, is quite enough.'[69]

Consideration of the treatment of neurasthenia and psychasthenia, whilst confirming the general lines of Gauchet and Swain's arguments, suggests some further points and qualifications. The manner in which neurasthenia was treated by Charcot's students suggests that moral treatment, rather than being reintroduced or reinvented by Déjerine and Dubois, had continued in a relatively unbroken manner since the time of Pinel and Esquirol.[70] Janet's text, which appeared before those of Déjerine and Dubois, also attests to this. It also gives some indication of the manner in which the practice of hypnotism and suggestion was incorporated into pre-existing medical and psychiatric models of treatment, such as moral treatment. The development of a critique of the use of hypnosis and suggestion in psychotherapy from the standpoint of moral treatment by Dubois and Déjerine can be seen as an attempt to restore the dimension of authority of the medical practitioner which was perceived to be threatened and undermined by suggestion therapy - or more exactly, the reflections raised concerning it by figures such as Joseph Delboeuf.[71]

The death of a disease

As we have seen, there were three main components of Janet's psychasthenia: it was a diagnostic category coupled with a system of dynamic psychology and linked with a conception of psychotherapy. These elements had different receptions.

Flournoy praised Janet's classificatory achievement. Janet had thrown a flash of light and introduced order into

> this inextricable mess of psychic anomalies - and nosological rubrics - which swarm under the confines of madness. Obsessions with consciousness, the reasoning monomanias of Esquirol, the manias and phobias, the emotional delirium of Morel, the madness of doubt and the delirium of contact, the famous cerebro-cardiac neuropathy of Krishaber, the *psychopathic inferiorities* of Koch, the psychic stigmatas of degeneration, the diverse anxiety neuroses of Freud and

376

Hartenberg, the disease of tics, etc., all these more or less discordant syndromes are found combined for the first time in a vast system of majestic order.[72]

Reflecting this view, a number of authors adopted the category, and articles on the subject followed in the journal that Janet himself founded with George Dumas in 1904, *Journal de psychologie normale et pathologique*, in the *Journal of Abnormal Psychology*, and elsewhere. In 1908, Bergson hailed Janet's study as 'profound' and 'original,' and welcomed his extension of his notion of the 'attention to life.'[73]

In 1910, Déjerine replaced Raymond at the Salpêtrière, who had died. Déjerine was hostile to Janet, and removed him from his position there. He did not have much more time for Janet's psychasthenia, and critised the concept. Whilst it might have a place among the psychoses, it was not a psychoneurosis.[74] Meanwhile, Déjerine continued to give pride of place to neurasthenia (one presumes that he rediagnosed some of Janet's patients as neurasthenics). He regarded this as being of psychic origin, and hence a psychoneurosis. All neurasthenias had emotional causes, and, in a manner that ironically recalls Charcot's concept of hysteria, they all went through three stages:

> a phase of simple emotional disturbance, a second phase of functional disturbances, and a third phase where the various consequences of the general invasion of the organism by previous functional disturbances finally appear.[75]

In a manner similar to Déjerine, Gilbert Ballet rejected Janet's psychasthenia, and continued to speak of neurasthenia[76]

As Ellenberger demonstrated, Janet had close linkages with American psychologists.[77] In 1904, he delivered lectures in America, and in 1906, he presented a series of lectures on hysteria at Harvard. Consequently, psychasthenia was taken up by the Emmanuel movement in Boston, a group of clergymen and doctors who did much to promote the use of psychotherapy, and it was also taken up by what Morton Prince called the Boston school of abnormal psychology.[78] Classing psychasthenia as one of the 'diseases of the subconscious,' Isador Coriat wrote in 1908:

> It is to the great credit of Janet, that he succeeded in unifying many diverse symptoms which had previously been described separately, and established that psychasthenia is really the mental state accompanying obsessions and fixed ideas.[79]

Hysteria, neurasthenia and psychasthenia were the 'great triad of the functional neuroses.'[80] Psychasthenia was also referred to by Adolf Meyer in several papers.[81]

In the diagnostic stakes, psychasthenia came up against the expansion of the psychoses. Thus in 1911, Eugen Bleuler claimed that Janet's cases were really hebephrenics and schizophrenics. In case one might think that Janet's psychological explanation was thus applicable to schizophrenia, he rejected it as a 'pseudo-explanation.'[82] This had implications for the prospects of psychotherapy. For if Janet's cases were really schizophrenic, as Bleuler claimed, they were suffering from a physical disease process, and so psychotherapy was of limited use.

C. G. Jung had attended Janet's lectures at the Collège de France in the winter of 1902-3, when Janet's work on psychasthenia appeared. Thereafter, he assimilated psychasthenia to dementia praecox, effectively nihilating Janet's nosological endeavours. Unlike Bleuler, however, he took over, with acknowledgement, the dynamics through which Janet explained psychasthenia - loss of the function of the real and lowering of the mental level - and considered these as fundamental mechanisms in both neuroses and psychoses. Thus in 1912, he argued that Freud's libido theory had failed to explain the loss of reality in schizophrenia, adding, 'we can hardly suppose that the normal *fonction du réel* (Janet) is maintained solely by erotic interest.'[83] In 1913, at the 17th International Medical Congress in London – where Janet presented his extended critique of psychoanalysis - Jung noted that his own conception of the neuroses as failures of adaptation in the present came very close to Janet's.[84]

Jung's response to Janet's work - disregarding his nosological endeavours, whilst utilising his general dynamic psychology to explain the neuroses - was part of a wider pattern. Around this time, a wide and general notion of neurosis and of the 'neurotic' developed, without precise reference to nosological frameworks. This development was coupled with the rise of private practice psychotherapy. Thus whilst Janet's nosography of psychasthenia was increasingly set to one side, the two other elements of his concept of psychasthenia did have a significant impact on establishing the notion that neuroses were of psychogenic origin and that psychotherapy was the treatment of choice.

German Berrios claims of psychasthenia that 'its speculative basis and the clinical over-inclusiveness have probably been the cause of its failure.'[85] However, in terms of over-inclusiveness, psychasthenia hardly matches Bleuler's schizophrenia, and farfetched speculations hardly checked the ascent of psychoanalysis. In 1935, William Alonson White noted that whilst the term psychasthenia still occurred, it had been superseded by Freud's terms.[86] Psychoanalysis increasingly took over the private practice marketplace for neuroses. The failure of psychasthenia to establish itself as a diagnostic category should not be sought on a realist level, as lying in its correspondence, or lack of it, to an independent reality. The same goes for other 'functional nervous disorders' or 'psychoneuroses.' Rather, comparison with the disorders promulgated by psychoanalysis (hysteria, obsessional neurosis, narcissism, etc.) suggests that what was significant was the fact that psychasthenia was not linked to an institution that trained patients and patient-practitioners (ie., analysts) to replicate it (one wonders what would have happened if Schreber, The Rat-Man or the Wolf-Man had been paraded as psychasthenics?). Thus a supply-side model goes a long way to accounting for the decline of psychasthenia. The training institutions of psychoanalysis enabled essentially nineteenth century categories to carry on up to the present day. How it achieved this is another story;[87] but no paper on psychasthenia would be complete without leaving a *'sentiment d'incomplétude.'*

Notes

1. There is a dearth of secondary literature on psychasthenia; see Georges Lanteri-Laura, 'La psychasthénie: histoire et évolution d'un concept de P. Janet', *L'Encéphale*, 20 (1994), 551–7; and Pierre-Henri Castel, *La Querelle de l'hystérie: la formation du discours psychopathologique en France, (1881-1913)* (Paris: PUF, 1998), 166–83.
2. Sonu Shamdasani, *Prisms of Psychology: Jung in History,* volume 1, forthcoming.
3. Tom Lutz, *American Nervousness, 1903: An Anecdotal History* (Ithaca: Cornell University Press, 1991).
4. Charles Rosenberg, 'Body and Mind in Nineteenth-Century Medicine: Some Clinical Origins of the Neurosis Construct', *Bulletin of the History of Medicine,* 63 (1989) 187–8.
5. *Ibid.,* 194.
6. John C. Burnham, *Psychoanalysis and American Medicine, 1894-1918: Medicine, Science and Culture* (New York: International Universities Press, 1967), 214.
7. Morton Prince, *Clinical and Experimental Studies in Personality* (Cambridge: Sci-Art, 1929), ix.

8. Pierre Janet, *Psychological Healing: A Historical and Clinical Study*, tr.
    E. & C. Paul, 2 vols (London: George Allen & Unwin, 1925),
    601–2.

9. Henri Ellenberger, *The Discovery of the Unconscious: The History and
    Evolution of Dynamic Psychiatry* (New York: Basic Books, 1970).

10. On the misreading of Janet by contemporary clinicians, see Ruth
    Leys, 'Traumatic Cures: Shell Shock, Janet, and the Question of
    Memory', *Critical Inquiry*, 20 (1994), 623–62; for a valuable
    account focusing on Janet's late work, see Jaan Valsiner and René van
    der Veer, *The Social Mind: Construction of the Idea* (Cambridge:
    Cambridge University Press, 2000).

11. On this period, see Jacqueline Carroy, 'Le docteur Gibert, ou le
    'Breuer' de Pierre Janet', in P. Fédida and F. Villa (eds), *Le cas en
    controverse* (Paris: PUF, 1999), 213–30.

12. Pierre Janet, *L'Automatisme psychologique: essais de psychologie
    expérimentale sur les formes inférieures de l'activité humaine*, 4th
    edition (Paris: Alcan, 1903).

13. Ernest Jones recalls a visit to Paris in 1908: 'I had greatly hoped to
    be able to work under Janet at the Salpêtrière, but although he
    received me kindly he explained that he always worked alone and
    had no student assistants'. *Free Associations: Memoirs of a Psycho-
    analyst* (London: Hogarth Press, 1959), 175. Freud was to prove
    somewhat more receptive to Jones...

14. Fernand Levillain, *La neurasthénie: maladie de Beard* (Paris: A.
    Maloine, 1891), 13.

15. Roy Porter, 'Nervousness, Eighteenth and Nineteenth Century
    Style: From Luxury to Labour,' this volume.

16. José López Piñero, *Historical Origins of the Concept of Neurosis*, tr. D.
    Berrios (Cambridge: Cambridge University Press, 1983), 73–4.

17. Levillain, *op. cit.* (note 14), 9.

18. J-M. Charcot, *Clinical Lectures on Diseases of the Nervous System*
    (1889), tr. T. Savill, (London: New Sydenham Society, 1889), 12.

19. *Ibid.*, 14.

20. *Ibid.*, 13.

21. Charcot, preface to Levillain, *op. cit.* (note 14), vii.

22. *Ibid.*, viii.

23. *Ibid.*.

24. *Ibid.*, ix.

25. *Ibid.*, xi.

26. Charcot, *op. cit.* (note 18), 236.

27. Levillain, *op. cit.* (note 14), 13. Charcot's work on neurasthenia is in
    need of further research. On the question of the differential

diagnosis of hysteria and neurasthenia, whilst noting the lack of sufficient documentation concerning Charcot's practice, Mark Micale suggests that 'private male patients with hysteria-like symptoms were more likely to be absorbed into the neighbouring diagnostic category of neurasthenia... than to be burdened with the dire and disreputable label of hysteria.' He puts forward the following profile: 'neurasthenia or hystero-neurasthenia for private upper-class patients; hysteria proper for working-class men; and hysteria and degeneration for the indigent.' ('Charcot and the idea of hysteria in the male: gender, mental science, and medical diagnosis in late nineteenth-century France', *Medical History*, 34 (1990), 363–411: 379). If this was the case, it would suggest a divergence between Charcot's theoretical desocialisation of neurasthenia and his actual practice, whilst also raising questions concerning Levillain's statistics (I thank Mikkel Borch-Jacobsen for drawing my attention to this point).

28. *Ibid.*, 73.
29. Daniel Hack Tuke. *Illustrations of the Influence of the Mind upon the Body in Health and Disease: Designed to Elucidate the Action of the Imagination* (London: J. & A. Churchill, 1872).
30. Hippolyte Bernheim, *De la suggestion et de ses applications à la thérapeutique* 3rd edition (Paris: Octave Dion, 1891), 296–7. This conjunction was noted by Marcel Gauchet and Gladys Swain, 'Du traitement moral aux psychothérapies: remarque sur la formation de l'idée contemporaine de psychothérapie', in Gladys Swain, *Dialogues avec l'insensé* (Paris: Gallimard, 1994), 237–262: 239. They unwittingly omitted the hyphen in their citation from Bernheim. On the development of psychotherapy in France, see Jacqueline Carroy, 'L'invention du mot de psychothérapie et ses enjeux', *Psychologie clinique*, 9 (2000), 11–30.
31. Hippolyte Bernheim, *New Studies in Hypnotism [Hypnotisme, suggestion, psychothérapie. Études nouvelles]* (New York: International Universities Press, 1980). 151.
32. *Ibid.*, 162–3.
33. *Ibid.*, 288–90. Bernheim later qualified his views on the utility of suggestion with neurasthenics in *Neurasthénies et psychonévroses* (Paris: Octave Doin, 1908).
34. Joseph Grasset, *L'Hypnotisme et la suggestion* (Paris: Octave Doin, 1909), 319.
35. Levillain, *op. cit.* (note 14), 226–7.
36. Léon Bouveret, *La neurasthénie: épuisement nerveux*, (Paris: J.-B. Baillière, 1891), 373.

37. A. Proust and Gilbert Ballet, *The Treatment of Neurasthenia*, tr. P. Cambell Smith (London: Henry Kimpton, 1902), 129.

38. Pierre Janet, 'J. M. Charcot: son oeuvre psychologique', *Revue Philosophique*, 34 (1895), 569–94, 575.

39. *Ibid.*, 576.

40. Pierre Janet, *Psychological Healing: A Historical and Clinical Study*, tr. E. & C. Paul (London: George Allen & Unwin, 1925), vol. 1, 186f.

41. Pierre Janet, 'Autobiography', in Carl Murchison (ed.), *A History of Psychology in Autobiography*, vol. I (1930), (New York: Russell and Russell, 1961) 123–33, 127.

42. Pierre Janet, *Mental State of Hystericals: A Study of Mental Stigmata and Mental Accidents*, tr. C. Corson (New York: G. P. Putnam's Sons, 1901) 519-21. Janet appears to have first introduced the term in 1893 in 'Quelques définitions récentes de l'hystérie,' *Archives de Neurologie*, 25 (1893), 417–38; 26 (1894), 1–29.

43. Pierre Janet, *Les obsessions et la psychasthénie* I (Paris: Alcan, 1903), x. The conception of hysteria in question being that which Janet had developed a few years previously.

44. *Ibid.*, 755.

45. *Ibid.*, 10–11.

46. *Ibid.*, 195. Janet had given an account of this case a few years earlier, without revealing that it was a priest. *Névroses et idées fixes* II (Paris: Alcan, 1898), 162–5. He did add there that the patient's religious dispositions led him to consider what was taking place as a diabolical temptation rather than as an illness. Janet recommended that he should pay less attention to his genitals, as this attention had led to the fixed idea becoming subconscious, leading to further symptoms.

47. *Ibid.*, 62, 114, 116.

48. *Ibid.*, 115.

49. Théodore Flournoy, review of Janet and Raymond, Les obsessions et la psychasthénie II, *Archives de Psychologie*, 2 (1903), 200.

50. Janet, *op. cit.* (note 43), 442.

51. *Ibid.*, 443.

52. *Ibid.*, 448.

53. Henri Bergson, *Matter and Memory (1896)*, tr. N. M. Paul and W. S. Palmer (New York: Zone books, 1991), 172ff. Bergson wrote 'Let us suppose we have to make a decision. Collecting, organising the totality of its experience in what we call its character, the mind causes it to converge upon actions in which we shall afterwards find, together with the past which is their matter, the unforeseen form which is stamped upon them by personality; but the action is not able to become real unless it succeeds in encasing itself in the actual

situation, that is to say, in that particular assemblage of circumstances which is due to the particular position of the body in time and space.' He also characterised insanity and dreams as consisting in a loss of this attention to life and the 'feeling of present reality'.

54. Janet, *op. cit.* (note 43), 491.

55. In his later work, Janet reformulated this as the feeling of emptiness (*sentiment du vide*), *op. cit.* (note 41), 129.

56. Mark Micale argues that 'Janet created the idea of psychasthenia essentially by splitting off the mental phenomena from the diagnoses of Beardian neurasthenia and Charcotian hysteria and combining them, somewhat arbitrarily, into a single diagnostic entity'. ('The "disappearance" of hysteria', *Isis*, 84 (1993) 496–526: 516). I argue here that its formation was somewhat more complicated.

57. Janet, *op. cit.* (note 43), 688.

58. On Janet and suggestion, see Jacqueline Carroy, *Hypnose, suggestion et psychologie* (Paris: PUF, 1991), 212–8.

59. Janet, *op. cit.* (note 43), 727.

60. *Ibid.*

61. *Ibid.*, 730.

62. Jean-Paul Sartre, *Being and Nothingness: An Essay on Phenomenological Ontology*, tr. H. Barnes (New York: Philosophical Library, 1957), 474.

63. Ellenberger, *op. cit.* (note 9); and Léon Chertok and Raymond de Saussure, *Naissance du psychanalyste (1973)* (Paris: Collection Les Empêcheurs de penser en rond, 1996).

64. Gauchet and Swain, *op. cit.* (note 30), 242. On the development of moral treatment in France, see Marcel Gauchet and Gladys Swain, *Madness and Democracy* [La pratique de l'esprit humain (1980)], tr. C. Porter (Princeton: Princeton University Press, 1999); and Jan Goldstein, *Console and Classify: The French Psychiatric Profession in the Nineteenth Century* (Cambridge: Cambridge University Press, 1987).

65. J. Déjerine and E. Glaucker, *The Psychoneuroses and their Treatment by Psychotherapy (1911)* [Les manifestations fonctionnelles des psychonévroses : leur traitement par la psychothérapie], tr. S. E. Jelliffe, (Philadelphia: J. B. Lippincott, 1918), vi.

66. Paul Dubois, *Psychic Treatment of Nervous Disorders*, [Les Psychonévroses et leur traitement moral] (1904), tr. S. E. Jeliffe and W. A. White (New York: Funk & Wagnalls, 1909), 221.

67. Déjerine and Glaucker, *op. cit.* (note 65), viii. As Catholics were used to confession, Déjerine and Glaucker felt that they were much

easier to treat in psychotherapy. They also claimed that women needed more frequent sessions than men, as they were more variable and emotional, and quickly forgot what was told to them (377–8).

68. Concerning direct suggestion, Déjerine and Glaucker claimed that 'the action of the physician is all powerful'. *Ibid.*, 278.

69. *Ibid,* 290. In a similar vein, Dubois wrote: 'I am not in any way opposed to Janet's education of the mind, but I would like to see less psychology and more ethics', *op. cit.* (note 66), viii.

70. On the continuity of moral therapy, see Michael Neve, 'Public Views of Neurasthenia in Britain 1880-1930', this volume.

71. See Joseph Delboeuf, 'Quelques considérations sur la psychologie de l'hypnotisme' (1893), in *Le sommeil et les rêves et autres textes* (Paris: Fayard, 1993), 405-22; Mikkel Borch-Jacobsen, 'L'effet Bernheim (fragments d'une théorie de l'artefact généralisé)', *Corpus des oeuvres philosophiques*, 32, (1997), 147-74; Jacqueline Carroy, 'L'effet Delboeuf, ou les jeux et les mots de l'hypnotisme', ibid., 89–118; and Sonu Shamdasani, 'Hypnose, médecine et droit: la correspondance entre Joseph Delboeuf et George Croom Robertson', *ibid.*, 71–88.

72. Flournoy, review of Janet, *Les Obsessions et la psychasthénie I, Archives de Psychologie* 2 (1903), 82.

73. Henri Bergson, 'Le souvenir du présent et la fausse reconnaissance,' in A. Robinet (ed.), *Oeuvres* (Paris, PUF, 1970), 897–930: **901, 906.**

74. Déjerine and Glaucker, *op. cit.* (note 65), 248.

75. *Ibid.*, 256.

76. Gilbert Ballet, *Neurasthenia [L'Hygiène du Neurasthénique]*, tr. P. Campbell Smith, 3rd ed. (London: Henry Kimpton, 1908), 117.

77. Henri Ellenberger, 'Pierre Janet and his American Friends', in George Gifford Jr. (ed.), *Psychoanalysis, Psychotherapy, and the New England Medical Scene, 1894-1944* (New York: Science History Publications, 1978), 63–72.

78. The work of the Boston school was reconstructed by Eugene Taylor in 'The Boston school of psychotherapy: Science, healing, and consciousness in 19th century New England'. Eight Lowell Lectures delivered for the Massachusetts Medical Society and the Boston Medical Library, March-April 1982, Boston Public Library, Boston, Mass, and in 'Psychotherapeutics and the problematic origins of clinical psychology in America'. *American Psychologist* (forthcoming).

79. Isador Coriat, in Elwood Worcester, Samuel McComb and Isador Coriat, *Religion and Medicine: The Moral Control of Nervous Disorders* (New York: Moffat Yard, 1908), 214.

80. Isador Coriat, *Abnormal Psychology* (London: Rider, 1911), 297.

There are also indications that psychasthenia spread to Britain, eg., W. H. B. Stoddart, *Mind and its Disorders: A Text-book for Students and Practitioners* (London: H. K. Lewis, 1908), 354ff.

81. See Alfred Lief (ed.), *The Commonsense Psychiatry of Dr. Adolf Meyer: Fifty-Two Selected Papers* (New York: McGraw Hill, 1948).

82. Eugen Bleuler, *Dementia Praecox, or the Group of Schizophrenias*, tr. J. Zinkin (New York: International Universities Press, 1950), 324, 380, 465.

83. C. G. Jung, 'An attempt at a Portrayal of Psychoanalytic Theory', *Collected Works* IV, Sir Herbert Read, Michael Fordham, Gerhard Adler and William McGuire (eds), tr. R. F. C. Hull (London/Princeton: Routledge/Bollingen Series, Princeton University Press, 1961), § 274. On Jung's relation to Janet, see John Haule 'From somnambulism to archetypes: the French roots of Jung's split from Freud', *Psychoanalytic Review*, 71 (1984), 635–59; and my 'De Genève à Zürich: Jung et la Suisse Romande', *Revue médicale de la Suisse Romande*, 116 (1996), 917-22.

84. Jung, 'Psychoanalysis and neurosis', *Collected Works* IV, *ibid.*, 569.

85. German Berrios, 'Obsessional Disorders during the Nineteenth Century: Terminological and Classificatory Issues', in W. F. Bynum, Roy Porter, and Michael Shepherd (eds), *The Anatomy of Madness*, vol. I (London: Tavistock, 1985), 186. Psychasthenia was recognised as a syndrome by Karl Jaspers, *General Psychopathology*, tr. J. Hoenig and M. Hamilton (Manchester: Manchester University Press, 1963), 442-3. On references to psychasthenia in psychiatry after Janet's death, see Lanteri-Laura, *op. cit.* (note 1), 556.

86. William Alonson White, *Outlines of Psychiatry*, 14th edition (New York: Nervous and Mental Disease Monographs, 1935), 365.

87. On this question, see Sonu Shamdasani, 'The Psychoanalytic Body', in Roger Cooter and John Pickstone (eds), *Medicine in the Twentieth Century* (Amsterdam: Harwood, 2000), 307–322.

List of Illustrations

Index

H

What is the Meaning of Human Life?

Raymond Angelo Belliotti

Amsterdam/Atlanta, GA 2001. VIII,176 pp.
(Value Inquiry Book Series 109)
ISBN: 90-420-1296-X   EUR 34,-/US-$ 32.-

This book examines core concerns of human life. What is the relationship between a meaningful life and theism? Why are some human beings radically adrift, without radical foundations, and struggling with hopelessness? Is the cosmos meaningless? Is human life akin to the ancient Myth of Sisyphus? What is the role of struggle and suffering in creating meaning? How do we discover or create value? Is happiness overrated as a goal of life? How, if at all, can we learn to die meaningfully?

Contents:
Foreword by Jan Narveson
Preface
ONE Meaning and Theism
TWO Nihilism, Schopenhauer, and Nietzsche
THREE The Myth of Sisyphus
FOUR The Meaning of Life
FIVE Value
SIX Why Happiness is Overrated
SEVEN Death
Notes
Bibliography
About the Author
Index

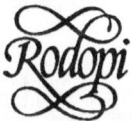

Editions Rodopi B.V.
USA/Canada: One Rockefeller Plaza, Ste. 1420, New York, NY 10020,
Tel. (212) 265-6360,
Call toll-free (U.S. only) 1-800-225-3998, Fax (212) 265-6402
All other countries: Tijnmuiden 7, 1046 AK Amsterdam, The Netherlands.
Tel. ++ 31 (0)20 611 48 21, Fax ++ 31 (0)20 447 29 79
Orders-queries@rodopi.nl   www.rodopi.nl

Theoretical Interpretations of the Holocaust

Ed. by Dan Stone
Amsterdam/Atlanta, GA 2001. IX,239 pp.
(Value Inquiry Book Services 108)
ISBN: 90-420-1505-5   EUR 45.-/US-$ 42.50

This book aims to show the many resources at our disposal for grappling with the Holocaust as the darkest occurrence of the twentieth century. These wide-ranging studies on philosophy, history, and literature address the way the Holocaust had led to the reconceptualization of the humanities. The scholarly approaches of Pierre Klossowki, Georges Bataille, and Maurice Blanchot are examined critically, and the volume explores such poignant topics as violence, evil, and monuments.

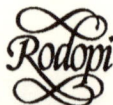

Rodopi

Editions Rodopi B.V.
USA/Canada: One Rockefeller Plaza, Ste. 1420, New York, NY 10020,
Tel. (212) 265-6360, Call toll-free (U.S. only) 1-800-225-3998, Fax (212) 265-6402
All other countries: Tijnmuiden 7, 1046 AK Amsterdam, The Netherlands.
Tel. ++ 31 (0)20 611 48 21, Fax ++ 31 (0)20 447 29 79
Orders-queries@rodopi.nl   www.rodopi.nl

Health, Science, and Ordinary Language

Lennart Nordenfelt
With contributions by George Khushf and K. W. M. Fulford:

Amsterdam/Atlanta, GA 2001.XII,235 pp.
(Value Inquiry Book Series 110)
ISBN: 90-420-1306-0   EUR 50,-/US-$ 47.-

This book is a contribution to the current philosophical discussion on the nature of health and illness. It contains a comparative analysis and reevaluation of four influential contemporary theories in this field. These are the biostatistical theory of Christopher Boorse which represents the mainstream thinking in medicine, and three versions of a holistic and normative understanding of health and illness which are the theories of Lawrie Reznek, K. W. M. Fulford, and Lennart Nordenfelt. In this unusual volume of assessment, Nordenfelt critically reexamines his own theory, and George Khushf and K. W. M. Fulford contribute critical responses.

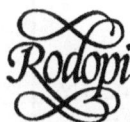

Editions Rodopi B.V.
USA/Canada: One Rockefeller Plaza, Ste. 1420, New York, NY 10020,
Tel. (212) 265-6360,
Call toll-free (U.S. only) 1-800-225-3998, Fax (212) 265-6402
All other countries: Tijnmuiden 7, 1046 AK Amsterdam, The Netherlands.
Tel. ++ 31 (0)20 611 48 21, Fax ++ 31 (0)20 447 29 79
Orders-queries@rodopi.nl   www.rodopi.nl

Exploding Aesthetics

Edited by Annette W. Balkema and Henk Slager
Amsterdam/Atlanta, GA 2001. 188 pp. (Lier en Boog Series 16)
ISBN: 90-420-1325-7   Bound   EUR   41,-/US-$ 38.-
ISBN: 90-420-1315-X   Paper   EUR   18,-/US-$ 17.-

Today, many visual artists are giving the cold shoulder to the static, isolated concept of visual art and searching instead for novel, dynamic connections to different image strategies. Because of that, visual art and aesthetics are both forced to reconsider their current positions and their traditional apparatus of concepts. In that process, many questions surface. To mention a few: Could the characteristics of an artistic image and its specific manner of signification be determined in a world which is entirely aesthetisized? What would be the consequences of a variety of image strategies for aesthetic experience? Would it be possible to develop a form of cultural criticism by means of artistic activities in a culture awash in images?

In order to answer such questions, aesthetics as a philosophy of art needs to transform its field into a critical philosophy of topical visual culture. As an impetus to such a reinterpretation of the visual working area, the L & B Series organized three symposia evenings under the title "Exploding Aesthetics", in cooperation with De Appel Center for Contemporary Art, Amsterdam. Besides the presentations and discussions from these symposia, this volume includes various arguments, positions, and statements in both articles and interviews by a variety of visual artists, designers, advertising professionals, theorists and curators. The participants are: Mieke Bal, Annette W. Balkema, Peg Brand, Experimental Jetset, Liam Gillick, Jeanne van Heeswijk, Martin Jay, KesselsKramer, Friedrich Kittler, Maria Lind, Wim Michels, Nicholas Mirzoeff, Planet Art, Joke Robaard, Annemieke Roobeek, Remko Scha, Rob Schröder, Henk Slager, Richard Shusterman, Pauline Terreehorst, Wolfgang Welsch and Marie-Lou Witmer.

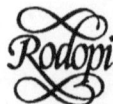

Rodopi

Editions Rodopi B.V.
USA/Canada: One Rockefeller Plaza, Ste. 1420, New York, NY 10020,
Tel. (212) 265-6360, Call toll-free (U.S. only) 1-800-225-3998, Fax (212) 265-6402
All other countries: Tijnmuiden 7, 1046 AK Amsterdam, The Netherlands.
Tel. ++ 31 (0)20 611 48 21, Fax ++ 31 (0)20 447 29 79
Orders-queries@rodopi.nl   www.rodopi.nl

INTERNATIONAL JOURNAL OF HEALTH SERVICES
Editor-in-Chief: Vicente Navarro

The *International Journal of Health Services* is one of the best known refereed quarterlies that covers health and social policy, political economy and sociology, history and philosophy, ethics and law, focusing on issues of health, social well being, and quality of life, with analyses of the socioeconomic and political interventions that affect them. Recent topics include studies on social inequalities and the impact of globalization on health and social policies. The *International Journal of Health Services* has been called one of the most stimulating and exciting journals in the health and social policy field.

RECENTLY PUBLISHED ARTICLES

A Review of Data on the Health Sector of the United States • *Ida Hellander*

On the "Efficiency" of Managed Care Plans • *Kip Sullivan*

Reforming Ontario's Primary Health Care System:
One Step Forward, Two Steps Back? • *Carole Suschnigg*

The National Plan for Britain's National Health Service:
Toward a Managed Market • *Steve Iliffe*

The National Health Service Plan:
Further Reform of British Health Care? • *Richard Lewis and Stephen Gillam*

Aging and the Market in the United States • *Ellen Frank*

Rethinking Difference:
A Feminist Reframing of Gender/Race/Class for the Improvement of
Women's Health Research • *K. Lisa Whittle and Marcia C. Inhorn*

Preventing Pathogenic Food Poisoning:
Sanitation, Not Irradiation • *Samuel S. Epstein and Wenonah Hauter*

Controversies at International Organizations over Asbestos
Industry Influence • *Barry I. Castleman*

On Joseph Mangano's Response to "Critical Assessment of Opposing
Views on Trends in Childhood Cancer" • *John A. Bukowski*

Complimentary sample issue available upon request

SUBSCRIPTION INFORMATION: Price per volume (4 issues yearly)
ISSN: 0020-7314, $192.00 Institutional, $53.00 Individual
postage and handling $7.50 U.S. and Canada, $13.50 elsewhere

BAYWOOD PUBLISHING COMPANY, INC.
26 Austin Avenue, PO Box 337, Amityville, NY 11701
call (631) 691-1270 • fax (631) 691-1770 • toll-free orderline (800) 638-7819
e-mail: baywood@baywood.com • web site: http://baywood.com

The Republic of Science
The Emergence of Popper's Social View of Science 1935-1945

Ian C. Jarvie

Amsterdam/Atlanta, GA 2001. 263 pp. (Series in the Philosophy of Karl R. Popper and Critical Rationalism 15)
ISBN: 90-420-1515-2   EUR 48.-/US-$ 45.-

This book offers a careful re-reading of Popper's classic falsificationist demarcation of science, stressing its institutional aspects. Popper's social thinking about science, individuals, institutions, and rationality is tracked through The Poverty of Historicism and The Open Society and Its Enemies as he criticises and improves his earlier work. New links are established between the works of the 1935-1945 period, revealing them as a source for criticism of the institutions and governance of science.

Contents: Preface. Chapter 1 Introduction: Science as an Institution. Chapter 2 Popper's 1935 Proto-constitution for the Republic of Science. Chapter 3 Problems in a Science of Social Institutions. Chapter 4 An Enriched View of Institutions. Chapter 5 Science and Society as Learning Institutions. Chapter 6 Conclusion: The Republic of Science. Sources and References. Index of Names. Index of Subjects.

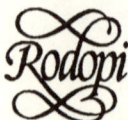

Editions Rodopi B.V.
USA/Canada: One Rockefeller Plaza, Ste. 1420, New York, NY 10020, Tel. (212) 265-6360,
Call toll-free (U.S. only) 1-800-225-3998, Fax (212) 265-6402
All other countries: Tijnmuiden 7, 1046 AK Amsterdam, The Netherlands.
Tel. ++ 31 (0)20 611 48 21, Fax ++ 31 (0)20 447 29 79
Orders-queries@rodopi.nl   www.rodopi.nl

INTERNATIONAL JOURNAL OF HEALTH SERVICES

EDITOR-IN-CHIEF: *Vicente Navarro*

The *International Journal of Health Services* is one of the best known refereed quarterlies that covers health and social policy, political economy and sociology, history and philosophy, ethics and law, focusing on issues of health, social well being, and quality of life, with analyses of the socioeconomic and political interventions that affect them. Recent topics include studies on social inequalities and the impact of globalization on health and social policies. The *International Journal of Health Services* has been called one of the most stimulating and exciting journals in the health and social policy field.

RECENTLY PUBLISHED ARTICLES

Are Pro-Welfare State and Full-Employment Policies Possible in the Era of Globalization? • *Vicente Navarro*

Excerpts from Joseph Stiglitz's Speech to the World Bank, April 1999 • *Abby Scher and Phineas Baxandall*

Competition and Containment in Health Care • *Ben Griffith*

The State, the Market, and General Practice: The Australian Case • *Kevin N. White*

New Labour and Britain's National Health Service: An Overview of Current Reforms • *Steve Iliffe and James Munro*

Does Social Policy Matter? Poverty Cycles in OECD Countries • *Olli Kangas and Joakim Palme*

Legislative Proposals for Reversing the Cancer Epidemic and Controlling Run-Away Industrial Technologies • *Samuel S. Epstein*

Critical Assessment of Opposing Views on Trends in Childhood Cancer • *John A. Bukowski*

Response to the Critique by John Bukowski • *Joseph J. Mangano*

The Construction of Gender and Mental Health in Nordic Psychotropic-Drug Advertising • *Ulrica Lövdahl and Elianne Riska*

Genetic Technologies and Achieving Health for Populations • *Patricia A. Baird*

Complimentary sample issue available upon request

SUBSCRIPTION INFORMATION: ISSN 0020-7314 price per volume (4 issues yearly) $192.00 Institutional; $53.00 Individual; P/H $7.50 U.S. and Canada, $13.50 elsewhere

BAYWOOD PUBLISHING COMPANY, INC.
26 Austin Avenue, PO Box 337, Amityville, NY 11701
call (631) 691-1270 **fax** (631) 691-1770 **orderline** (800) 638-7819
e-mail: baywood@baywood.com **web site:** http://baywood.com

Theodor Fontane and the European Context

Literature, Culture and Society in Prussia and Europe
Proceedings of the Interdisciplinary Symposium at the
Institute of Germanic Studies, University of London in March
1999.
Edited by Patricia Howe and Helen Chambers
Amsterdam/Atlanta, GA 2001. 270 pp. (Internationale
Forschungen zur Allgemeinen und Vergleichenden Literatur-
wissenschaft 53)
ISBN: 90-420-1236-6   EUR 50,-/US-$ 47.-

On the centenary of Fontane's death and at the turn of the century
these essays take a new look at this supreme chronicler of Prussia
and of the Germany that emerges after 1871. Written by scholars
from different countries and disciplines, they focus on novels and
theatre reviews from the perspectives of philosophy, sociology,
comparative literature and translation theory, and in the contexts of
topography and painting. Connections and crosscurrents emerge to
reveal new aspects of Fontane's poetics and to produce contrasting
but complementary readings of his novels. He appears in the
company of predecessors and contemporaries, such as Scott,
Thackeray, Saar, Ibsen, Turgenev, but also in that of writers he has
rarely, if ever, been seen beside, such as E.T.A. Hoffmann,
Stendhal, Trollope, Henry James and Edith Wharton, Beckett and
Faulkner. The historical novel and the social position of women are
each a recurring focus of interest. Fontane emerges as receptive to
other voices, as a precursor of developments in modern narrative,
and confirmed as the novelist who brings the nineteenth-century
German novel closest to the broad traditions of European realism.

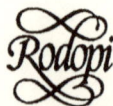

Rodopi

Editions Rodopi B.V.
USA/Canada: One Rockefeller Plaza, Ste. 1420, New York, NY
10020,
Tel. (212) 265-6360, Call toll-free (U.S. only) 1-800-225-3998, Fax
(212) 265-6402
All other countries: Tijnmuiden 7, 1046 AK Amsterdam, The
Netherlands.
Tel. ++ 31 (0)20 611 48 21, Fax ++ 31 (0)20 447 29 79
Orders-queries@rodopi.nl   www.rodopi.nl

The Positivist and the Ontologist
Bergmann, Carnap and Logical Realism

Herbert Hochberg
Amsterdam/Atlanta, GA 2001. VI,400 pp. (Studien zur
Österreichischen Philosophie 32)
ISBN: 90-420-1434-2   EUR 73,-/US-$ 68.-

The book contains the first systematic study of the ontology and
metaphysics of Gustav Bergmann, tracing their development from
early (1940s) criticisms of Carnap's semantical theories in
Introduction to Semantics, to their culmination in his 1992 *New
Foundations of Ontology* . This involves a detailed study of the implicit
metaphysical doctrines in Carnap's important, but long neglected,
1942 book and their connection to his influential views on reference,
truth and modality, (including, contrary to current opinion, Carnap's
initiating the development of predicate modal logic) that culminated
in *Meaning and Necessity*. In dealing with various fundamental
issues in ontology and metaphysics tbe book discusses relevant
views of major philosophers, such as Russell, Moore, Bradley,
Wittgenstein, Meinong, Brentano, Husserl, Broad, McTaggart, and
Quine, and of contemporary and recent figures, including D. M.
Armstrong, D. Lewis, S. Kripke, J. Searle, W. Sellars, D. Davidson, J. J.
C. Smart, and H. Feigl. Building on the critical studies of Bergmann,
Carnap and such other philosophers, the author argues for a form of
Logical Realism derived from important, but long misunderstood and
ignored, aspects of Russell's theories of descriptions, reference and
truth.

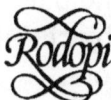

Rodopi

Editions Rodopi B.V.
USA/Canada: One Rockefeller Plaza, Ste. 1420, New York, NY
10020,
Tel. (212) 265-6360,
Call toll-free (U.S. only) 1-800-225-3998, Fax (212) 265-6402
All other countries: Tijnmuiden 7, 1046 AK Amsterdam, The
Netherlands.
Tel. ++ 31 (0)20 611 48 21, Fax ++ 31 (0)20 447 29 79
Orders-queries@rodopi.nl   www.rodopi.nl

Moving Subjects
Processional Performance in the Middle Age and the
Renaissance

Ed. by Kathleen Ashley and Wim Hüsken

Amsterdam/Atlanta, GA 2001. 257 pp. (Ludus 5)
ISBN: 90-420-1265-X   Bound EUR 59,-/US-$ 55.-
ISBN: 90-420-1255-2   Paper EUR 23,-/US-$ 21.-

Procession, arguably the most ubiquitous and versatile public
performance mode until the seventeenth century, has
received little scholarly or theoretical attention. Yet, this form
of social behaviour has been so thoroughly naturalised in our
accounts of western European history that it merited little
comment as a cultural performance choice over many
centuries until recently, when a generation of cultural
historians using explanatory models from anthropology called
attention to the processional mode as a privileged vehicle for
articulation in its society. Their analyses, however, tended to
focus on the issue of whether processions produced social
harmony or reinforced social distinctions, potentially leading
to conflict. While such questions are not ignored in this
collection of essays, its primary purpose is to reflect upon
salient theatrical aspects of processions that may help us
understand how in the performance of "moving subjects" they
accomplished their often transformative cultural work.

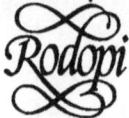

Rodopi

Editions Rodopi B.V.
USA/Canada: One Rockefeller Plaza, Ste. 1420, New York, NY 10020,
Tel. (212) 265-6360,
Call toll-free (U.S. only) 1-800-225-3998, Fax (212) 265-6402
All other countries: Tijnmuiden 7, 1046 AK Amsterdam, The Netherlands.
Tel. ++ 31 (0)20 611 48 21, Fax ++ 31 (0)20 447 29 79
Orders-queries@rodopi.nl   www.rodopi.nl

The Seeing Century
Film, Vision, and Identity

Edited by Wendy Everett

Amsterdam/Atlanta, GA 2000. 210 pp.
(Critical Studies 14)

ISBN: 90-420-1494-6   Bound EUR 50,-/US-$ 47.-
ISBN: 90-420-1484-9   Paper EUR 23,-/US-$ 21.-

The twentieth century, with all its turbulence and change, its conflicts and its discoveries was, perhaps above all, the century of cinema, and *The Seeing Century* offers an innovative, international, and interdisciplinary exploration of the role cinema plays in contemporary life and culture, and the complex and fascinating relationship between screen images and our changing concepts of personal and national identity.

Rejecting the compartmentalisation that has traditionally marked film studies, and confronting an impressively eclectic range of material, fifteen essays by leading academics from around the world cut across 'divergent' cultures, languages, and genres: mainstream Hollywood rubs shoulders with low-budget Icelandic or Sicilian cinema, and the popular and the esoteric feature alongside each other. In this way, the reader is offered a stimulating overview which directly addresses the contradictions and ambiguities inherent in the relationship between film and identity, and reveals the vibrancy of contemporary film debate, to which *The Seeing Century* makes an important and thought-provoking contribution.

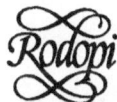

Rodopi

Editions Rodopi B.V.
USA/Canada: One Rockefeller Plaza, Ste. 1420, New York, NY 10020,
Tel. (212) 265-6360, Call toll-free (U.S. only) 1-800-225-3998, Fax (212) 265-6402
All other countries: Tijnmuiden 7, 1046 AK Amsterdam, The Netherlands.
Tel. ++ 31 (0)20 611 48 21, Fax ++ 31 (0)20 447 29 79
Orders-queries@rodopi.nl   **www.rodopi.nl**

National Stereotypes in Perspective
Americans in France, Frenchmen in America

Ed. by William L. Chew, III

Amsterdam/New York, NY 2001. X,433 pp.
(Studia Imagologica 9)
ISBN: 90-420-1365-6   EUR 82,-/US-$ 77.-

Since the late 18th century, when they first entered into an alliance during the American Revolution, the French and Americans have had a long and sometimes stormy relationship based on a complex mix of mutual admiration, cultural criticism, and sometimes downright disgust for the "other." The relatively new interdisciplinary field of imagology, or image studies, allows us to place the dynamics of such a relationship into perspective by grounding its analysis firmly in the study of national stereotypes, in the process providing new insights into the mentality of the observer. For if anything, image studies demonstrate again and again that national character is not–as assumed uncritically for centuries–an innate essence of the "other", but rather a self-serving functional construct of the observer.

For the table of contents please refer to our website

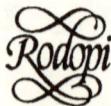

Editions Rodopi B.V.
USA/Canada: One Rockefeller Plaza, Ste. 1420, New York, NY 10020,
Tel. (212) 265-6360, Call toll-free (U.S. only) 1-800-225-3998, Fax (212) 265-6402
All other countries: Tijnmuiden 7, 1046 AK Amsterdam, The Netherlands.
Tel. ++ 31 (0)20 611 48 21, Fax ++ 31 (0)20 447 29 79
Orders-queries@rodopi.nl   www.rodopi.nl

Essays on the Song Cycle and on Defining the Field

Essays on the Song Cycle and on Defining the Field. Proceedings of the Second International Conference on Word and Music Studies at Ann Arbor, MI, 1999.

Edited by Walter Bernhart and Werner Wolf in collaboration with David Mosley Amsterdam/Atlanta, GA 2001. XII,253 pp. (Word and Music Studies 3)

ISBN: 90-420-1575-6   EUR 57.-/US-$ 53.-

ISBN: 90-420-1565-9   EUR 23.-/US-$ 21.-

This volume assembles twelve interdisciplinary essays that were originally presented at the Second International Conference on Word and Music Studies at Ann Arbor, MI, in 1999, a conference organized by the International Association for Word and Music Studies (WMA).

The contributions to this volume focus on two centres of interest. The first deals with general issues of literature and music relations from culturalist, historical, reception-aesthetic and cognitive points of view. It covers issues such as conceptual problems in devising transdisciplinary histories of both arts, cultural functions of opera as a means of reflecting postcolonial national identity, the problem of verbalizing musical experience in nineteenth-century aesthetics and of understanding reception processes triggered by musicalized fiction.

The second centre of interest deals with a specific genre of vocal music as an obvious area of word and music interaction, namely the song cycle. As a musico-literary genre, the song cycle not only permits explorations of relations between text and music in individual songs but also raises the question if, and to what extent words and/or music contribute to creating a larger unity beyond the limits of single songs. Elucidating both of these issues with stimulating diversity the essays in this section highlight classic nineteenth- and twentieth-century song cycles by Franz Schubert, Robert Schumann, Hugo Wolf, Richard Strauss and Benjamin Britten and also include the discussion of a modern successor of the song cycle, the concept album as part of today's popular culture.

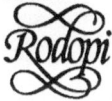

Rodopi

Editions Rodopi B.V.

USA/Canada: One Rockefeller Plaza, Ste. 1420, New York, NY 10020,

Tel. (212) 265-6360, Call toll-free (U.S. only) 1-800-225-3998, Fax (212) 265-6402

All other countries: Tijnmuiden 7, 1046 AK Amsterdam, The Netherlands.

Tel. ++ 31 (0)20 611 48 21, Fax ++ 31 (0)20 447 29 79

Orders-queries@rodopi.nl   www.rodopi.nl

Marteaus Europa oder der Roman, bevor er Literatur wurde

Eine Untersuchung des deutschen und englischen Buchangebots der Jahre 1710 bis 1720.

Olaf Simons

Amsterdam/Atlanta, GA 2001. 765 pp. (Internationale Forschungen zur Allgemeinen und Vergleichenden Literaturwissenschaft 52)
ISBN: 90-420-1226-9   EUR 136,-/US-$ 127.50

Bewähren sich vor 1720 noch die Wissenschaften der Nationen als der ursprüngliche Gegenstand der Literaturkritik, so ändert sich dies im Lauf des Jahrhunderts: Die Literaturbesprechung wendet sich Romanen, Dramen und Gedichten zu und etabliert am Ende die Literaturgeschichten, die uns noch heute beschäftigen.

Die Literaturbetrachtung gewinnt mit den poetischen und fiktionalen Schriften einen Gegenstand, mit dem sie sich bis in den Schulunterricht ausbreiten kann. Gleichzeitig verändert sie den Markt, dem sie sich zuwendet. Im Blick auf das Romanangebot des frühen 18. Jahrhunderts wird dies deutlich: Einen skandalösen, aktuellen, ungemein europäischen Markt nehmen die Leser in Leipzig wie in London vor 1720 wahr, wenn sie den Romanmarkt berühren - einen Markt, der sich gegenwärtig als historischer und politischer unter kaum erträglichen Manieren den privatesten Nutzungen anbot.

Die vorliegende Untersuchung unterstellt, daß die Literaturbetrachtung diesen Markt - an seiner Reform interessiert - von Anfang an disqualifizierte. Ein breites Aufgebot an Zeitzeugnissen, unter denen sie das Angebot überblickt, stellt sie dazu den späteren Literaturgeschichtsschreibungen gegenüber. Romane, die wir gewohnt sind, getrennten nationalen Literaturen und Epochen zuzuordnen, werden dabei als Produktionen eines größeren europäischen Marktes greifbar.

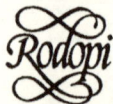

Rodopi

Editions Rodopi B.V.
USA/Canada: One Rockefeller Plaza, Ste. 1420, New York, NY 10020,
Tel. (212) 265-6360, Call toll-free (U.S. only) 1-800-225-3998, Fax (212) 265-6402
All other countries: Tijnmuiden 7, 1046 AK Amsterdam, The Netherlands.
Tel. ++ 31 (0)20 611 48 21, Fax ++ 31 (0)20 447 29 79
Orders-queries@rodopi.nl   www.rodopi.nl

www.ingramcontent.com/pod-product-compliance
Lightning Source LLC
Chambersburg PA
CBHW021931220326
41598CB00061BA/912